Essentials in Cytopathology

Series Editor

Momin T. Siddiqui
Pathology and Laboratory Medicine
Emory University Hospital
Georgia, USA

The subspecialty of Cytopathology is 60 years old and has become established as a solid and reliable discipline in medicine. As expected, cytopathology literature has expanded in a remarkably short period of time, from a few textbooks prior to the 1980's to a current library of texts and journals devoted exclusively to cytomorphology that is substantial. Essentials in Cytopathology does not presume to replace any of the distinguished textbooks in Cytopathology. Instead, the series will publish generously illustrated and user-friendly guides for both pathologists and clinicians.

More information about this series at http://www.springer.com/series/6996

César R. Lacruz • Javier Saénz de Santamaría
Ricardo H. Bardales

Central Nervous System Intraoperative Cytopathology

Second Edition

Springer

César R. Lacruz
Professor of Pathology
Complutense University School of Medicine
Madrid, Spain

Ricardo H. Bardales
Pathologist
Director Ultrasound-guided Fine Needle Aspiration Service
Outpatient Pathology Associates / Precision Pathology
Sacramento, CA, USA

Javier Saénz de Santamaría
Professor of Pathology
University Hospital Extremadura Medical School
Badajoz, Spain

ISSN 1574-9053 ISSN 1574-9061 (electronic)
Essentials in Cytopathology
ISBN 978-3-319-98490-2 ISBN 978-3-319-98491-9 (eBook)
https://doi.org/10.1007/978-3-319-98491-9

Library of Congress Control Number: 2018954225

This Springer imprint is published by the registered company Springer Nature Switzerland AG
The registered company address is: Gewerbestrasse 11, 6330 Cham, Switzerland

Preface to the Second Edition

Since the well-received *First Edition*, the advances in radiological, clinical, morphological, and molecular aspects of CNS diseases, as well as the increasing options for different treatment modalities, require updating of textbooks and revision of diagnostic algorithms. Accordingly, in this *Second Edition*, we have focused our efforts on updating and refining the text in light of recent knowledge, while adding new entities and histologic variants according to the 2016 updated WHO classification of CNS tumors. Throughout, additional emphasis has been placed on cytomorphologic characteristics and differential diagnosis, which are often summarized in tables making the explanation of certain topics even more powerful. Likewise, since pathology is one of the most visually oriented medical specialties, the illustrations have been evaluated carefully; some have been deleted and hundreds of new generously sized high-quality ones acquired. This fully updated edition also includes expanded clinical and radiological approach and recent biomarkers. Also, great efforts have been made to include all findings and other information likely to be relevant in clinical practice and cytomorphologic interpretation.

In summary, the textbook has been extensively revised and largely rewritten to offer the practicing pathologists, clinicians, and trainees a concise guide of the current critical information needed to recognize, understand, and interpret this demanding field of surgical neuropathology. Our efforts will be doubly rewarded if this book continues to find acceptance as a practical diagnostic aid.

Madrid, Spain — César R. Lacruz
Badajoz, Spain — Javier Saénz de Santamaría
Sacramento, CA, USA — Ricardo H. Bardales

Acknowledgment

Wayte, DM in his manuscript “A Christmas lesson: biopsy techniques for the young clinician” (J Clin Pathol 1992:45:1045–6) expresses the following …“Do not anticipate the need for an intraoperative diagnosis by ascertaining whether the pathologist will be available. Surprise him: ring him after you have got the biopsy specimen in hand. You must remember that the pathologist and his staff are just sitting waiting at all times for your specimen. After all, they have no other commitments or responsibilities except to you and your unexpected demands. Never tell the pathologist that the tissue may be infected. Remember, he will only panic and delay the diagnosis. Do not tell the pathologist that the patient has been previously diagnosed. He will have so much pleasure attempting to confirm your diagnosis on a minute fragment of tissue. And, is one way of auditing the pathologist’s ability.”

These remarks, that seem to be ironic and a comic caricature of the reality, unfortunately describe a real situation confronted daily by many pathology services all over the world. We would like to dedicate this book with outmost solidarity to our colleagues who face this sad situation.

Contents

Part I Introduction

1 Introduction to CNS Intraoperative Cytopathology 3
Advantages of the Smear Technique. 4
Disadvantages of the Smear Technique 4
Historical Background 6
Accuracy of CNS Intraoperative Cytopathology 7
Histologic Types of Central Nervous System Neoplasia 9
Suggested Reading 12

2 Clinical and Radiological Approach to CNS Intraoperative Diagnosis 15
Clinical Considerations for Pathologists. 15
Age and Location 16
Medical History 16
Family History 17
Neuroimaging Considerations for Pathologists 17
Principal Neuroimaging Modalities 17
Neuroimaging Evaluation 23
Suggested Reading 30

3 Specimen Handling and Optimal Processing 31
Specimen Identification and Transportation 31
Tissue Sampling 32
Smear Technique. 32
Fixation 34
Staining Methods 35
Fast Hematoxylin and Eosin Method 35
Fast Papanicolaou Method 37
Modified Fast Romanowsky Stain 37
Fast Toluidine Blue Method 38
Suggested Reading 39

4 Algorithmic Approach to CNS Intraoperative Cytopathology 41
Sample Triage ... 41
Smear Evaluation ... 42
Type of Smearing ... 44
Type of Background ... 44
Type of Blood Vessels ... 46
Specific Cell Groups ... 48
Type of Cell ... 48
Specific Cellular Elements ... 48
General-Category Interpretation ... 57
Abnormal ... 57
Neoplastic ... 57
Glial Versus Non-glial ... 59
Low Versus High Grade ... 59
Nonneoplastic ... 59
Final Recommendations ... 59
Suggested Reading ... 60

5 Normal Brain and Gliosis ... 61
White Matter Pattern ... 61
Gray Matter Pattern ... 62
Cerebellar Cortex Pattern ... 65
Choroid Plexus Pattern ... 65
Leptomeningeal Pattern ... 65
Pineal Pattern ... 68
Gliosis ... 68
Piloid Gliosis ... 71
Contaminants ... 74
Suggesting Reading ... 76

Part II Neoplastic

6 Astrocytic Tumors ... 79
Diffuse Astrocytomas ... 79
General Diagnostic Approach ... 82
Cytologic Features of Diffuse Astrocytoma ... 84
Differential Diagnosis Considerations of Diffuse Astrocytoma ... 88
Cytologic Features of Anaplastic Astrocytoma ... 89
Differential Diagnosis Considerations of Anaplastic Astrocytoma ... 89
Cytologic Features of Glioblastoma ... 89
Differential Diagnosis Considerations of Glioblastoma ... 95
Diffuse Midline Glioma ... 100
Gliomatosis Cerebri ... 100
Cytologic Features ... 103
Differential Diagnosis Considerations ... 103
Pilocytic Astrocytoma ... 103

Cytologic Features 106
Differential Diagnosis Considerations 106
Subependymal Giant Cell Astrocytoma 110
Cytologic Features 111
Differential Diagnosis Considerations 111
Pleomorphic Xanthoastrocytoma 111
Cytologic Features 113
Differential Diagnosis Considerations 115
Suggesting Reading 115

7 Oligodendroglial Tumors 119
Cytologic Features 120
Differential Diagnosis Considerations 125
Suggested Reading 128

8 Ependymal Tumors 129
Ependymoma 130
Cytologic Features 132
Differential Diagnosis Considerations 134
Subependymoma 139
Cytologic Features 139
Differential Diagnosis Considerations 139
Myxopapillary Ependymoma 141
Cytologic Features 141
Differential Diagnosis Considerations 143
Suggested Reading 143

9 Other Gliomas 145
Astroblastoma 145
Cytologic Features 147
Differential Diagnosis Considerations 147
Angiocentric Glioma 147
Cytologic Features 148
Differential Diagnosis Considerations 148
Chordoid Glioma 150
Cytologic Features 150
Differential Diagnosis Considerations 152
Suggested Reading 152

10 Choroid Plexus Tumors 155
Cytologic Features 156
Differential Diagnosis Considerations 160
Suggested Reading 164

11 Neuronal and Mixed Neuronal-Glial Tumors 165
Dysembryoplastic Neuroepithelial Tumor 165
Cytologic Features 166
Ganglion Cell Tumors (Ganglioglioma/Gangliocytoma) 166

Cytologic Features ... 169
Desmoplastic Infantile Astrocytoma and Ganglioglioma ... 169
Cytologic Features ... 172
Central Neurocytoma ... 172
Cytologic Features ... 175
Rosette-Forming Glioneuronal Tumor ... 175
Cytologic Features ... 175
Spinal Paraganglioma ... 179
Cytologic Features ... 179
Differential Diagnosis Considerations of Neuronal and Mixed Neuronal-Glial Tumors ... 179
Suggested Reading ... 182

12 Embryonal (Primitive) Tumors ... 185
Medulloblastoma ... 186
General Diagnostic Approach ... 189
Cytologic Features ... 189
CNS Embryonal Tumors Replacing PNET ... 189
Cytologic Features ... 194
Differential Diagnosis Considerations of Medulloblastoma/CNS Embryonal Tumors Replacing PNET ... 197
Atypical Teratoid/Rhabdoid Tumor ... 199
Cytologic Features ... 203
Differential Diagnosis Considerations ... 203
Suggested Reading ... 205

13 Meningiomas ... 207
Cytologic Features of Common Meningioma Variants ... 211
Cytologic Features of Uncommon Meningioma Variants ... 211
Cytologic Features of Grade II Meningiomas ... 215
Cytologic Features of Grade III Meningiomas ... 222
Cytologic Features of Extracranial Meningiomas ... 228
Differential Diagnosis Considerations ... 228
Suggested Reading ... 230

14 Non-meningothelial Mesenchymal Tumors ... 233
Hemangioblastoma ... 233
Cytologic Features ... 236
Differential Diagnosis Considerations ... 236
Solitary Fibrous Tumor/Hemangiopericytoma ... 236
Cytologic Features ... 237
Differential Diagnosis Considerations ... 239
Lipoma ... 239
Cytologic Features and Differential Diagnosis ... 241
Rhabdomyosarcoma ... 243
Cytologic Features and Differential Diagnosis ... 243

Ewing Sarcoma . . . 243
Cytologic Features and Differential Diagnosis . . . 245
Fibrosarcoma . . . 245
Cytologic Features and Differential Diagnosis . . . 248
Chordoma . . . 248
Cytologic Features and Differential Diagnosis . . . 248
Osteosarcoma . . . 250
Cytologic Features and Differential Diagnosis . . . 250
Suggested Reading . . . 252

15 Germ Cell Tumors . . . 255
Germinoma . . . 256
Cytologic Features . . . 258
Differential Diagnosis Considerations . . . 258
Teratoma . . . 258
Cytologic Features . . . 261
Differential Diagnosis Considerations . . . 263
Non-germinomatous (Malignant) Germ Cell Tumors . . . 263
Cytologic Features . . . 266
Differential Diagnosis Considerations . . . 266
Suggested Reading . . . 268

16 Lymphomas and Histiocytic Tumors . . . 269
Primary Central Nervous System Lymphomas . . . 269
General Diagnostic Approach . . . 271
Cytologic Features . . . 271
Differential Diagnosis Considerations . . . 276
Histiocytic Tumors . . . 276
General Features of Histiocytic Disorders . . . 276
Cytologic Features . . . 278
Suggested Reading . . . 280

17 Nerve Sheath Tumors of the Craniospinal Axis . . . 283
Schwannoma . . . 283
Cytologic Features . . . 284
Differential Diagnosis Considerations . . . 286
Melanotic Schwannoma . . . 289
Cytologic Features . . . 290
Differential Diagnosis Considerations . . . 290
Neurofibroma . . . 290
Cytologic Features . . . 293
Differential Diagnosis Considerations . . . 293
Malignant Peripheral Nerve Sheath Tumors . . . 295
Cytologic Features . . . 295
Differential Diagnosis Considerations . . . 297
Ganglioneuroma . . . 297
Suggested Reading . . . 299

18 Metastatic Tumors . . . 301
General Diagnostic Approach . . . 304
Cytologic Features . . . 304
Differential Diagnosis Considerations . . . 305
Suggested Reading . . . 315

Part III Nonneoplastic

19 Benign Cystic Lesions . . . 319
Squamous Epithelium-Lined Cysts . . . 319
Epidermoid Cyst . . . 319
Dermoid Cyst . . . 320
Cytologic Features and Differential Diagnosis . . . 322
Columnar to Cuboidal Epithelium-Lined Cysts . . . 322
Colloid Cyst of the Third Ventricle . . . 322
Rathke Cleft Cyst . . . 322
Endodermal (Enterogenous) Cyst . . . 323
Ependymal Cyst . . . 323
Choroid Plexus Cyst . . . 324
Cytologic Features and Differential Diagnosis . . . 324
Nonepithelial-Lining Cysts . . . 325
Arachnoid Cyst . . . 325
Glial Cyst . . . 326
Pineal Cyst . . . 326
Suggested Reading . . . 328

20 Infectious, Inflammatory, and Reactive Lesions . . . 331
General Diagnostic Approach . . . 331
Acute Inflammatory-Cell-Rich Lesions . . . 332
Brain Abscess . . . 332
Subdural Empyema . . . 334
Epidural Abscess . . . 334
Perivascular Chronic Inflammatory Cell-Rich Lesions . . . 334
Infectious Encephalitis . . . 335
Noninfectious Perivascular Chronic Inflammation . . . 336
Epithelioid-Cell-Rich Lesions (Granulomatous Inflammation) . . . 336
Neurosarcoidosis . . . 337
Mycobacterial Infections . . . 337
Macrophage-Rich Lesions . . . 341
Tumorlike Demyelinating Lesion “A Potential Litigation Diagnosis” . 341
Cerebral Infarction . . . 345
Infectious-Inflammatory Lesions in AIDS . . . 345
Toxoplasmosis . . . 347
Progressive Multifocal Leukoencephalopathy . . . 349
Cytomegalovirus Encephalitis . . . 353
Suggested Reading . . . 353

Part IV Regions

21 Pineal Region . . . 359
Pineocytoma . . . 360
Cytologic Features . . . 362
Differential Diagnosis Considerations . . . 362
Pineoblastoma . . . 362
Cytologic Features . . . 365
Differential Diagnosis Considerations . . . 368
Papillary Tumor of the Pineal Region . . . 368
Cytologic Features and Differential Diagnosis . . . 369
Suggested Reading . . . 371

22 Sellar Region . . . 373
Pituitary Adenoma . . . 373
Cytologic Features . . . 377
Differential Diagnosis Considerations . . . 377
Craniopharyngioma . . . 380
Cytologic Features . . . 382
Differential Diagnosis Considerations . . . 382
Other Lesions of the Sellar Region . . . 384
Neoplastic Lesions . . . 384
Nonneoplastic Lesions . . . 387
Suggested Reading . . . 388

23 Spine and Epidural Space . . . 391
Neoplastic Lesions . . . 391
Metastatic Carcinoma . . . 392
Lymphoma . . . 392
Myeloma . . . 394
Chordoma . . . 394
Other Regional Tumors . . . 397
Nonneoplastic Lesions . . . 397
Prolapsed Disc . . . 398
Epidural Abscess . . . 398
Tuberculosis . . . 399
Other Regional Nonneoplastic Processes . . . 401
Suggested Reading . . . 402

Appendix A: Diagnoses that May Change the Surgical Approach . . . 405

Appendix B: Troubleshooting with CNS Intraoperative Consultation . . . 407

Index . . . 409

Part I
Introduction

Chapter 1
Introduction to CNS Intraoperative Cytopathology

> *Nothing can be a greater value to a neurosurgeon than the ability to visualize, immediately, from the gross appearances of a tumor what will be its histological nature. Too great emphasis cannot be laid on this.*

These words, expressed more than 80 years ago by Harvey Cushing, one of the pioneers of modern neurosurgery, are still fully relevant today. At present, the extraordinary development of neuroimaging modalities has enabled us to locate intracranial lesions with great precision, no matter how small, and to establish their degree of circumscription, vascularization, calcification, and even metabolic activity. Likewise, modern stereotactic and neuroendoscopic techniques enable the neurosurgeon to access these lesions safely and with minimum trauma, even if they are located in deep regions once thought to be inaccessible, such as the brainstem, cerebral centrum, third ventricle, and pineal regions. However, even in the current age of advanced neuroimaging and image-guided biopsies, rational treatment of intracranial lesions still requires the diagnostic certainty that only pathology can offer. Infectious, inflammatory, and reactive processes must be distinguished from neoplastic processes, while defining the type of the neoplastic process involved is a crucial factor in determining surgical strategy. Similarly, intraoperative consultation is essential to avoid non-diagnostic biopsies by confirming that the specimen obtained is adequate for an accurate final diagnosis.

Aware of the need for intraoperative consultation, in spite of the current technological breakthroughs, we must decide on a rational basis for the method that should be used. Two main techniques are available for the rapid diagnosis of biopsies from the central nervous system (CNS); these are frozen sections and the smear technique. Unlike other organs, the CNS involves several factors that make it difficult to perform this rapid diagnosis by using cryostat sections. On the one hand, the inherit soft nature of nerve tissue, with its high content of water and lipids, renders poor-quality frozen sections giving rise to freezing artifact and distortion of the tissue that may result in misdiagnosis. On the other hand, samples obtained through stereotactic

C. R. Lacruz et al., *Central Nervous System Intraoperative Cytopathology*, Essentials in Cytopathology 13, https://doi.org/10.1007/978-3-319-98491-9_1

surgery, extremely small and usually rather soft, are difficult to handle in the cryostat. In contrast, smear preparations sidestep these issues quickly and simply, yielding beautiful nuclear and cytoplasmic details, without any freezing artifact, of a very small amount of tissue (Fig. 1.1a, b). We can see in the following list a summary of the advantages and disadvantages of the smear technique when compared to frozen sections.

Advantages of the Smear Technique

- Improved cost-effectiveness.
- More rapid and technically simpler
- Only a small amount of tissue needed
- Far better preservation of cellular detail
- Best in demonstrating fibrillary cytoplasmic processes
- Provides additional information to the permanent sections
- If the case turns out to be infectious, contamination of the cryostat and subsequent defrosting and sterilization can be avoided
- Abrogate the risk of distorting valuable diagnostic material during freezing, which compromise permanent sections and immunomarkers

Disadvantages of the Smear Technique

- Low-magnification architecture is lost
- Some lesions do not smear well (especially those having extensive reticulin or collagen)
- Specific training needed (many pathologists are more familiar with frozen section techniques and interpretation)

It is not our intention to argue in favor of the superiority of one method over the other, as no technique ensures absolute accuracy, but there is no doubt that the positive factors outweigh the negative, and that is why we believe that the smear technique is the best alternative for the intraoperative study of brain biopsies, especially when dealing with small stereotactic or neuroendoscopic biopsy specimens. We suggest to those pathologists who are not familiar with this technique that they start using it as an adjunct to frozen sections, because they can only reap benefits from doing so. As authoritative voices have already stated, histology and cytology are not two competitive fields of pathology – quite the opposite – both are part of pathology's resources, and they complement each other magnificently. As the pathologist becomes experienced, the smears become self-explanatory and present a clear pic-

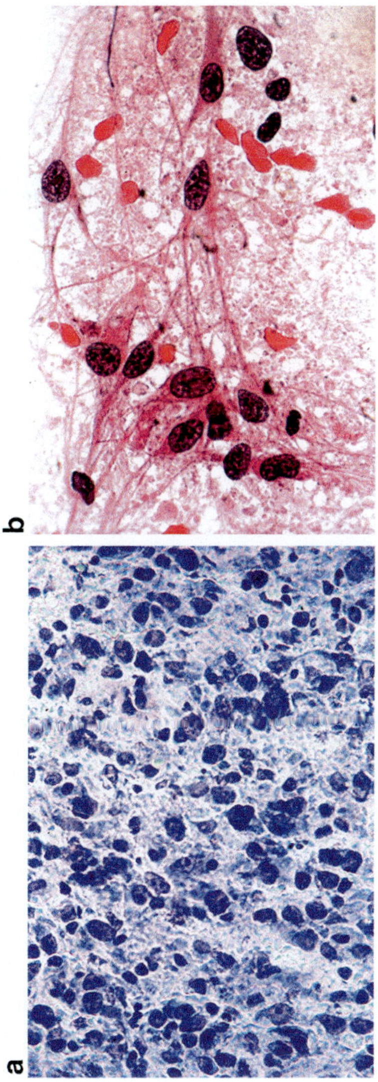

Fig. 1.1 *Anaplastic astrocytoma*. (**a**) Cryostat section showing freezing artifact, nuclear distortion, and effacement of the fibrillary background (Methylene blue). (**b**) Cytologic preparation from the same tumor showing beautifully preserved nuclear and cytoplasmic details. Note the characteristic multipolar astrocytic processes (Smear, H&E)

Table 1.1 CNS lesions in which the smear technique is an especially useful procedure

Astrocytoma
Oligodendroglioma
Ependymoma
Glioblastoma
Ganglion cell tumors
Meningioma
Lymphoma
Germinoma
Pituitary adenoma
Metastases
Reactive gliosis
Cerebral infarction
Inflammatory processes
Demyelinating disorders
Cranial and spinal bone masses

ture in lesions often obscured in frozen sections. Table 1.1 lists the processes in which the smear technique is particularly recommended.

Historical Background

We should keep in mind, from a historical perspective, the difficult early times of this technique, its development which was full of uncertainty, and its consolidation phase culminating in the publication of the first article acknowledging its high degree of reliability.

The beginnings of the cytologic method were clearly conditioned by a marked skepticism or obvious rejection in all fields of surgical pathology. Most physicians considered that performing diagnostic cytopathology was a waste of time. In such an adverse, if not markedly hostile, environment, Professor Leonard S. Dudgeon, who was the Dean of St. Thomas's Hospital Medical School of London and pioneer in the development of intraoperative cytology on surgical specimens, published in 1927, together with C.V. Patrick, an initial study of 200 cases which included some examples of brain tumors. This study showed that his preparations, made by scraping of the surfaces of surgical specimens with a scalpel and smearing the scrapings on glass slides, were of great value for the diagnosis of the disease process. The smears were fixed immediately – without being allowed to dry – for 2 to 10 minutes in Schaudinn's fluid (a fixative mixture of 2 parts of saturated mercuric chloride solution, 1 part of absolute ethanol, and enough glacial acetic acid to form a 4% solution) and then stained by hematoxylin and eosin. He called his preparations "wet films" and stated – "we wish to emphasize that this method of fixation provides a very beautiful method of demonstrating the appearances of malignant and other cells, showing the structural details of the individual cells in a manner not seen in the corresponding sections." Influenced by this paper, Louise Eisenhardt and Harvey Cushing published an article in 1930 demonstrating the usefulness of the cytologic method for the rapid diagnosis of brain tumors. The procedure used by these authors was the performance of squash preparations, stained supravitally with neutral red. Thus, the "wet film" technique managed to survive and to show its usefulness in the field of surgical neuropathology. A few years later, supported by this paper, the technique returned to the United Kingdom, where it was used successfully by Russell, Krayenbühl, and Cairns, who reported their favorable conclusions in 1937. These authors appear to have introduced toluidine blue as staining method instead of neutral red, because the supravital technique, while effective, did not allow the specimens to be retained for subsequent review.

The development of this initial work continued a decade later with new contributions and modifications of the technique. In 1947, Morris developed a procedure that replaced supravital stains with air-dried slides, staining them with eosin and methylene blue dyes. In 1960, wet fixation in 95% alcohol was introduced by McMenemey; this makes possible the use of the more common cytologic stains such as hematoxylin and eosin or Papanicolaou.

The consolidation phase took place during the 1960s and early 1970s when based on the toluidine blue method, the Morris method, or the conventional cytologic stains on wet-fixed slides that were much more familiar to a majority of pathologists, the "squash technique" becomes more popular in a few neurosurgical centers. Thus, Jane and Bertrand in 1962, and Jane and Yashon in 1969 and 1972 based on their experience in the interpretation of smears, published detailed descriptions, including an atlas, of the cytologic aspects of most common brain tumors, whereas the accuracy of smear diagnosis of brain biopsies was first published by Marshall and colleagues in 1973. They found that 93.6% of 184 specimens were diagnosed correctly by intraoperative cytology. This publication basically marked the end of the historical phase for the establishment of a technique that continues to be alive, as shown by its wide use throughout the world.

At present, because the use of minimally invasive neurosurgical techniques has increased exponentially, with the resulting drastic decrease in sample size, the interest in smear preparations has increased even more, to the point that, in some centers, they are now used exclusively for the intraoperative diagnosis of brain lesions.

Accuracy of CNS Intraoperative Cytopathology

There is little doubt that the use of the smear technique alone in experienced hands is capable of great diagnostic accuracy. Since the aforementioned paper by Marshall and colleagues in 1973, many series dealing with accuracy in CNS intraoperative cytopathology have been reported, and all tend to agree that it is an accurate diagnostic test (Table 1.2).

Table 1.2 Accuracy of intraoperative neurocytopathology

Authors	(%)
Marshall et al. (1973)	93.6
Ostertag et al. (1980)	95.0
Liwnicz et al. (1982)	92.0
Willems and Alva-Willems (1984)	87.0
Cahill and Hidvegi (1985)	90.6
Silverman et al. (1986)	91.0
Zhang et al. (1987)	91.7
Mouriquand et al. (1987)	87.5
Martinez et al. (1988)	95.0
Guarda (1990)	97.6
Reyes et al. (1991)	91.0
Torres and Collaço (1993)	92.2
Shah et al. (1998)	89.7
Di Stefano et al. (1998)	95.3
Firlik et al. (1999)	90.0
Lacruz and Escalona (2000)	91.5
Savargaonkar and Farmer (2001)	94.0
Bleggi-Torres et al. (2001)	97.3
Roessler et al. (2002)	95.0
Iqbal et al. (2006)	95.4
Goel et al. (2007)	85.0
Mitra et al. (2010)	88.5
Ghosal et al. (2011)	93.0
Sharma and Deb (2011)	93.3
Krishnani et al. (2012)	94.9
Jaiswal et al. (2012)	83.7
Agrawal et al. (2014)	95.0
Nanarng et al. (2015)	89.2
Kishore et al. (2016)	95.3
Hamasaki et al. (2017)	95.3

In general, the yield is more than 90% (average rate, 92.2%), being somewhat higher for open than for stereotactic biopsies. This discrepancy seems to be due mainly to sampling problems during stereotactic biopsy. Taking up to four biopsies also increases the diagnostic yield of stereotactic biopsy to 90%. This figure compares favorably with that for frozen sections, because the errors resulting from this technique in neurosurgery may reach more than 10%. Analysis of the available data shows that the main problem was the failure to classify a malignant tumor correctly; however, it was unlikely to affect immediate management decisions. It also may be ascertained with a more detailed analysis of the published series that the diagnostic accuracy increased with operator and smear interpretation experience and when cases of partial correlation, mainly due to grading deviations, were included.

As shown by these data, the technique is not infallible, which is why prudence is called for. To demand from intraoperative cytology the same diagnostic capability as from permanent-section biopsy is a great mistake. We are not dealing here with a method of absolute precision, but rather with the fact that its validity resides in its ability, within a minimum span of time and a scant amount of tissue, to give the neurosurgeon sufficient information to enable him to take a concrete position during the surgical act that impacts patient management.

Histologic Types of Central Nervous System Neoplasia

One of the main usefulness of intraoperative consultation on lesions of the CNS is to confirm or rule out the presence of neoplasia and to define the neoplastic cell type according to consensus classification. CNS tumors, with their huge variety of types and subtypes, each with its own clinical peculiarities and different cytohistologic characteristics, presented a great challenge from the start. Because of this reason, since Bailey and Cushing provided the first widely accepted nomenclature in 1926, more than 12 classifications have been brought forth, which include that of Kernohan et al. in 1949, that of Zülch in 1965, and that of Russell and Rubinstein in 1971, just to mention those that are better known. This profusion of classifications gave rise to a rather confusing situation, in which the same tumor could have more than one name depending on the classification used. In 1979, the situation began to improve with the publication of the World Health Organization (WHO) classification, which represented a reconciliation of the previous conflicting terminologies. Since 1979, three more editions of the WHO classification have been brought forth – 1993 second edition, 2000 third edition, and 2007 fourth edition – based solely on morphology. Currently, molecular features are becoming increasingly important in predicting patient prognosis and outcome and have been incorporated, for the first time, in addition to histology into the 2016 updated fourth edition. Thus, most of the new entities/variants in the WHO 2016 classification are defined based on a combination of histologic features and molecular alterations. A summary, including grades of tumors, is listed in Table 1.3; very uncommon tumor types or subtypes (e.g., melanocytic tumors, most mesenchymal, non-meningothelial tumors) were not considered for the sake of simplicity.

Table 1.3 The 2016 WHO classification of tumors of the CNS

Tumors	WHO grade
Diffuse astrocytic and oligodendroglioma tumors	
Diffuse astrocytoma (IDH-mutant; IDH-wildtype; NOS)	II
Gemistocytic astrocytoma, IDH-mutant	II
Anaplastic astrocytoma (IDH-mutant; IDH-wildtype; NOS)	III
Glioblastoma, IDH-wildtype	IV
Giant cell glioblastoma	IV
Gliosarcoma	IV
Epithelioid glioblastoma	IV
Glioblastoma (IDH mutant; NOS)	IV
Diffuse midline glioma, H3 K27 M-mutant	IV
Oligodendroglioma (IDH-mutant and 1p/19q-codeleted; NOS)	II
Anaplastic oligodendroglioma (IDH-mutant and 1p/19q-codeleted; NOS)	III
Oligoastrocytoma, NOS	II
Anaplastic oligoastrocytoma, NOS	III
Other astrocytic tumors	
Pilocytic astrocytoma	I
Pilomyxoid astrocytoma	a
Subependymal giant cell astrocytoma	I
Pleomorphic xanthoastrocytoma	II
Anaplastic pleomorphic xanthoastrocytoma	III
Ependymal tumors	
Subependymoma	I
Myxopapillary ependymoma	I
Ependymoma	II
Ependymoma, *RELA* fusion-positive	II/III
Anaplastic ependymoma	III
Other gliomas	
Chordoid glioma of the third ventricle	II
Angiocentric glioma	I
Astroblastoma	a
Choroid plexus tumors	
Choroid plexus papilloma	I
Atypical choroid plexus papilloma	II
Choroid plexus carcinoma	III
Neuronal and mixed neuronal-glial tumors	
Dysembryoplastic neuroepithelial tumor	I
Gangliocytoma and ganglioglioma	I
Anaplastic ganglioglioma	III
Dysplastic cerebellar gangliocytoma	I
Desmoplastic infantile astrocytoma and ganglioglioma	I
Papillary glioneuronal tumor	I
Rosette-forming glioneuronal tumor	I
Diffuse leptomeningeal glioneuronal tumor	a
Central and extraventricular neurocytoma	II
Cerebellar liponeurocytoma	II
Paraganglioma	I
Tumors of the pineal region	

(continued)

Table 1.3 (continued)

Tumors	WHO grade
Pineocytoma	I
Pineal parenchymal tumor of intermediate differentiation	II/III
Pineoblastoma	IV
Papillary tumor of the pineal region	II/III
Embryonal tumors	
Medulloblastoma (genetically defined; histologically defined; NOS)	IV
Embryonal tumor with multilayered rosettes (C19MC-altered; NOS)	IV
Medulloepithelioma	IV
CNS neuroblastoma	IV
CNS ganglioneuroblastoma	IV
CNS embryonal tumor, NOS	IV
Atypical teratoid/rhabdoid tumor	IV
CNS embryonal tumor with rhabdoid features	IV
Tumors of the cranial and paraspinal nerves	
Schwannoma	I
Melanotic schwannoma	a
Neurofibroma	I
Malignant peripheral nerve sheath tumor	II/III/IV
Meningiomas	
Meningioma	I
Atypical meningioma	II
Anaplastic (malignant) meningioma	III
Mesenchymal, non-meningeal tumors	
Hemangioblastoma	I
Solitary fibrous tumor/ Hemangiopericytoma	I/II/III
Lymphomas	
Diffuse large B-cell lymphoma of the CNS	a
Immunodeficiency-associated CNS lymphomas	a
Intravascular large B-cell lymphoma	a
Low-grade B-cell lymphoma of the CNS	a
T-cell and NK/T-cell lymphomas of the CNS	a
Anaplastic large cell lymphoma (ALK-positive; ALK-negative)	a
MALT lymphoma of the dura	a
Germ cell tumors	
Germinoma	a
Embryonal carcinoma	a
Yolk sac tumor	a
Choriocarcinoma	a
Teratoma (mature; immature; with malignant transformation)	a
Mixed germ cell tumor	a
Tumors of the sellar region	
Craniopharyngioma	I
Granular cell tumor of the sellar region	I
Pituicytoma	I
Spindle cell oncocytoma	I
Metastatic tumors	a

Modified from Louis et al. (2016a)
NOS insufficient information to assign a more specific code, *a* no WHO grading of tumors

Suggested Reading

Agrawal M, Chandrakar SK, Lokwani D, Purohit MR. Squash cytology in neurosurgical practice: a useful method in resource-limited setting with lack of a frozen section facility. J Clin Diagn Res. 2014;8:FC09–FC012.

Bleggi-Torres LF, de Noronha L, Schneider Gugelmin E, Martins Sebastião AP, et al. Accuracy of the smear technique in the cytological diagnosis of 650 lesions of the central nervous system. Diagn Cytopathol. 2001;24:293–5.

Brainard JA, Prayson RA, Barnett GH. Frozen section evaluation of stereotactic brain biopsies. Diagnostic yield at the stereotactic target position in 188 cases. Arch Pathol Lab Med. 1997;121:481–4.

Brommeland T, Lindal S, Straume B, Dahl IL, Henning R. Does imprint cytology of brain tumors improve intraoperative diagnoses? Acta Neurol Scand. 2003;108:153–6.

Cahill EM, Hidvegi DF. Crush preparations of lesions of the central nervous system. A useful adjunct to the frozen section. Acta Cytol. 1985;29:279–85.

Di Stefano D, Scucchi LF, Cosentino L, Bosman C, Vecchione A. Intraoperative diagnosis of nervous system lesions. Acta Cytol. 1998;42:346–56.

Dudgeon LS, Patrick CV. A new method for the rapid microscopical diagnosis of tumors: With an account of 200 cases so examined. Brit J Surg. 1927;15:250–61.

Eisenhardt L, Cushing H. Diagnosis of intracranial tumors by supravital technique. Am J Pathol. 1930;6:541–2.

Firlik KS, Martinez AJ, Lundsford LD. Use of cytological preparations for the intraoperative diagnosis of stereotactically obtained brain biopsies: A 19-year experience and survey of neuropathologists. Neurosurgery. 1999;91:454–8.

Folkerth RD. Smears and frozen sections in the intraoperative diagnosis of central nervous system lesions. Neurosurg Clin North Am. 1994;5:1–18.

Ghosal N, Hegde AS, Murthy G, Furtado SV. Smear preparation of intracranial lesions: A retrospective study of 306 cases. Acta Cytopathol. 2011;39:582–92.

Goel D, Sundaram C, Paul TR, Uppin SG, et al. Intraoperative cytology (squash smear) in neurosurgical practice - pitfalls in diagnosis experience based on 3057 samples from a single institution. Cytopathology. 2007;18:300–8.

Guarda LA. Intraoperative cytologic diagnosis: evaluation of 370 consecutive intraoperative cytologies. Diagn Cytopathol. 1990;6:235–42.

Hamasaki M, Chang KHF, Nabeshima K, Tauchi-Nishi PS. Intraoperative squash and touch preparation cytology of brain lesions stained with H+E and Diff-Quik™. A 20-year retrospective analysis and comparative literature review. Acta Cytol. 2018;62:44–53.

Hayden R, Cajulis RS, Frias-Hidvegi D, Brody BA, Yu G, Levy R. Intraoperative diagnostic techniques for stereotactic brain biopsies: cytology versus frozen-section histopathology. Stereotact Funct Neurosurg. 1995;65:187–93.

Iqbal M, Shah A, Wani MA, Kirmani A, Ramzan A. Cytopathology of the central nervous system. I. Utility of crush smear cytology in intraoperative diagnosis of central nervous system lesions. Acta Cytol. 2006;50:608–16.

Ironside JW. Update on central nervous system cytopathology. II. Brain smear technique. J Clin Pathol. 1994;47:683–8.

Jaiswall S, Mukul V, Jaiswal AK, Behari S. Intraoperative squash cytology of central nervous system lesions. A single center study of 326 cases. Diagn cytopathol. 2012;40:104–12.

Jane JA, Bertrand G. A cytological method for the diagnosis of tumors affecting the central nervous system. J Neuropath Exp Neurol. 1962;21:400–9.

Jane JA, Yashon D. Cytology of tumors affecting the nervous system. Springfield, Illinois: Charkles C Thomas; 1969.

Kishore S, Bhardwaj A, Kusum A, Thakur B, Kaushik S, Sharma N. Intraoperative squash cytology of central nervous system and spinal cord lesions with histological correlation. Ann Pathol Lab Med. 2016;3:61–72.

Krishnani N, Kumari N, Behari S, Rana C, Gupta P. Intraoperative squash cytology: accuracy and impact on immediate surgical management of central nervous system tumors. Cytopathology. 2012;23:308–14.

Lacruz CR, Escalona J. Diagnóstico citológico de los tumores del sistema nervioso central. Barcelona: César Viguera; 2000.

Liwnicz BH, Henderson KS, Masukawa T, Smith RD. Needle aspiration cytology of intracranial lesions: A review of 84 cases. Acta Cytol. 1982;26:779–86.

Louis DN, Ohgaki H, Wiestler OD, Cavenee WK, editors. WHO classification of tumours of the central nervous system (Revised 4th ed). Lyon: International Agency for Research on Cancer (IARC); 2016a.

Louis DN, Perry A, Reifenberger G, von Deimling A, et al. The 2016 world health organization classification of tumors of the central nervous system: a summary. Acta Neuropathol. 2016b;13:803–20.

Marshall LF, Adams H, Doyle D, Graham DI. The histological accuracy of the smear technique for neurosurgical biopsies. J Neurosurg. 1973;39:82–8.

Martinez AJ, Pollack I, Hall WA, Lunsford LD. Touch preparations in the rapid intraoperative diagnosis of central nervous system lesions. A comparison with frozen sections and paraffin-embedded sections. Mod Pathol. 1988;1:378–84.

McMenemey WH. An appraisal of smear diagnosis in neurosurgery. Am J Clin Pathol. 1960;33:471–9.

Mitra S, Kumar M, Sharma V, Mukhopadhyay D. Squash preparation. a reliable diagnostic tool in the intraoperative diagnosis of central nervous system tumors. J Cytol. 2010;27:81–5.

Morris AA. The use of the smear technique in the rapid histological diagnosis of tumors of the central nervous system. Description of a new staining method. J Neurosurg. 1947;4:497–504.

Mouriquand C, Benabid AL, Breyton M. Stereotaxic cytology of brain tumors. Review of an eight year experience. Acta Cytol. 1987;31:756–65.

Nanarng V, Jacob S, Mahapatra D, Mathew JE. Intraoperative diagnosis of central nervous system lesions: comparison of squash smear, touch imprint, and frozen section. J Cytol. 2015;32:153–8.

O'Neill KS, Dyer PV, Bell BA, Wilkins PR, Uttley D, Marsh HT. Is perioperative smear cytology necessary for CT-guided stereotaxic biopsy? Br J Neurosurg. 1992;6:421–7.

Ostertag CB, Mennel HD, Kiessling M. Stereotaxic biopsy of brain tumors. Surg Neurol. 1980;14:275–83.

Plesec TP, Prayson RA. Frozen section discrepancy in the evaluation of central nervous system tumors. Arch Pathol Lab Med. 2007;131:1532–40.

Plesec TP, Prayson RA. Frozen section discrepancy in the evaluation of nonneoplastic central nervous system samples. Ann Diagn Pathol. 2009;13:359–66.

Reyes MG, Homsi FM, McDonald LW, Glick RPI. smears, and frozen sections of brain tumors. Neurosurgery. 1991;29:575–9.

Roessler K, Dietrich W, Kitz K. High diagnostic accuracy of cytologic smears of central nervous system tumors. A 15-years' experience based on 4172 patients. Acta Cytol. 2002;46:667–74.

Russell DS, Krayenbühl H, Cairns H. The wet film technique in the histological diagnosis of intracranial tumors; a rapid method. J Path Bac.t. 1937;45:501–5.

Savargaonkar P, Farmer PM. Utility of intra-operative consultations for the diagnosis of central nervous system lesions. Ann Clin Lab Sci. 2001;31:133–9.

Shah AB, Muzumdar GA, Chitale AR, Bhagwati SN. Squash preparation and frozen section in intraoperative diagnosis of central nervous system tumours. Acta Cytol. 1998;42:1149–54.

Sharma S, Deb P. Intraoperative neurocytology of primary central nervous system neoplasia: a simplified and practical diagnostic approach. J Cytol. 2011;28:147–58.

Silverman JF, Timmons RL, Leonard JR, Hardy IM, et al. Cytologic results of fine-needle aspiration aspiration biopsies of the central nervous system. Cancer. 1986;58:1117–21.

Torres LFB, Collaço LM. Smear technique for the intraoperative examination of nervous system lesions. Acta Cytol. 1993;37:34–9.

Wilkerson JA, Bonnin JM. Intraoperative cytology. An adjunct to frozen sections. New York: Igaku-Shoin; 1987.
Willems JGMS, Alva-Willems JM. Accuracy of cytologic diagnosis of central nervous system neoplasms in stereotactic biopsies. Acta Cytol. 1984;28:243–9.
Zhang YX, Luo KS, Liv JC, Chen Y, Chen YH, Lai RS. Cytological diagnosis of 500 cases of intracranial tumors during craniotomy. Chin J Clin Cytol. 1987;3:19–27.

Chapter 2
Clinical and Radiological Approach to CNS Intraoperative Diagnosis

The more information, the better the understanding

Intraoperative consultation in neurosurgery is not an exception to this rule, but quite the opposite – whoever attempts to make intraoperative diagnoses aided only by microscopic findings will be making a big mistake. The variety and range of possibilities are so great that we must propose making the intraoperative consultation in two consecutive phases: As first step, to get clinical and radiological information is critical to narrow the clinical differential diagnosis for a certain patient given the gender, age, lesion location, neuroimaging findings, pertinent clinical course, and prior history. The clinico-radiologic correlation makes the subsequent microscopic interpretation easier. This interpretation is the second part of the process and deals with the purely microscopic differential diagnosis of a certain number of entities that are already limited by the prior clinico-radiologic assessment. In selected cases (e.g., emergent cases), direct communication with the neurosurgeon may be the only source of patient history.

Unequivocal understanding of the need to combine these two phases of the consultation correctly is essential if good results are to be achieved.

Clinical Considerations for Pathologists

The clinical information that must reach the pathologist must be logically limited but useful and should include age of the patient, lesion location, current and prior medical history, and relevant family history.

C. R. Lacruz et al., *Central Nervous System Intraoperative Cytopathology*, Essentials in Cytopathology 13, https://doi.org/10.1007/978-3-319-98491-9_2

Age and Location

The histologic type of an intracranial tumor is intimately related to the age of the patient and to its location, although exceptions do occur. This way, by pooling together topographic criteria and age, we can arrive at the following systematization:

In adults, both intra- and extra-axial supratentorial tumors predominate, with malignant gliomas, meningioma, and metastases being the most frequent. In the posterior fossa, meningioma, schwannoma, hemangioblastoma, and epidermoid cyst are predominant.

In children and adolescents, posterior fossa and midline tumors predominate, being the most common medulloblastoma, ependymoma of the posterior fossa, craniopharyngioma, and astrocytomas of the cerebellum, brain stem, and optical tract. Less frequent, but also expected tumors are germ cell tumors (pineal/suprasellar), and ganglion cell tumors (superficial hemispheric based). Other histologic types, such as choroid plexus tumors (ventricles) and atypical teratoid/rhabdoid tumor (supra and infratentorial regions), are uncommon but distinctive neoplasms affecting infants and young children.

Medical History

The medical history should include the nature and duration of symptoms and whether the patient has other significant medical problems or previous history of CNS disease and/or treatment.

Patients may have symptoms either due to focal destruction of neural tissue or due to edema, distortion of intracranial structures, and raised intracranial pressure. Focal clinical signs, such a hemiparesis, dysphasia, or seizures, depend on the anatomic location of the lesion and reflect impaired regional cerebral function (Table 2.1).

Frequently, however, the initial symptoms result only from mass effect, local pressure, and distortion of adjacent structures. These symptoms consist of headache, irritability, emotional lability, drowsiness, forgetfulness, and lethargy. In general, tumors present with progressive symptoms, as opposed to the sudden onset of focal neurologic signs of patients with a stroke.

A history of neoplasms, even if they are not related to the CNS, is also a critical point. Obviously, if the patient has had a CNS tumor, it is fundamental to know the histologic type and the nature of any treatment received, especially if it was radiotherapy (the changes induced by radiotherapy may be mistaken for a recurrent tumor). On the other hand, due to the high rate of neurologic complications in AIDS, at times, the first manifestation of the disease, HIV testing should be considered for all patients with unexplained cerebral mass lesions.

Table 2.1 Lesional topography and related symptoms and signs

Location	Symptoms/Sings
Cerebral hemispheres	Seizures
Left hemisphere	Dysphasia/aphasia
Frontal/temporal lobes	Emotional/behavioral changes
Parietal lobes	Dyspraxia; sensory abnormalities
Occipital lobes	Visual disturbances
Sellar/suprasellar	Hydrocephalus; impaired vision; Pituitary/hypothalamic dysfunction
Pineal region	Hydrocephalus; Parinaud's syndrome[a]
Cerebellum	Hydrocephalus; disturbed gait; Ataxia; dysmetria; nystagmus
Pons	Cranial nerve palsies; hemiparesis
Cerebellopontine angle	Hearing loss; tinnitus; vertigo
Spinal cord	Back pain; sensory-motor deficits; paraparesis/paraplegia

[a]Paralysis of extraocular movements due to involvement of the tectal plate

Family History

Certain CNS tumors occur in the context of genetic disorders, and it is of great interest to know whether the patient has a neuroectodermal dysplasia or some other type of genetic disorder related to CNS neoplasms (Table 2.2).

Neuroimaging Considerations for Pathologists

Neuropathology, much like bone pathology, is better done in correlation with the radiologic features. In particular, cross-sectional imaging modalities – computerized tomography (CT) and magnetic resonance imaging (MRI) – are essential tools in compiling a preoperative differential diagnosis. Therefore, at a minimum, one should be familiar with the findings described in the neuroimaging report and the radiologist's opinion of the lesion.

Principal Neuroimaging Modalities

Basics Principles

- CT uses X-rays
- MRI uses not ionizing radiation but a magnetic field to excite protons in the nuclei of hydrogen atoms, which emit signal (echo) upon relaxation. Image appearance is dependent upon time interval between time excitation (TE) and

Table 2.2 Genetic disorders and related CNS tumors

Disorder	Tumors and tumor-like lesions
Tuberous sclerosis complex	Subependymal giant cell astrocytoma
	Cortical tubers
	Subependymal nodules
Neurofibromatosis type 1	Neurofibromas
	Malignant peripheral nerve sheath tumors
	Optic nerve glioma
	Pilocytic or diffuse astrocytomas
Neurofibromatosis type 2	Vestibular schwannoma (often bilateral)
	Meningioma (often multiple)
	Spinal ependymoma (often multiple)
	Meningioangiomatosis
	Glial micro-hamartomas
Schwannomatosis	Non-vestibular schwannomas
	Meningiomas
Von Hippel-Lindau disease	Hemangioblastoma
	Endolymphatic sac tumor
Li-Fraumeni syndrome	Medulloblastoma
	Glioblastoma
	Choroid plexus carcinoma
Gorlin syndrome	Medulloblastoma (SHH-activated)
	Meningioma
Turcot syndrome type 1	Glioblastoma
Turcot syndrome type 2	Medulloblastoma (WNT-activated)
Cowden disease	Dysplastic gangliocytoma of the cerebellum
	Ganglioneuroma
RTPS	Atypical teratoid/rhabdoid tumor
Carney complex	Psammomatous melanotic schwannoma
	Somatotrophic pituitary adenoma
Familial retinoblastoma	Retinoblastoma (often bilateral)
	Pineoblastoma
DICER 1 syndrome	Pineoblastoma
	Pituitary blastoma
Wermer syndrome (MEN 1)	Pituitary adenoma
	Ependymoma
Aicardi syndrome	Choroid plexus papilloma
	Choroid plexus cysts
Sturge-Weber syndrome	Meningeal angiomatosis
Melanoma-astrocytoma syndrome	Diffuse astrocytomas
	Pleomorphic xanthoastrocytoma
	Nerve sheath tumors
	Meningioma

RTPS rhabdoid tumor predisposition syndrome, *DICER 1* syndrome, an autosomal dominant disorder caused by heterozygous germline mutation in the *DICER 1* gene, *MEN 1* multiple endocrine neoplasm type 1

time relaxation (TR). Two basic "weights" of images are obtained based upon TE and TR (T1 and T2).

- Both CT and MRI operate with digital images – during the actual scanning a huge amount of digital data is being acquired, which is then processed by a powerful computer and converted into images on the scanner.

Computed Tomography (CT)

- Interpretation/terminology:
  - White areas (hyperdense): areas that absorb or "attenuate" the passage of X-ray beam (bone, calcium, acute hematoma).
  - Black areas (hypodense): areas that do not absorb or "attenuate" the passage of X-ray beam (air, fat, edema, CSF).
  - Normal brain tissue (isodense) is intermediate between these two extremes.
- Used as screening tool, particularly in the emergency room (critically ill, pediatric, or unstable patients) and immediate postoperative studies. (Fig. 2.1).
- Essential in the imaging of patients who cannot have MRI (pacemakers, certain cerebral aneurysm clips, and other indwelling metallic devices).
- It is superior in detecting calcification and hemorrhage.

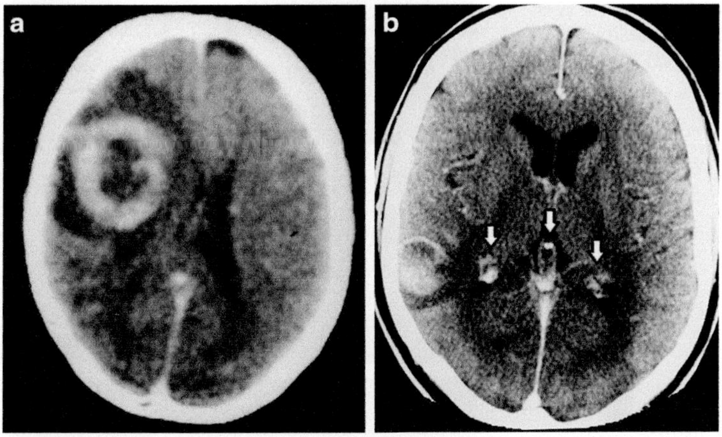

Fig. 2.1 *Emergency CT scans*. (**a**) Axial post contrast brain CT showing a large rim-enhancing lesion with prominent surrounding edema in the right hemisphere, which proved to be *Toxoplasma abscess* after biopsy. Also note marked midline shift to the left due to mass effect with complete compression of the adjacent ventricle. (**b**) Axial post contrast brain CT. In this case, in the setting of new-onset seizures status, a heterogeneous enhancing mass in the right hemisphere involving gray and white matter is revealed, which proved to be *glioblastoma* after biopsy. In addition to bone, CT shows other calcified structures, such as the pineal gland and choroid plexus in the atria of both lateral ventricles (*arrows*)

- A better evaluation of bony pathology (skull base, calvarium, spine) and bone changes related to the tumor.
- Intravenous iodinated contrast improves the visibility of cerebral vessels and highlights lesions in which there is a breakdown of the blood-brain barrier (enhancing lesions).

Magnetic Resonance Imaging (MRI)

- Interpretation/terminology (lesion description terminology is slightly different from CT): brighter is hyperintense (of increased signal), and darker is hypointense (with decreased signal) compared to normal anatomic structures (Figs. 2.2, 2.3 and 2.4).

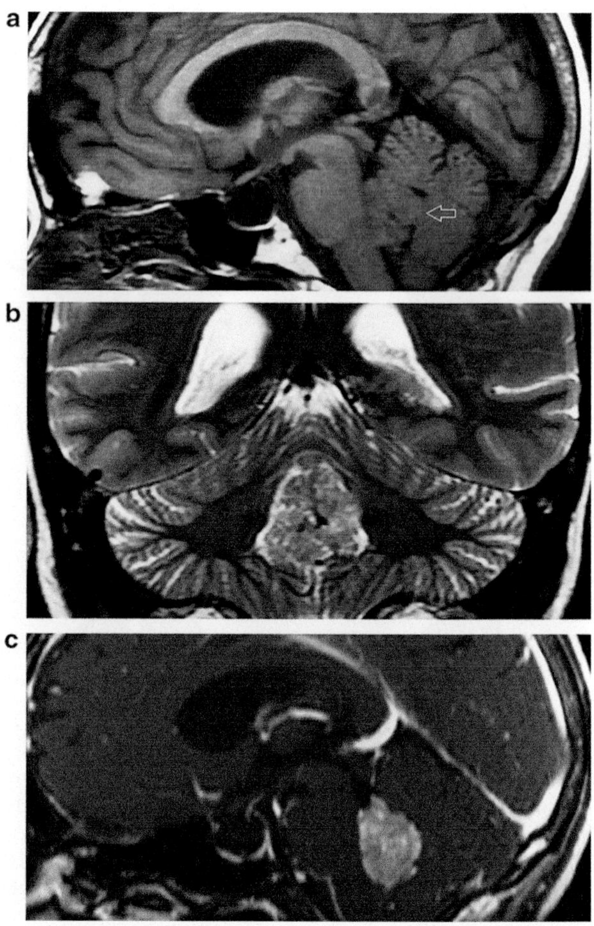

Fig. 2.2 *Ependymoma on MRI*. Sagittal T1 (**a**), coronal T2 (**b**), and sagittal post contrast T1 (**c**) images show a well-demarcated tumor (arrow) with heterogeneous enhancement filling the fourth ventricle. (Courtesy, Dr. Mar Jimenez; Quirónsalud University Hospital, Madrid)

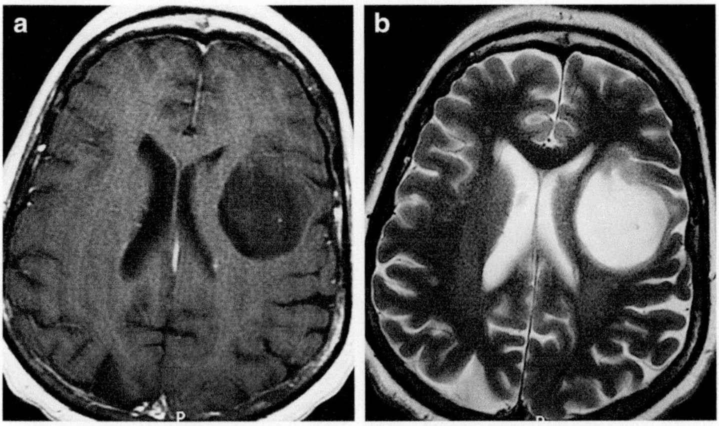

Fig. 2.3 *Infiltrative astrocytoma, WHO grade II on MRI.* (**a**) An axial T1 image with gadolinium shows a partially cystic, non-enhancing mass in the left hemisphere. There is compression of the adjacent ventricle due to mass effect. (**b**) This same region is much better visualized by its increased signal intensity on T2 image. Also CSF in the ventricular system and subarachnoid space are hyperintense. (Courtesy, Dr. Mar Jimenez; Quirónsalud University Hospital, Madrid)

- Commonly used MRI sequences:
  - T1-weighted (short TE and TR): best demonstrate normal anatomic structures (excellent for anatomic portrayal). On T1 image, white matter is brighter than the gray matter, and the CSF is very dark.
  - T2-weighted (long TE and TR): highlight tissues and lesions with high water content (edema, tumor, and fluids). On T2, the white matter is darker than the gray matter, and the CSF is very bright.
  - Fluid-attenuated inversion recovery (FLAIR): is basically a T2 sequence with water suppression. Also emphasized free water changes observed in pathologic conditions (edema, tumor, infection), but the CSF is dark (Fig. 2.5a).
  - Diffusion-weighted imaging (DWI): to evaluate decreased movement of protons (water molecules) throughout tissue, which may be seen in early (acute) infarcts, abscesses, epidermoids, and dense cell packing tumors (Fig. 2.5b).
- Improved soft tissue characterization (the technique of choice for studying the brain).
- Evaluation of most brain and spinal tumors.
- High sensitivity to tissue edema.
- Multiplanar capability (axial, coronal, and sagittal) without the need of repositioning the patient.
- Capacity to delineate small tumors in site near bone, such as the posterior and pituitary fossas, where beam-hardening artifacts limit the utility of CT.
- Intravenous contrast agent gadolinium to highlight lesions with disrupted blood-brain barrier (enhancing lesions) (Fig. 2.6).

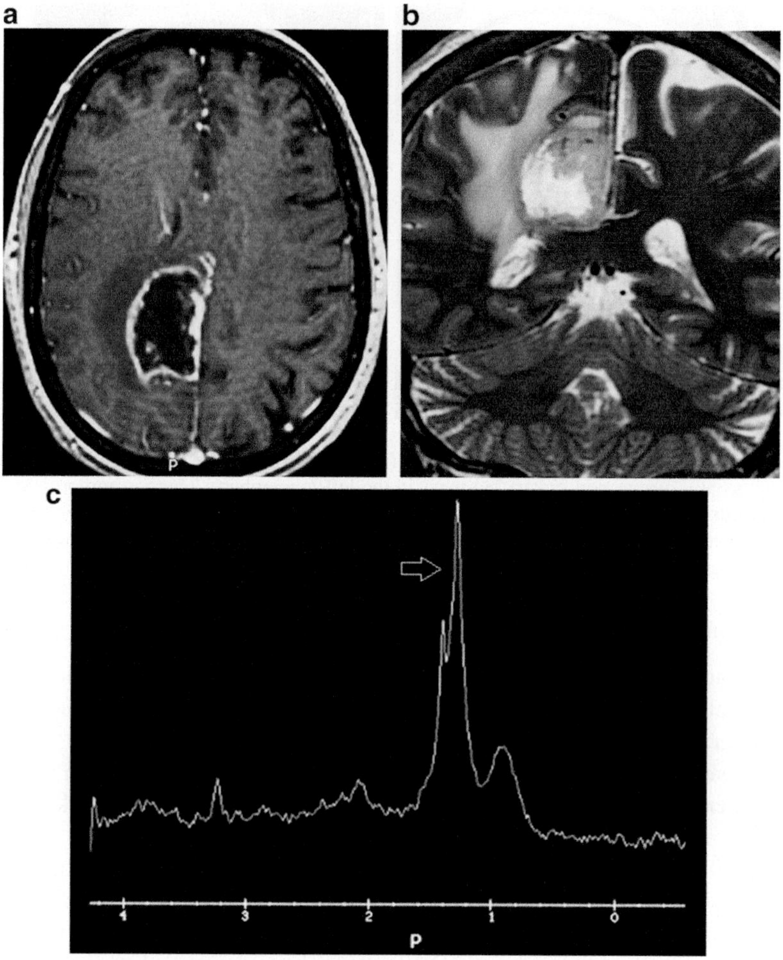

Fig. 2.4 *Glioblastoma, WHO grade IV on MRI.* (**a**) An axial T1 image with gadolinium reveals a deep-seated, irregularly "shaggy" ring-enhancing mass in the right hemisphere. (**b**) This same region and associated vasogenic edema are better visualized by its increased signal intensity on coronal T2 sequence. Note preserved cortical gray matter, which is not affected by vasogenic edema. (**c**) The corresponding magnetic resonance spectroscopy (MRS) shows an elevated choline peak (means increased cell turnover) suggesting a neoplastic process (*arrow*). (Courtesy, Dr. Mar Jimenez; Quirónsalud University Hospital, Madrid)

Proton Magnetic Resonance Spectroscopy (MRS)

- Provides information about the activity of specific metabolites that can supplement the information obtained for routine anatomic sequences. The following list summarizes some of the most important metabolites encountered in MRS and their clinical significance: (Table 2.3).

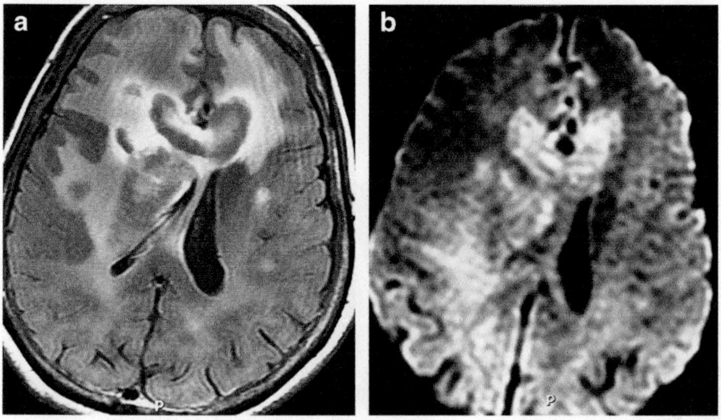

Fig. 2.5 *CNS lymphoma on MRI.* (**a**) A T2 fluid-attenuated inversion recovery (FLAIR) image reveals a heterogeneous lesion situated straddling the corpus callosum, creating a "butterfly" appearance. This sequence demonstrates hyperintense vasogenic edema surrounding the mass, but CSF is dark. (**b**) A diffusion-weighted image (DWI) demonstrates extensive reduced diffusion within the mass (bright signal), suggesting dense cell packing tumor (i.e., lymphoma). (Courtesy, Dr. Mar Jimenez; Quirónsalud University Hospital, Madrid)

- Can be used to predict tumor grade, to evaluate response to treatment, and to help distinguish tumor recurrence from treatment-induced tissue injury (Fig. 2.4c).

Positron Emission Tomography (PET)

- Tumors take up the tracer to a greater degree than normal tissues.
- Like MRS, PET is used to evaluate response to treatment and to identify recurrent tumor.

Thallium-201 Single-Photon Emission Computed Tomography (SPECT)

- Appropriate in patients with AIDS to help in differentiating toxoplasmosis (low radionuclide uptake) from primary CNS lymphoma (high radionuclide uptake).

Neuroimaging Evaluation

A consistent approach is to start evaluation by knowing the exact anatomic location of the lesion. The tendency of CNS tumors/processes to occur with a similar morphology in certain areas and compartments is well known; therefore, the first step is to determinate whether the lesion resides inside the neural tissue (*intra-axial*) or

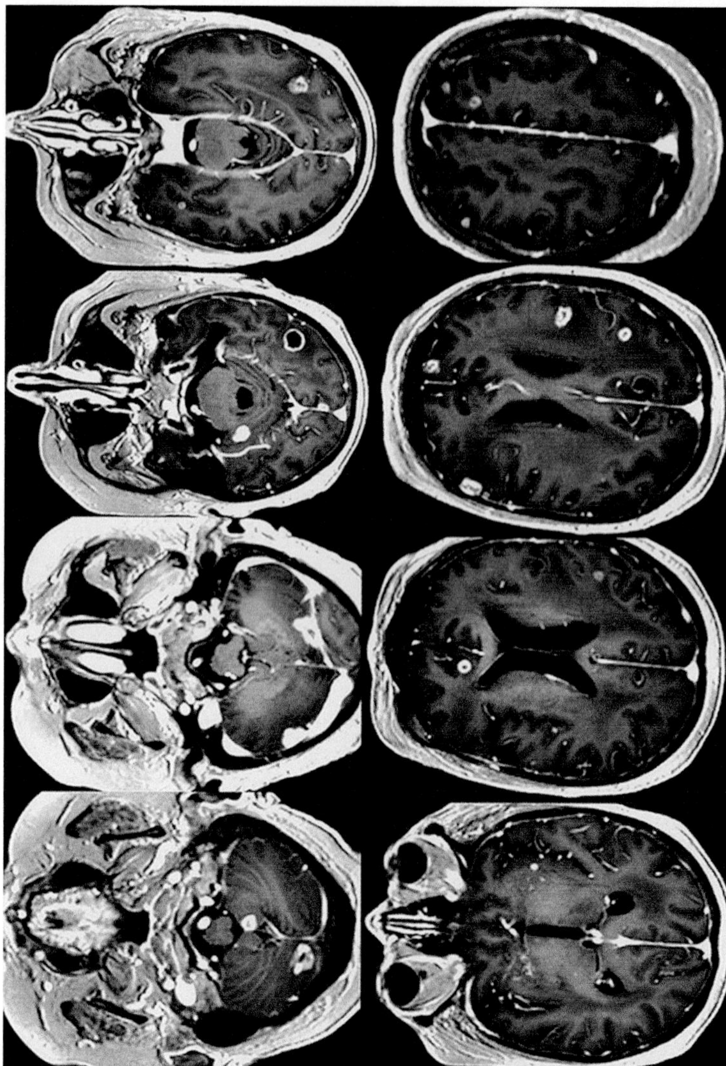

Fig. 2.6 *Metastasis on MRI*. Post contrast T1 slices from this patient reveal a large number of variably sized lesions suggesting metastases. Multifocality is a feature that is characteristically associated with hematogenously spreading processes. (Courtesy, Dr. Mar Jimenez; Quirónsalud University Hospital, Madrid)

Table 2.3 Important metabolites in MRS and their clinical significance

Metabolites	Clinical significance
Choline	Marker for turnover in the membrane
N-acetyl aspartate	Surrogate for neuronal integrity
Creatine	Marker for energy metabolism
Lactate	Nonoxidative glycolysis. Also seen in necrosis and hypoxia
Lipid	Marker for cellular necrosis

outside the brain/cord (*extra-axial*). If the lesion is intra-axial, the next step is to determine whether it is *intraparenchymal* or *intraventricular* (Tables 2.4 and 2.5). At times, this distinction may be difficult or even impossible, usually when aggressive lesions invade the other compartment.

At each of these locations, lesions can appear as well-circumscribed (discrete) or as ill-defined (diffuse) masses. These basic types of development may be modified as a result of the existence of secondary features such as *calcifications* and *cysts,* frequently related to long-standing lesions (Table 2.6), or *edema*, *necrosis*, and *bleeding,* usually associated with high-grade tumors or active lesions (Table 2.7). Regarding edema, two main types can be distinguished: vasogenic and cytotoxic. *Vasogenic edema* surrounds masses and extends into the white matter, sparing the (cortical) gray matter and hence having a finger-like appearance (Fig. 2.5a). In addition, there is increased diffusion of water molecules in this area, seen as hypointense (dark) signal on DWI (Fig. 2.5b). In contrast, *cytotoxic edema*, which is characteristic for infarctions, homogenously involves a well-delineated area including the gray and white matter extending to the brain surface. Additionally, the diffusion of water is decreased, and infarcts are hyperintense (bright) on DWI.

On the other hand, processes may be solitary or multiple (multifocal). *Multifocality* can be associated with demyelinating, vascular and infectious diseases, or neoplasms. Regarding neoplasms, the "M-rule" for differential diagnosis of common multiple tumors includes metastatic carcinoma, malignant CNS lymphoma, and melanoma (Fig. 2.6). However, beware of "multifocal glioblastoma."

By knowing the location, the manner of growth, the density (CT), or signal intensity (MRI), the presence and type of secondary features, the uni- or multifocality, as well as the *pattern of contrast enhancement* of a particular process (Table 2.8), one can reduce the number of potential diagnoses considerably. For example, a cystic intra-axial lesion with an enhancing mural nodule in the posterior fossa will lead us to suspect the presence of pilocytic astrocytoma or hemangioblastoma, whereas the presence of multiple intra-axial lesions with ring-enhancement and prominent vasogenic edema, of an AIDS-related CNS lymphoma or an infectious process.

Table 2.4 Location of different brain lesions

Intra-axial, intraparenchymal	*Extra-axial*
Astrocytoma	Meningioma
Oligodendroglioma	SFT/HPC
Extraventricular ependymoma	Schwannoma
CNS lymphoma	Metastasis
Embryonal tumors	Inflammatory pseudotumor
Ganglion cell tumors	Rosai-Dorfman disease
Hemangioblastoma[a]	Epidermoid cyst
Pleomorphic xanthoastrocytoma[a]	Dermoid cyst
Astroblastoma	Arachnoid cyst
Angiocentric glioma	Endodermal cyst
DNT	*Extra-axial (sellar/suprasellar)*
DIG/DIA[a]	Pituitary adenoma
Metastasis	Craniopharyngioma
Bacterial abscess	Germ cell tumors
Infarction	Chiasmatic/optic nerve glioma
Demyelinating disease	Pituicytoma
Parasite	Granular cell tumor
Tuberculoma	Spindle cell oncocytoma
Intra-axial, intraventricular	Meningioma
Ependymoma (F, L, T)	Chordoma
Subependymoma (L, F)	Metastasis
SEGA (L, T)	Rathke cleft cyst
Choroid plexus tumors (L, T, F)	Langerhans cell histiocytosis
Central neurocytoma (L)	Sarcoidosis
Meningioma (L, T, F)	*Extra-axial (pineal region)*
Chordoid glioma (T)	Germinoma
Colloid cyst (T)	Pineal parenchymal tumors
Exophytic tumor pattern[b]	Teratoma
Cerebellopontine angle	Glial tumors
Schwannoma	Meningioma
Meningioma	PTPR
Atypical teratoid/rhabdoid tumor	Pineal anlage tumor
Epidermoid cyst	Pineal cyst

[a]Frequent involvement of the overlying meninges

[b]Any parenchymal-based tumor can grow in an exophytic pattern into the ventricle (e.g., pilocytic astrocytoma); *DNT*, dysembryoplastic neuroepithelial tumor; *DIG/DIA*, desmoplastic infantile ganglioglioma/astrocytoma; SEGA, subependymal giant cell astrocytoma; *F/L/T*, fourth, lateral, and third ventricles; *SFT/HPC*, solitary fibrous tumor/hemangiopericytoma; *PTPR*, papillary tumor of the pineal region

Table 2.5 Location of different spinal cord lesions

Intra-axial	*Epidural*
Ependymoma	Metastasis
Pilocytic astrocytoma	Lymphoma
Hemangioblastoma[a]	Neurofibroma
Diffuse astrocytoma	Myeloma
Ganglion cell tumor	Chordoma
Oligodendroglioma	Other bone tumors
Metastasis	Hemangioma
Nonneoplastic disorders	Lipoma
Extra-axial, intradural	Nonneoplastic disorders
Meningioma	Bacterial abscess
Schwannoma	Tuberculosis
SFT/HPC	Prolapsed disc
Paraganglioma (filum terminale)	Extramedullary hematopoiesis
Drop metastasis (subarachnoid)	Vascular malformations
Endodermal/arachnoid cysts	Synovial cyst
Vascular malformations	Postoperative scar

[a]Frequent involvement of the overlying leptomeninges, *SFT/HPC* solitary fibrous tumor/hemangiopericytoma

The task of integrating all of these data belongs to an expert neuroradiologist, who usually suggests a family of lesions – often referred to as *gamuts* – that may have similar imaging appearances. For example, "the ring-enhancing mass," "the cystic mass," or "the hemorrhagic mass." In addition to the imaging appearance of a lesion, a *gamut* may be further characterized by the pertinent clinical information, eventually generating the differential diagnostic list that must be used as a starting point and as a basis for the intraoperative consultation. However, since neuroimaging provides the most relevant "gross pathology" for biopsy interpretation, a review of the scans personally is especially valuable, particularly if, as is the case, one must decide if the small biopsy specimen submitted for intraoperative consultation is a representative sample of a large or heterogeneous lesion.

Table 2.6 Likelihood of cysts, calcifications, and fat content in different lesions

Tumors with cystic change	*Calcification*
Pilocytic astrocytoma[a]	Oligodendroglioma
Ganglioglioma[a]	Pilocytic astrocytoma
Hemangioblastoma[a]	Meningioma
DIG/DIA[a]	Ependymoma
Extraventricular neurocytoma	Subependymoma
Pleomorphic xanthoastrocytoma	Choroid plexus papilloma
Craniopharyngioma	Diffuse astrocytoma
Teratoma	Supratentorial embryonal tumors
Ependymoma (supratentorial)	Neurocytoma
Pineocytoma	Ganglion cell tumors
Choroid plexus tumors	SEGA
Diffuse astrocytoma (occasional)	Craniopharyngioma
Meningioma (occasional)	Pineocytoma
Pituitary adenoma (occasional)	Metastatic mucinous ADC
Schwannoma (large lesions)	CAPNON
Nonneoplastic cysts	Associated to radionecrosis
Arachnoid	Tuberculoma
Choroid plexus	Vascular malformations
Colloid third ventricle	Epidermoid/dermoid cysts
Dermoid	Meningioangiomatosis
Endodermal	*Fat content*
Ependymal	Lipoma
Epidermoid	Adipocytic (lipomatous) meningioma
Parasitic	Teratoma
Pineal	Dermoid Cyst
Rathke cleft	Liponeurocytoma

[a]Often a cystic lesion with a mural nodule, *DIG/DIA* desmoplastic infantile ganglioglioma/astrocytoma, *SEGA* subependymal giant cell astrocytoma, *ADC* adenocarcinoma, *CAPNON* calcifying pseudoneoplasm of the neuraxis

Table 2.7 Likelihood of bleeding and edema in different lesions

Hemorrhagic mass	Edema
Neoplastic	*Prominent vasogenic edema*
Glioblastoma	AIDS-related CNS lymphoma
Oligodendroglioma	High-grade gliomas
Central neurocytoma	Atypical/anaplastic meningiomas
Choriocarcinoma	Metastasis
Metastatic melanoma	Abscesses
Metastatic renal cell carcinoma	Toxoplasmosis
Metastatic lung carcinoma	Granulomas
Nonneoplastic	PML

(continued)

Table 2.7 (continued)

Hemorrhagic mass	Edema
Hypertension	*Absent to minimal edema*
Infarction (hemorrhagic)	DNT
Aneurysm/vascular malformations	Low-grade gliomas
Coagulopathy	Ganglioglioma
Vasculitis	Focal cortical dysplasia
Amyloid angiopathy	*Cytotoxic edema*
Fungal infection	Infarction

PML progressive multifocal leukoencephalopathy, *DNT* dysembryoplastic neuroepithelial tumor

Table 2.8 Patterns of contrast enhancement in different lesions

Enhancing process	*Non-enhancing process*
Pilocytic astrocytoma	Low-grade diffuse gliomas
Ependymoma	Chronic/cystic infarction
High-grade diffuse gliomas	PML
Meningioma (with "dura tail")	*Little, if any, enhancing process*
Embryonal tumors	Subependymoma
CNS Lymphoma	DNT
Craniopharyngioma	Angiocentric glioma
Nerve sheath tumors	Gliomatosis (initially)
Ganglion cell tumors	*Ring-enhancing process*
Choroid plexus tumors	Glioblastoma
Pineal parenchymal tumors	Necrotic metastasis
Pituitary adenoma[a]	Necrotic lymphoma
Pleomorphic xanthoastrocytoma	Abscess
SEGA	Toxoplasmosis
Astroblastoma	Tumefactive demyelination
Neurocytoma	Radiation necrosis
Hemangioblastoma	Resolving infarction
SFT/Hemangiopericytoma	Resolving hematoma
Teratoma	*Leptomeningeal enhancement*
Germinoma	Meningeal carcinomatosis,
Paraganglioma	Lymphomatosis, melanomatosis
Chordoid glioma	Meningitis
Metastatic tumors	Meningioangiomatosis
Vascular malformations	*Dural enhancement*
Inflammatory pseudotumor	Meningioma
Rosai-Dorfman disease	Metastatic disease
Sarcoidosis	Secondary lymphoma
Infarct (first few days)	Granulomatous disease

[a]Less and delayed than normal pituitary gland, *SEGA* subependymal giant cell astrocytoma, *SFT* solitary fibrous tumor, *PML* progressive multifocal leukoencephalopathy, *DNT* dysembryoplastic neuroepithelial tumor

Suggested Reading

Abul-Kasim K, Thurnher MM, McKeever P, Sundgren PC. Intradural spinal tumors: current classification and MRI features. Neuroradiology. 2008;50(4):301–14.
Bakshi R. Advances in neuroimaging technology: state of the art. Rev Neurol Dis. 2007;4:97–9.
Burger PC, Nelson JS, Boyko OB. Diagnostic synergy in radiology and surgical neuropathology: neuroimaging techniques and general interpretative guidelines. Arch Pathol Lab Med. 1998;122:609–19.
Burger PC, Nelson JS, Boyko OB. Diagnostic synergy in radiology and surgical neuropathology: radiographic findings of specific pathologic entities. Arch Pathol Lab Med. 1998;122:620–32.
Byrne TN. Imaging of gliomas. Semin Oncol. 1994;21:162–71.
Cha S. Update on brain tumor imaging: from anatomy to physiology. Am J Neuroradiol. 2006;27:475–87.
Cha S. Neuroimaging in neuro-oncology. Neurotherapeutics. 2009;74:1319–22.
Drevrelegas A, editor. Imaging of brain tumors with histological correlations. 2nd ed. Berlin/Heidelberg: Springer; 2011.
Farrell CJ, Plotkin SR. Genetic causes of brain tumors: neurofibromatosis, tuberous sclerosis, von Hippel-Lindau, and other syndromes. Neurol Clin. 2007;25:925–46. viii
Gilman S. Imaging the brain. First of two parts. N Engl J Med. 1998;338:812–20.
Gilman S. Imaging the brain. Second of two parts. N Engl J Med. 1998;338:889–96.
Hoffman JM. New advances in brain tumor imaging. Curr Opin Oncol. 2001;13:148–53.
Solomon DA, Perry A. Familial tumor syndromes. In: Perry A, Brat DJ, editors. Practical surgical neuropathology. A diagnostic approach. Philadelphia: Elsevier; 2018. p. 505–45.

Chapter 3
Specimen Handling and Optimal Processing

The microscopic interpretation of any type of smear depends largely on the excellence of the preparations

Ruth M. Graham

Proper handling and processing of surgical specimens are crucial for an accurate intraoperative diagnosis. Indeed, in many instances diagnostic errors are due to inadequate tissue sampling and/or subpar preparations. Thus, the correct performance of the whole process should include proper identification and appropriate specimen transportation, adequate tissue sampling, careful performance of the smear, and quick, but optimal, fixation and staining.

Specimen Identification and Transportation

The specimen must be carried out from the operating room to the pathology department in a sterile container on a saline-moistened lens paper or *telfa* pad (never gauze) to prevent drying, accompanied by a request form which summarizes the relevant clinico-radiologic data and the precise site from which the biopsy was taken.

It is also very useful, in order to hone better our response, to specify the reason for which the intraoperative diagnosis was sought – adequacy or guidance – as well as the technique used for obtaining the specimen: open biopsy, stereotactic-guided needle aspiration biopsy with intraoperative CT monitoring, or fine-needle aspiration biopsy performed freehand under CT guidance without stereotactic instrumentation (can be done in the CT suite).

C. R. Lacruz et al., *Central Nervous System Intraoperative Cytopathology*, Essentials in Cytopathology 13, https://doi.org/10.1007/978-3-319-98491-9_3

Tissue Sampling

There are three types of specimens that account for most neurosurgical intraoperative consultations; from largest to smallest, they are irregular tissue fragments from open biopsy/resections, tissue cores from stereotactic needle biopsies, and tiny endoscopic biopsies. A careful gross examination is necessary to select the zones most likely to be diagnostic – a magnifying lens may be helpful – by noting any deviations from normal appearance. Normal brain can often be identified even in small core biopsies; the tissue is slightly firm with a distinctive white or gray homogeneous appearance and will maintain its shape. By the contrary, lesional tissue usually shows a more variegated appearance with hemorrhagic, friable, gelatinous, or fragmented solid quality and soft or firm consistency, which provides some clues about the abnormal nature of the tissue (Fig. 3.1). In bone curettage specimens, diagnostic areas tend to stand out among the hemorrhagic bone fragments as soft or friable zones. With experience, the pathologist is soon able to recognize the more abnormal tissue for smearing. As a general rule, it is advisable to sample "everything that looks different," particularly the softest and darkest regions of the specimen. To overcome sampling errors, multiple smears from different regions, particularly in large or heterogeneous specimens, should be obtained. It is also advisable to retain the remainder of the biopsy unfixed until the first batch of smears has been examined, because if these are negative, further smears can be prepared from the same biopsy specimen.

Smear Technique

Due to inherent soft nature of nerve tissue, cytologic technique suits CNS lesions better than any other lesions elsewhere in the body. Of the three ways of obtaining intraoperative cytological preparations, i.e., touch/imprint technique, scraping technique, and the squash/smear technique, the last is the technique of choice for the study of the CNS. As against the other techniques, the squash/smear is really a "microbiopsy" in which, within reasonable limits, an architectural evaluation may be performed by recognizing complex cellular associations such as papillae, rosettes or fascicles, or even relationships between the cells with surrounding blood vessels, stromal tissue, or extracellular matrix.

The biopsies must be handled gently as there is little supporting tissue and they are easily distorted (avoid the use of forceps, the edge or point of a sterile blade will often suffice). It's also advisable not to smear too large specimens which may yield a slide too thick for optimal cellular detail. Thus, the selected fragment is placed on a glass slide and then divided into smaller pieces (1–2 mm^3), each of which is transferred to a new labeled slide. The single specimen is squashed gently by a second glass slide, and this second slide is moved down to smear the tissue onto the first slide (like smearing a FNA specimen). Crushing and overstretching artifacts, from

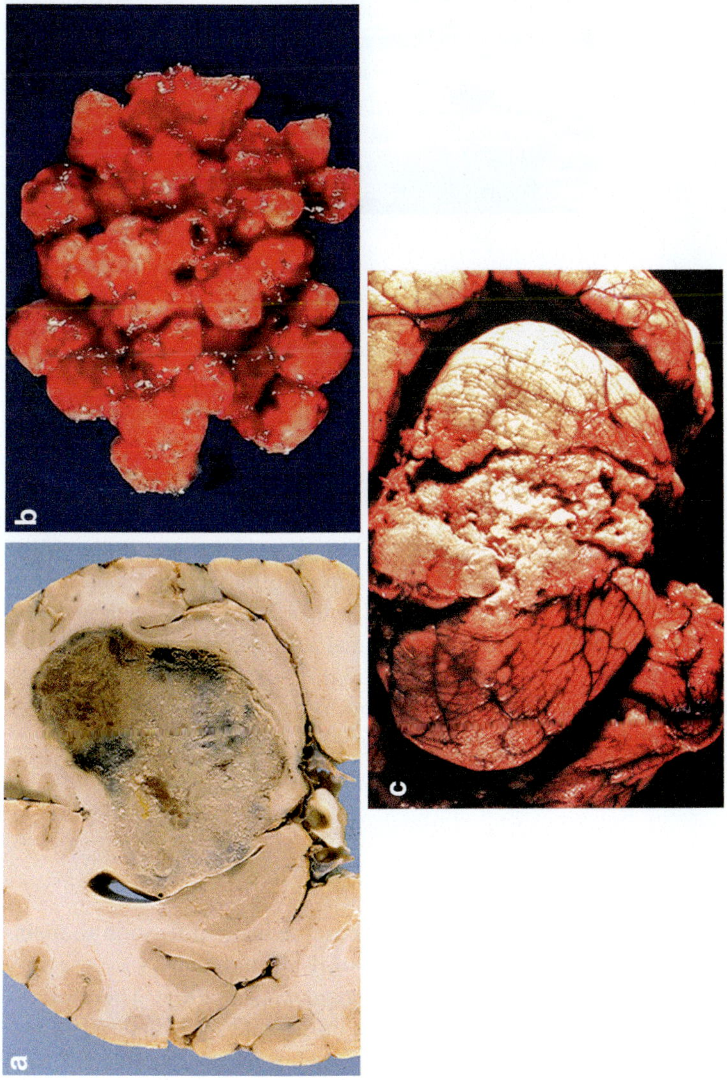

Fig. 3.1 *Macroscopic appearances*. (**a**) *Prototypical glioblastoma multiforme* (autopsied brain). Distinctive variegated "geographic" appearance with tan-grayish tumor tissue, yellowish areas of necrosis, and darkest zones of hemorrhage. Compare with the gray or white homogeneous aspect of the normal brain. (**b**) *Intraventricular ependymoma*. This resection specimen shows a characteristic fleshy and mamelonated "placenta-like" appearance. (**c**) *Medulloblastoma* (autopsied brain). This tumor involving vermis displays subarachnoid space invasion. Note a whitish granular "sugar-coating" appearance of the pia-arachnoid

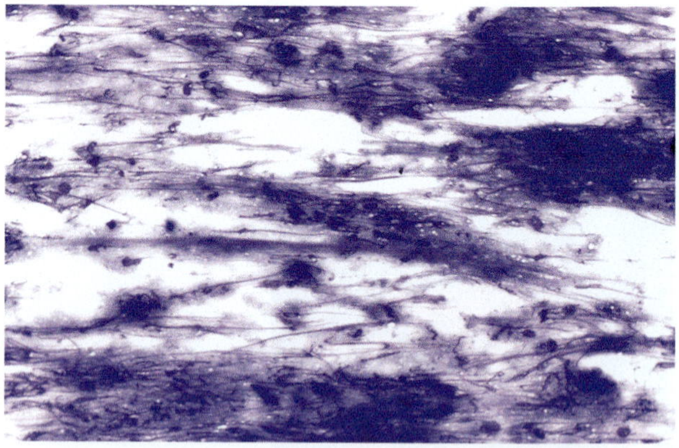

Fig. 3.2 *Crush artifact, CNS lymphoma.* Due to excessive pressure, most nuclei have streaked out during the smear (Romanowsky stain)

Table 3.1 Comparison of tissue smearing

Easily	Poorly
Normal brain/cord	Reactive gliosis
Most primary/secondary tumors	Schwannoma
	Hemangioblastoma
	Subependymoma
	Desmoplastic tumors
Nonneoplastic disorders	Vascular malformations

applying excessive pressure and rapidly pulling the glass slides apart, should be avoided (Fig. 3.2). With experience, the skill of applying the appropriate level of pressure for different types of lesions is acquired. If a lesion does not smear well and if single cells are not separable, then the cytological information obtained will be limited, but the way it smears (or doesn't smear) will, in itself, be a valuable piece of information and aids diagnosis. Only some types of tissue defy smearing, especially those having extensive reticulin, collagen, or glial fibers (Table 3.1).

Fixation

The most critical step in making preparations is the immediacy of fixation to maintain morphology. A fresh smear will rapidly dry out if left unfixed for even a very short period of time, which tends to ruin cytological preservation. Therefore, it should be fixed immediately *while still moist*. This immediate wet fixation of fresh specimens is the appropriate one, contrary to what is believed, independently of the staining method used. Even fast Romanowsky stains, i.e., Diff-Quik, usually employed with air-dried preparations, benefit from wet fixation in the case of the brain/cord. The fixative of choice is 95% ethanol; in the case of fast Romanowsky stains, the same fixative (absolute methanol) supplied by the manufacturer can be used without noticeable morphologic differences. The fixation time is 1–2 min depending on the thickness of the smear.

Staining Methods

A wide variety of staining techniques can be used: hematoxylin and eosin, the Papanicolaou method, toluidine blue, methylene blue, crystal violet, Romanowsky-type stains, Morris's method, etc. Each method, in turn, may be used with different protocols, times, and types of reagents, which is why it may be said, without fear of making a mistake, that there are as many fast intraoperative staining methods as there are pathology laboratories in the world. If any one of these laboratories has problems with the method employed, we suggest that they use the following protocols that we have chosen based on their simplicity and good results.

Fast Hematoxylin and Eosin Method

Recommended Procedure

A fast hematoxylin (Harris, Gill II, or similar) should be used, instead of a slower hematoxylin (Mayer, Caracci, or similar). Adding acetic acid to eosin Y solution (0, 5 ml/100 ml) promotes a fast eosin uptake in cells. Standing rinses are discouraged (dipping smears in each rinse promotes the exchange of solutions). Stain and rinse duty cycles should be assessed.

Steps

1. Fix in 95% ethanol	1–2 min
2. Tap water	5–10 dips until surface is smooth
3. Fast Hematoxylin	30 s with 10 initial dips
4. Tap water	Rinse until clear
5. Bluing reagent	5 dips
6. Tap water	5 dips
7. Eosin Y (alcoholic)	15 dips

8. The smear is rapidly dehydrated, cleared, and mounted

Results

Nuclei stain blue and cytoplasmic structures with varying shades of pink to red. Cells containing a large number of intermediate filaments are particularly striking (i.e., keratinized cells, gemistocytes). The fibrillary background of gliomas shows through well. Metachromatic substances are hardly visualized (Fig. 3.3a).

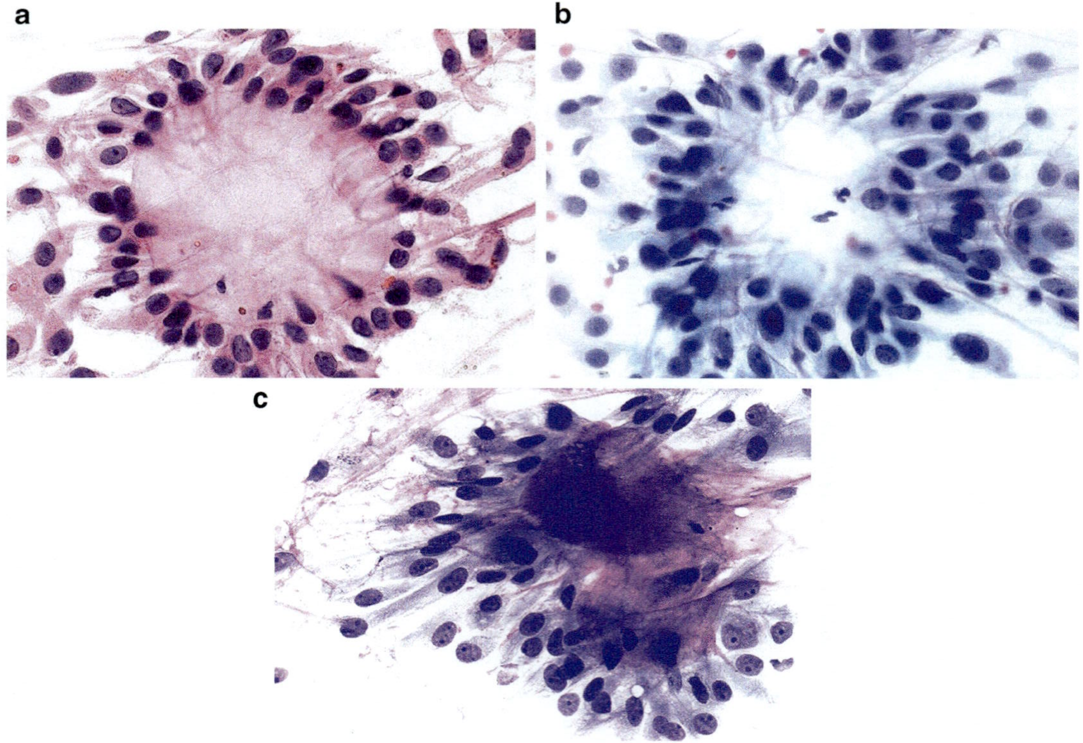

Fig. 3.3 *Myxopapillary ependymoma*. (**a**) *H&E-stained smear* showing a clump of radially arranged tumor cells. (**b**) *Papanicolaou-stained smear* also shows the characteristic morphology of ependymal cells; however, the myxoid stromal component is not shown. (**c**) *Romanowsky stain* provides key information about matrix-containing lesions: the myxoid blebs not clearly seen with Papanicolaou- and H&E-stained smears are nicely revealed here. Also note that nuclear smudging is avoided in wet-fixed preparations

Fast Papanicolaou Method

Recommended Procedure

Same as for the H&E method.

Steps

Steps 1–6	Same as for the H&E method
7. OG-6	15 dips
8. 95% ethanol	10 dips
9. EA-50	30 s with 10 initial dips

10. The smear is rapidly dehydrated, cleared, and mounted

Results

Nuclei stain just the same as with H&E. The cytoplasm stains turquoise blue, except for keratinized cells which stain orange (orangeophilia). The fibrillary background of gliomas appears bluish green in great detail. Somas and cytoplasmic processes, rich in filaments of GFAP, tend to stain eosinophilic. Metachromatic substances are hardly visualized (Fig. 3.3b).

Modified Fast Romanowsky Stain

Recommended Procedure

Perform *wet fixation.* Only in the case of rather fluid specimens, it is necessary to let the slide air-dry to promote cell adhesion before fixation in methanol (air-dry per se does not fix cells). The same commercial reagents (i.e., Diff-Quik, MGG-Quik) are used.

Steps

1. Dip smear, *while still moist*, in fixative solution for 1–2 min. Allows excess to drain
2. Dip slide in xanthene dye (pink-orange) solution for 10 s (10 1-second dips). Allows excess to drain
3. Dip slide in thiazine dye (dark blue) solution for 12 s (12 1-second dips). Allows excess to drain.

4. Rinse slide with distilled or deionized water until clear
5. Wet mounting for a rapid diagnosis
6. After diagnosis allow to dry completely (no alcohol dehydration!)
7. Dip in xylene and coverslip using permanent mounting medium

Results

Nuclei stain purple and the cytoplasmic structures with varying shades of blue. Cells with a large amount of intermediate filaments (i.e., keratinized cells, gemistocytes) stain a brilliant sky blue. Metachromatic substances reveal themselves clearly in purple or intense pink. The fibrillary background of gliomas can be seen in detail (Fig. 3.3c). With this modified procedure, the problems caused by the air-drying of the preparation are avoided, such as nuclear enlargement, chromatin smudging, and quick deterioration (smears less suitable for keeping as a part of the permanent record); but all of the qualities of the so-called Romanowsky effect are preserved (metachromatic cellular staining and identification of stromal matrix).

Fast Toluidine Blue Method

Recommended Procedure

Toluidine blue solution: dissolve toluidine blue (1 g) in 95% ethyl alcohol (20 mL) and add distilled water (80 mL). Filter and store in a dark bottle in the refrigerator.

Steps

1. Fix in 95% ethanol	1–2 min
2. 1% toluidine blue solution	1 min with 10 initial dips
3. Tap water	Rinse until clear

6. Wet mounted for a rapid diagnosis
7. After diagnosis the smear is dehydrated, cleared, and mounted with a permanent mounting medium.

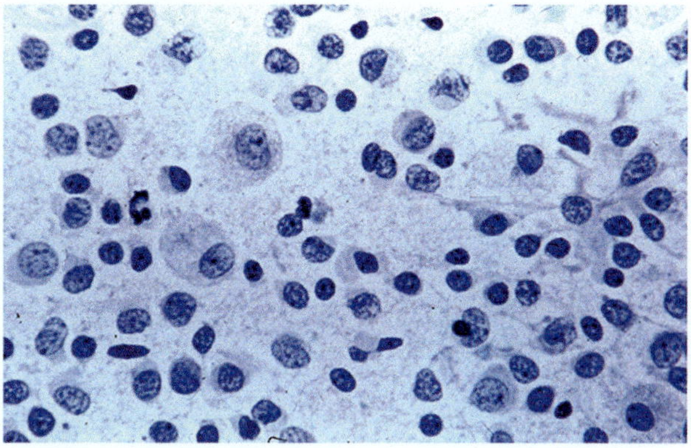

Fig. 3.4 *CNS ganglioneuroblastoma. Toluidine blue-stained smear* showing a mixed population of neuroblastic, neurocytic, and gangliocytic cells. In contrast to the Romanowsky methods, nuclei stain not purple (metachromatic) but dark blue

Results

Nuclei stain dark blue and the cytoplasm light blue. The fibrillary background is outlined. Mucins stain in purple/red. Coloration is very striking in wet-mount smears but turns pale after dehydration (Fig. 3.4).

We have tried all of these techniques, and our recommendation is to use the wet-fixed stain you are most familiar with, usually H&E or Papanicolaou, together with a fast Romanowsky stain in alcohol-fixed slides, because this provides very valuable complementary information about the cytoplasmic details, background elements, mucins, and stromal matrix components of the lesion examined, avoiding the problems caused by air-drying.

Suggested Reading

Bezrukov AV. Romanowsky staining, the Romanowsky effect and thoughts on the question of scientific priority. Biotech histochem. 2017;92:29–35.

Boom ME, Drijver JS. Routine cytological staining techniques. London: MacMillan; 1986.

Burger PC, Nelson JS. Stereotactic brain biopsies: specimen preparation and evaluation. Arch Pathol Lab Med. 1997;121:477–80.

Gill GH. Cytopreparation: principles & practice. In: Essentials in cytopathology series. New York, NY: Springer; 2013.

Meyer M, Keith-Rokosh J, Reddy H, Megyesi J, Hammond RR. Sources of error in neuropathology intraoperative diagnosis. Can J Neurol Sci. 2010;37:620–4.

Seliem RM, Assaad MW, Gorombey SJ, Moral LA, Kirkwood JR, Otis CN. Fine-needle aspiration biopsy of the central nervous system performed freehand under computed tomography guidance without stereotactic instrumentation. Cancer. 2003;99:277–84.

Yachnis AT. Intraoperative consultation for nervous system lesions. Semin Diagn Pathol. 2002;19:192–206.

Chapter 4
Algorithmic Approach to CNS Intraoperative Cytopathology

Complicated algorithms are not useful, whereas
simple algorithms are often false.

The aim of CNS intraoperative cytopathology is to allow reliable preliminary diagnoses and guidance during targeting and resecting of lesions in neurosurgery. To facilitate this objective, it is advisable to use algorithms that make it easier to perform a sample triage as well as a smear evaluation and general-category interpretation. It has been said that complicated algorithms are not useful, whereas simple algorithms are often false. In order to avoid this, we use three simple algorithms for each of these steps, which, when employed together, complement each other and make it possible to perform an adequate evaluation of the disease process. In this way, we make sure that we do not forget anything essential at a most demanding diagnostic moment.

Sample Triage

Tissue triaging depends on the neurosurgical procedure employed because the degrees of accuracy and detail required are different. For the "closed" stereotactic technique, to state that the sample is adequate and representative is enough, whereas "open" surgical resections require a more detailed diagnostic approach that can guide the neurosurgeon. Therefore, we should take into account the following possibilities:

1. The smear provides enough information to satisfy the degree of accuracy required (adequacy or guidance).
    - The residual tissue is processed for routine paraffin sections.
    - In cases in which a differed diagnosis requires electron microscopy studies, flow cytometry, FISH, or some other ancillary technique, tissue/preparations are taken for those studies.

C. R. Lacruz et al., *Central Nervous System Intraoperative Cytopathology*, Essentials in Cytopathology 13, https://doi.org/10.1007/978-3-319-98491-9_4

- If infectious disorder, recommend the surgeon to obtain samples for cultures from sterile operating field.
- If stereotactic biopsy, report presence of large vessels to neurosurgeon.

2. The smear does not provide an adequate response for these demands.

   - Further smears/frozen sections.
   - If these are not conclusive either, it is recommended to obtain more tissue (the pathologist must not be tempted to "overcall" minimal abnormalities lest the surgeon believes there is adequate diagnostic material when there is not).
   - The final decision as to whether to obtain more tissue and from where additional biopsy specimens are to be taken must be made by the surgeon.

3. Cases in which it is recommended to obtain further smears to overcome sampling or diagnostic errors:

   - Normal tissue.
   - To prevent grading errors in large diffuse gliomas.
   - When pathologic diagnosis is not consistent with clinical and neuroimaging findings.

4. Brain biopsies in AIDS patients require extreme precautions to prevent accidental infection (gloves, complete immersion of smears in alcohol, washing work area with a bleach solution, no cryostat utilization).
5. Brain biopsies done for suspected prion disease should never be examined through cytologic technique or cryostat sections, because of the biohazard risk to laboratory personnel. Snap-frozen tissue is saved for potential Western blotting and remaining tissue treated with formic acid before processing by hand.

Special precaution is recommended when the pathologic diagnosis is not consistent with clinical and radiologic findings. Often, in approaching the lesion, the surgeon takes samples of the periphery that are not truly representative. This can lead to error by confusing, for example, perilesional gliosis with a glioma or the inflammatory reaction characteristic of some tumors (i.e., germinoma) with a nonneoplastic process.

Smear Evaluation

A complete evaluation of the smear requires the study of six parameters: type of smearing, type of background, type of blood vessels, presence of specific cell groups, predominant type of cell, and presence of specific cellular elements. All of this, which may seem complicated and tedious, with practice, is done reflexively in a few seconds and facilitates the interpretation of smears. Therefore, we should take into account the following:

1. Type of smearing
   - Normal tissue pattern (uniform/smooth)
   - Lesional tissue pattern (speckled/granular)
2. Type of background
   - Finely granular (feltlike)
   - Clear (empty)
   - Fibrillary (threadlike)
   - Necrotic (dirty)
   - Granular-vacuolated
   - Myxoid-mucoid
3. Type of blood vessels
   - Thin-walled
   - Thick-walled (hyalinized)
   - Endothelial cell proliferation (microvascular hyperplasia)
   - Network of vascular channels
4. Specific cell groups
   - Whorls
   - Papillae
   - True rosettes (Flexner-Wintersteiner)
   - Pseudorosettes (Homer-Wright)
   - Perivascular pseudorosettes
5. Type of cell
   - Glial (fine processes)
   - Ganglion/ganglion-like
   - Round
   - Epithelial/epithelial-like
   - Fusiform
   - Small poorly differentiated
   - Mixed/polymorphic
6. Specific cellular elements
   - Rosenthal fibers
   - Eosinophilic granular bodies
   - Lymphoglandular bodies
   - Keratin
   - Melanin
   - Mucin

Type of Smearing

Normal brain/cord smears easily and evenly with preparations displaying a uniform/smooth pattern to the naked eye. On the contrary, in reactive states and in neoplasms, tissues tend to smear with an irregular consistency producing preparations with a speckled/granular pattern, which microscopic appearance will depend on the nature and degree of intercellular adhesion and the varying proportions of stromal elements. For example, tumors with strong attachments and cohesive stroma (i.e., schwannoma) will spread little, if any, yielding tissue fragments, whereas those with little cohesion and stroma (i.e., lymphoma) will spread into single cells. Tumors whose cells have widespread but relatively weak attachments and scant, less cohesive stroma (i.e., meningioma, carcinoma) will result in a mixed pattern with cell sheets, smaller cell clusters, and individual cells (Fig. 4.1).

Type of Background

The pressure needed for performing the squash technique breaks apart the tissue, thereby creating a space between the cells and cell groups or background. In normal neuroglial tissue, the neuropil components translate into a finely granular (feltlike) background, which represents the microscopic counterpart of the uniform-smooth smear pattern. In the case of lesional tissue, this intercellular space may be empty (clear background), or it may be occupied by various cell products or components, such as fine cytoplasmic processes (fibrillary background); necrotic debris (necrotic background); released intracytoplasmic components of a proteinaceous, lipidic, or glycogenic nature (granular/vacuolated background); or stromal or mucinous matrix (myxoid/mucoid background). Thus, five fundamental types of abnormal background are produced, each one of them related to different processes (Table 4.1). In order to observe granular/vacuolated and myxoid/mucoid backgrounds clearly, it is advisable to use Romanowsky-type stains.

It is characteristic for some tumors to produce smears with mixtures of different backgrounds, such as a fibrillary-necrotic background (glioblastoma) or fibrillary-myxoid background (pilocytic/pilomyxoid astrocytoma). A special type of granular/vacuolated background is the so-called striped "tigroid" background that originates by the released intracytoplasmic contents of glycogen-rich tumors during the squash technique.

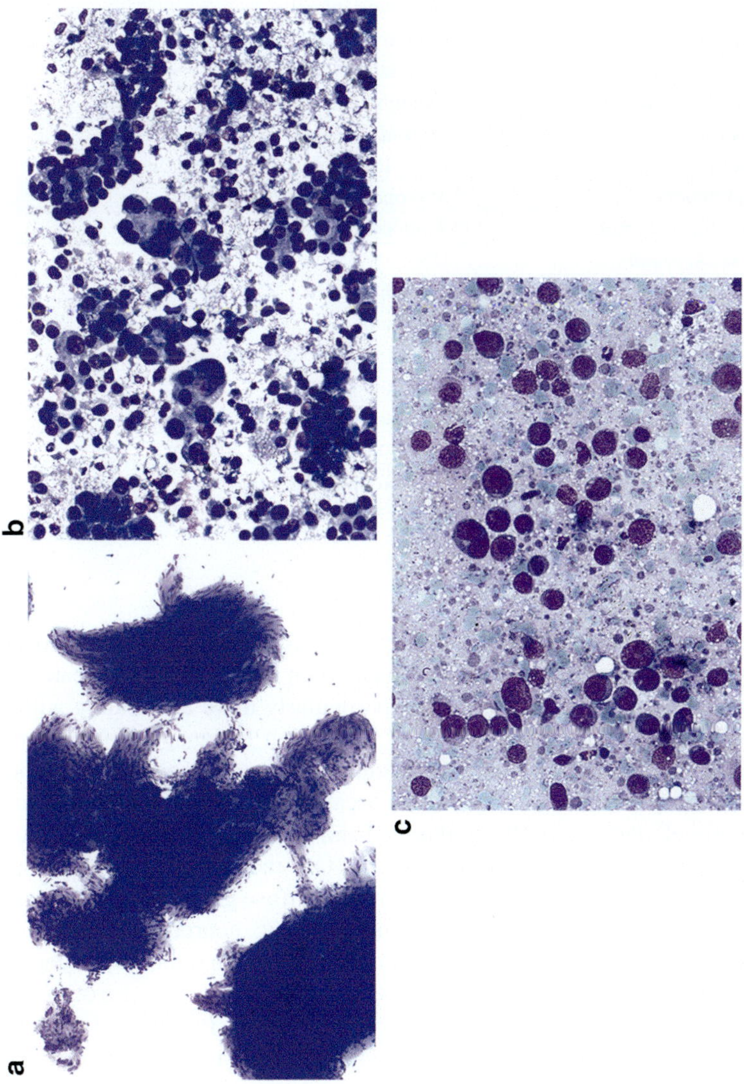

Fig. 4.1 *Type of smearing*. (**a**) Schwannoma smear reveals only tissue fragments without single cells. (**b**) Smear from metastatic carcinoma showing a mixed pattern with cell sheets, smaller cell clusters, and individual cells. (**c**) Smear from lymphoma showing single cells without cell aggregates. Note the numerous lymphoglandular bodies in the background (**a–c**; Smears, Romanowsky)

Table 4.1 Type of background and related processes

Clear (empty) background	*Granular/vacuolated background*
Schwannoma	Oligodendroglioma
Meningioma	Hemangioblastoma
Pineocytoma	Demyelinating lesions
SFT/Hemangiopericytoma	Resolving infarct
Choroid plexus papilloma	Pituitary adenoma (if squash/smear)
Pituitary adenoma (if imprints)	Germinoma ("tigroid")
Fibrillary (thread-like) background	Ewing's sarcoma ("tigroid")
Astrocytic tumors	*Myxoid/mucoid background*
Ependymal tumors	Pilocytic/pilomyxoid astrocytoma
Mixed glioneural tumors	Myxopapillary ependymoma
Neuronal tumors (fine neuropil)	Angiocentric glioma
Necrotic (dirty) background	DNT
Necrotic primary tumors	Neurofibroma
Necrotic metastasis	Chordoma
Necrotic CNS lymphoma	Chordoid/myxoid meningioma
Cerebral infarction	Chordoid glioma
Necrotizing infections	Gliomas with mucinous degeneration
Radiation necrosis	Mucinous metastatic carcinoma

SFT solitary fibrous tumor, *DNT* dysembryoplastic neuroepithelial tumor

Type of Blood Vessels

Blood vessels are structures that can often blend into the background on a frozen section but are easy to identify on smears. Thus, when evaluating the smear, one should pay attention to the blood vessel type, particularly if we are dealing with a glioma. Microvascular proliferation (MVP) is a criterion for anaplasia in diffuse astrocytoma and, to a lesser degree, in oligodendroglioma and ependymoma, but not in pilocytic astrocytoma. MVP may be also occasionally seen in metastatic cancer (mainly small-cell and renal cell carcinomas) and nonneoplastic processes (surrounding resolving infarctions and abscesses). On the contrary, thin-walled capillaries are the characteristic vessels of low-grade diffuse gliomas (astrocytoma, oligodendroglioma), neurocytoma, and dysembryoplastic neuroepithelial tumor. Thick-walled (hyalinized) vessels are frequently encountered in tumors with degenerative changes, such as schwannoma, ganglioglioma, and pilocytic astrocytoma, and in the setting of radiation. Lastly, an intricate network of thin-walled vascular channels is the characteristic pattern of hemangioblastoma and hemangiopericytoma. It is also useful to be aware that, in contrast to normal tissue, tumor vessel caliber doesn't decrease as the vessels branch (Fig. 4.2).

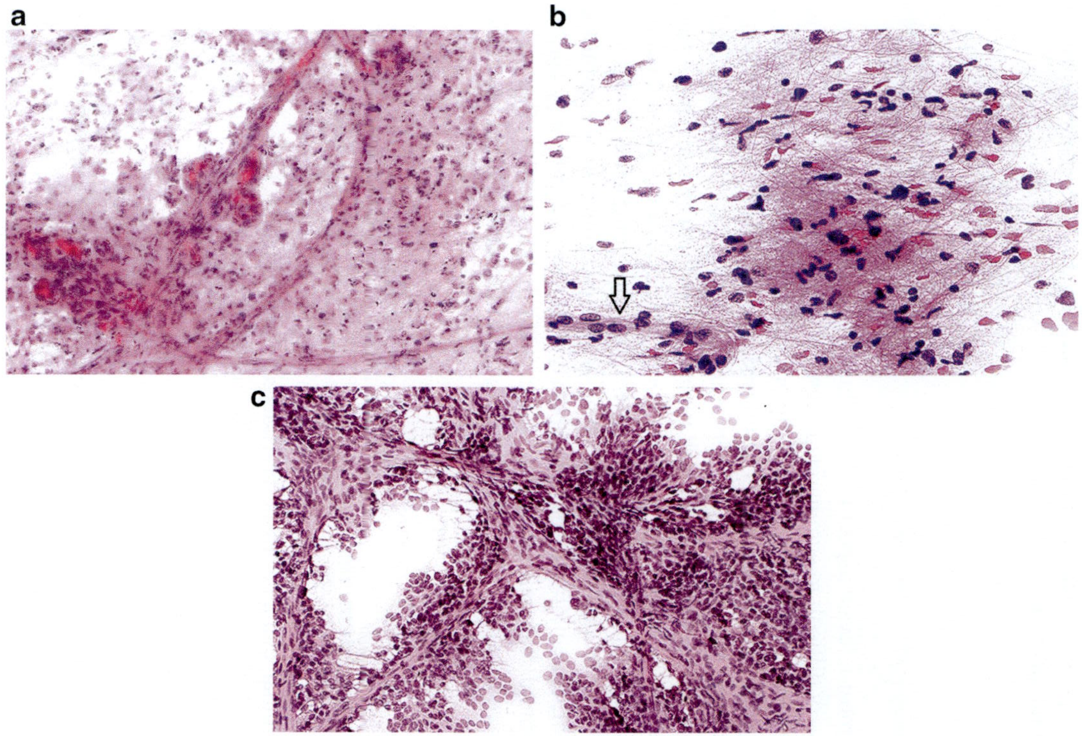

Fig. 4.2 *Type of blood vessels.* (**a**) Glioblastoma. Characteristic microvascular hyperplasia displaying a “glomeruloid” appearance. (**b**) Diffuse astrocytoma, WHO grade II. Thin-walled, capillary vessels are usually found in low-grade diffuse gliomas (*arrow*). (**c**) Hemangiopericytoma. Network of vascular channels with tumor cell aggregates (**a**–**c**; Smears, H&E)

Specific Cell Groups

As mentioned above, the squash technique enables us to preserve tissue structures such as whorls (Fig. 4.3a), papillae (Fig. 4.3b), rosettes (Fig. 4.4a), pseudorosettes (Fig. 4.4b), and perivascular pseudorosettes (Fig. 4.4c) on the smears. These specific cell groups possess great defining power because they are characteristic of certain types of tumors (Table 4.2).

Type of Cell

The obviously most relevant aspect in the evaluation of smears is the predominant cell type. It is very difficult to summarize in few cellular patterns the vast array of individual cell types and subtypes of CNS tumors, but this can be done by dividing them into seven different types: tumors composed of glial cells with fine cytoplasmic processes, tumors with ganglion cell appearance, tumors consisting of epithelial-like cells, tumors made up of large or small round cells without apparent processes, tumors composed of spindle-shaped cells, tumors whose cells are small and poorly differentiated, and polymorphic tumors with two or more conspicuously different types of cells. Clear examples of the last type are glioblastoma, in which on the same smear glial, epithelial-like and small poorly differentiated cells may coexist and atypical teratoid/rhabdoid tumor that may contain rhabdoid cells, often primitive neuroectodermal cells, and cells with divergent differentiation along epithelial, mesenchymal, or glial lines (Table 4.3).

Specific Cellular Elements

The specific cellular elements to be considered should include Rosenthal fibers (RFs) and eosinophilic granular bodies (EGBs) in astrocytic cells and lymphoglandular bodies (LGBs), keratin, melanin, and mucin in non-glial cells (stromal mucinous degeneration may also occur in gliomas). All these elements are preserved better in cytologic preparations than in frozen sections. RFs are intensely eosinophilic, wormlike cords of aggregated proteins composed of GFAP, ubiquitin, and alpha B-crystallin (Fig. 4.5a). EGBs, of lysosomal derivation, are brightly eosinophilic, spherical protein droplets that occur in aggregates or as larger single globules. They are composed of ubiquitinated α1-chymotrypsin and α1-antitrypsin (Fig. 4.5b). LGBs represent small, membrane-delimited cytoplasmic fragments of lymphoid cells produced by the squash technique, which is why they appear in smears but not in frozen sections. They are observed in detail, against the background, with a grayish-blue coloration when Romanowsky-type stains are used (Fig. 4.1c). LGBs are not entirely specific for lymphoid tissue or lymphomas since

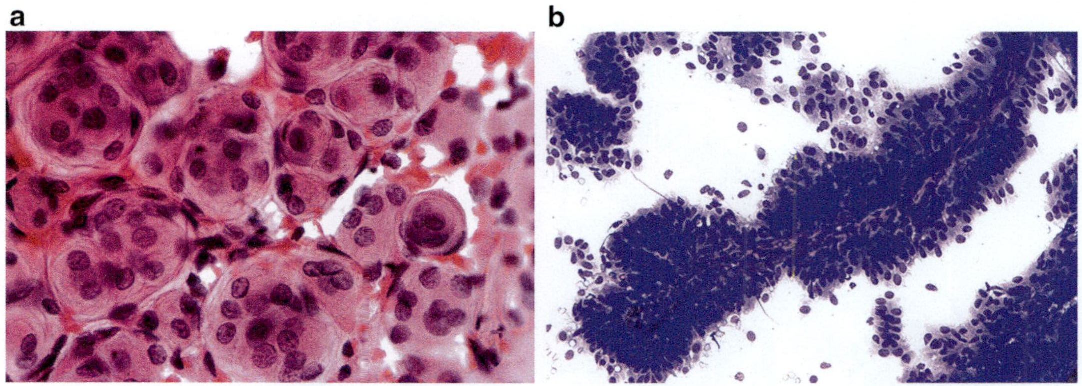

Fig. 4.3 *Specific cell groups*. (**a**) Transitional meningioma. Typical cell whorls showing tight concentric arrangements (Smear, H&E). (**b**) Choroid plexus papilloma. Characteristic papilla with a vascular stromal core (Smear, Romanowsky)

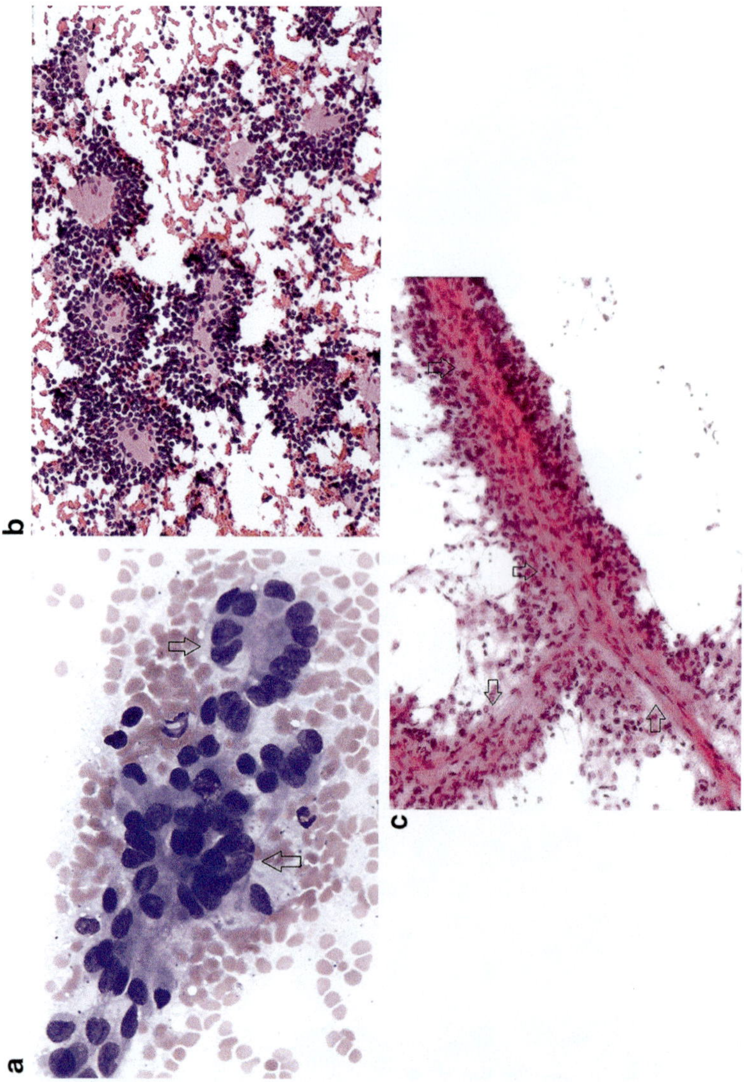

Fig. 4.4 *Specific cell groups*. (**a**) Flexner-Wintersteiner rosettes from ependymoma, with prismatic cells arranged around a small luminal structure (*arrows*). In smears, often there are one or more cells overlying the center of the rosette and obscuring the lumen (Smear, Romanowsky). (**b**) Homer-Wright rosettes from neuroblastoma, with central tangles of fibrillary processes (Smear, H&E). (**c**) Perivascular pseudorosettes from ependymoma, with tumor cell processes radiating toward a central vessel (arrows; Smear, H&E)

Table 4.2 Specific cell groups and types of tumors

Whorls	*Pseudorosettes (Homer-Wright)*
Meningioma	Neuroblastoma
Craniopharyngioma	Ganglioneuroblastoma
Epidermoid carcinoma	Neurocytoma
Schwannoma	Pineocytoma
Papillae	PPTID
Choroid plexus tumors	Medulloblastoma
Papillary/myxopapillary ependymoma	Rosette-forming glioneural tumor
Papillary meningioma	*Perivascular pseudorosettes*
Papillary craniopharyngioma	Ependymoma
Papillary tumor of the pineal region	Astroblastoma
Metastatic papillary carcinomas	Subependymal giant cell astrocytoma
True rosettes (Flexner-Wintersteiner)	Pilomyxoid astrocytoma
Ependymoma	Papillary glioneural tumor
Subependymoma	Rosette-forming glioneural tumor
ETANTR	Angiocentric glioma
Pineoblastoma	Anaplastic astrocytoma
Medulloepithelioma	Glioblastoma

PPTID pineal parenchymal tumor of intermediate differentiation, *ETANTR* embryonal tumor with abundant neuropil and true rosettes

they may also be seen in small-cell carcinoma, melanoma, germinoma, and “small round blue cell tumors” of childhood. However, in all of these tumors, their number is considerably less than in smears of lymphoid proliferations. Cells with keratin show a pink (H&E stain), orange (Papanicolaou stain), or sky-blue (Romanowsky stain) dense hyaline cytoplasm (Fig. 4.6). Melanin pigment forms finely granular dark-brown intracytoplasmic aggregates with H&E and Papanicolaou stains, or black aggregates with Romanowsky stain (Fig. 4.7). Mucin forms intracytoplasmic globular deposits or else is observed as amorphous extracellular aggregates. Mucin stains light with Papanicolaou or H&E stain but intensely (magenta) with Romanowsky-type stains (Fig. 4.8). Table 4.4 summarizes these specific cellular elements and related processes.

A consistent approach is to start the smear examination at low/intermediate magnification to evaluate the first four parameters and then confirm ones impression of a lesion at high magnification evaluating the remaining two (type of cell and specific cellular elements); for example:

- Mixed smear pattern with cell sheets, smaller cell clusters, and individual cells; clear background; whorls; epithelioid cells; oval, bland nuclei with pseudoinclusions – Meningioma?
- Discohesive pattern of single cells; necrotic background; atypical round cells; apoptosis, and LGBs – Lymphoma?

Table 4.3 Predominant cell types in the various tumors

Glial cells (fine cytoplasmic processes)	*Spindle-shaped cells*
Astrocytic tumors	Nerve sheath tumors
Ependymal tumors	Fibrous meningioma
Ganglion/ganglioid cells	Solitary fibrous tumor
Gangliocytoma	Pituicytoma
Dysplastic gangliocytoma (cerebellum)	Fusiform melanoma/melanocytoma
Hypothalamic hamartoma	Fusiform sarcomas
Gangliocytic paraganglioma	Spindle cell oncocytoma
Subependymal giant cell astrocytoma	Angiocentric glioma
Ganglioneuroma	*Small, poorly differentiated cells*
Round cells	Medulloblastoma
Oligodendroglioma	Other CNS embryonal tumors
DNT	PNET-like AT/RT
Neurocytoma	Pineoblastoma
Pineocytoma	Small-cell glioblastoma
Pituitary adenoma	Hemangiopericytoma
Germinoma	Ewing sarcoma
Lymphoma	small-cell carcinoma
Epithelial/epithelial-like cells	Melanoma (occasionally)
Metastatic carcinoma/melanoma	*Mixed/polymorphous cell pattern*
Most meningiomas	Glioblastoma
Choroid plexus tumors	Gliosarcoma.
Craniopharyngioma	Neuronal-glial mixed tumors
Embryonal carcinoma	Teratoma
Paraganglioma	Atypical teratoid/rhabdoid tumor
Epithelioid glioblastoma	Choriocarcinoma
Chordoma	MPNST with divergent differentiation

DNT dysembryoplastic neuroepithelial tumor, *PNET* primitive neuroectodermal tumor, *AT/RT* atypical teratoid/rhabdoid tumor, *MPNST* malignant peripheral nerve sheath tumor

- Only cohesive tissue fragments, no single cells; clear background; fusiform cells; club-shaped, tapered or curved nuclei – Schwannoma?
- Discohesive tissue fragments and single cells; fibrillary/myxoid background; "glomeruloid" vessels; "piloid" cells; RFs, and EGBs – Pilocytic astrocytoma?

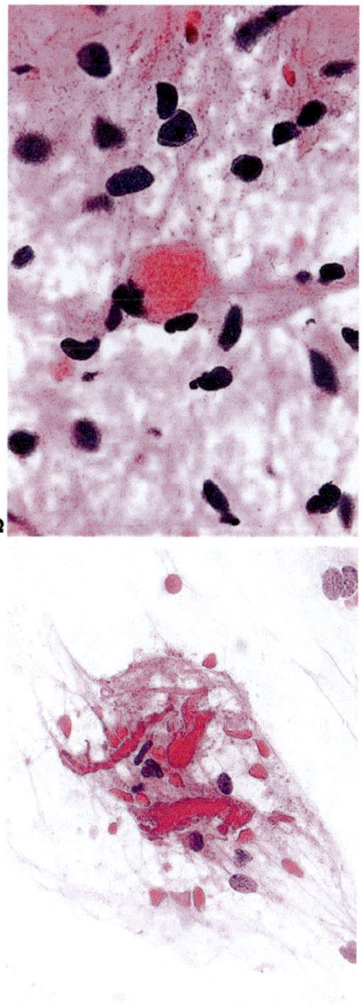

Fig. 4.5 *Specific glial cellular elements*. Clump of Rosenthal fibers (**a**) and eosinophilic granular body (**b**, *center of frame*) from a pilocytic astrocytoma (**a**, **b**; Smears, H&E)

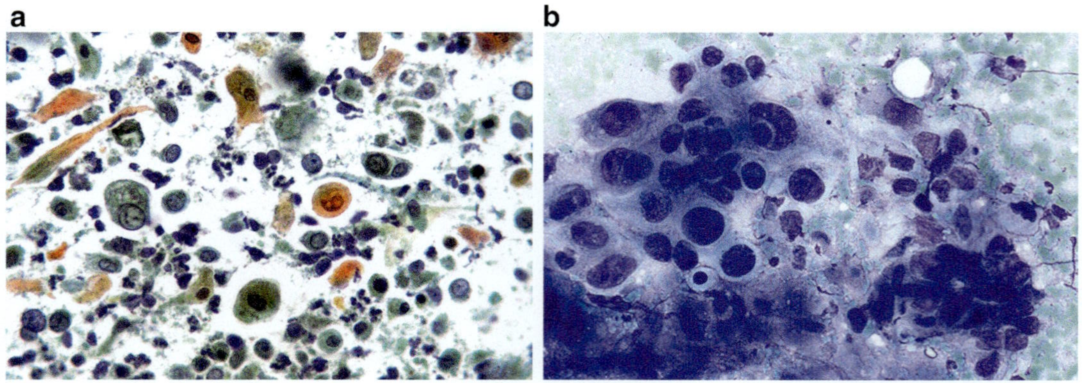

Fig. 4.6 *Specific cellular elements, keratin*. These smears from a metastatic epidermoid carcinoma show orange hyaline cytoplasm with Papanicolaou stain (**a**) and sky-blue hyaline aspect with Romanowsky stain (**b**)

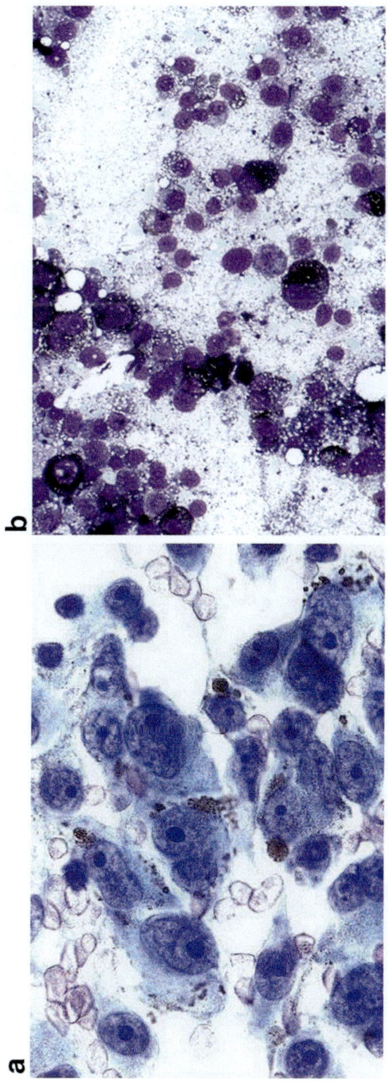

Fig. 4.7 *Specific cellular elements, melanin*. These smears from a metastatic melanoma show dark-brown cytoplasmic granules with Papanicolaou stain (**a**) and black granules with Romanowsky stain (**b**)

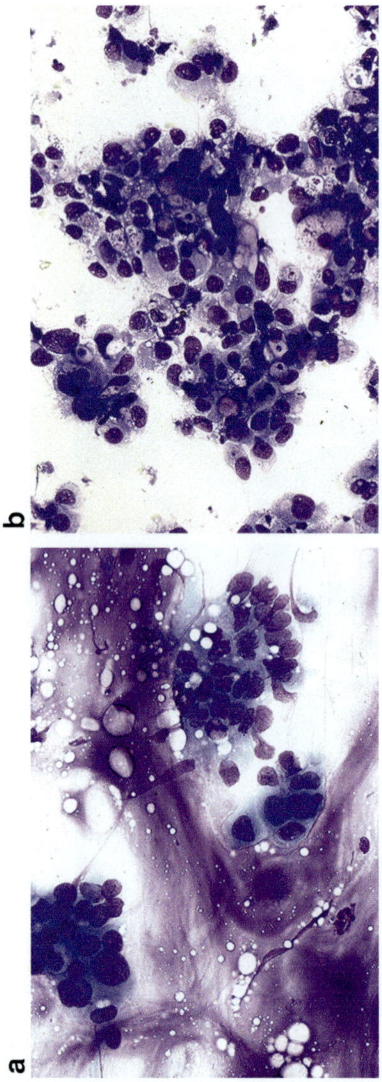

Fig. 4.8 *Specific cellular elements, mucin*. (**a**) Metastatic mucinous colonic adenocarcinoma with abundant thick mucoid background. (**b**) Metastatic lung adenocarcinoma displays numerous intracytoplasmic vacuolar purple granules or "magenta bodies" (**a–b**; Smears, Romanowsky)

Table 4.4 Specific cellular elements and related processes

Rosenthal fibers	*Melanin*
Pilocytic astrocytoma	Melanoma/Melanocytoma
Ganglioglioma	Neurocutaneous melanosis
Chronic "piloid" gliosis	Teratoma
Rosette-forming glioneural tumor	Pineal anlage tumor
Alexander's disease	Melanotic schwannoma
Eosinophilic granular bodies	Melanotic medulloblastoma
Pilocytic astrocytoma	Melanotic ependymoma
Ganglion cell tumors	Melanotic paraganglioma
Pleomorphic xanthoastrocytoma	Melanotic progonoma
Rosette-forming glioneural tumor	*Mucin*
DNT (occasionally)	Mucinous metastatic carcinoma
Keratin	Nonneoplastic cysts of the neuroaxis
Craniopharyngioma	Glandular component in teratoma
Teratoma	Gliomas with mucinous degeneration
Epidermoid cyst	*Lymphoglandular bodies*
Dermoid cyst	Lymphomas
Metastatic epidermoid carcinoma	Nonneoplastic lymphoid infiltrations

DNT dysembryoplastic neuroepithelial tumor

General-Category Interpretation

The correlation of the clinical, radiological, and cytological information (synthesizing) serves as a basis for classifying the disease process by using the following flow chart (Fig. 4.9).

Now, some useful advice to evaluate this flow chart:

Abnormal

For a case to fit this definition, it is fundamental to determine the degree of cellularity. Any biopsy specimen of the CNS that releases a large number of cells in the smears probably contains lesional tissue. An exception to this is the cerebellar cortex, whose smears are very cellular. On the other hand, there are few tumors that can yield hypocellular smears basically schwannoma, hemangioblastoma, and subependymoma, if the technique employed is touch/imprint instead squash/smear cytology.

Neoplastic

Tumors tend to exfoliate cells that are very similar to each other and, with the exception of mixed tumors, which have a small contribution from other cell types. In comparison, nonneoplastic processes are usually more polymorphic.

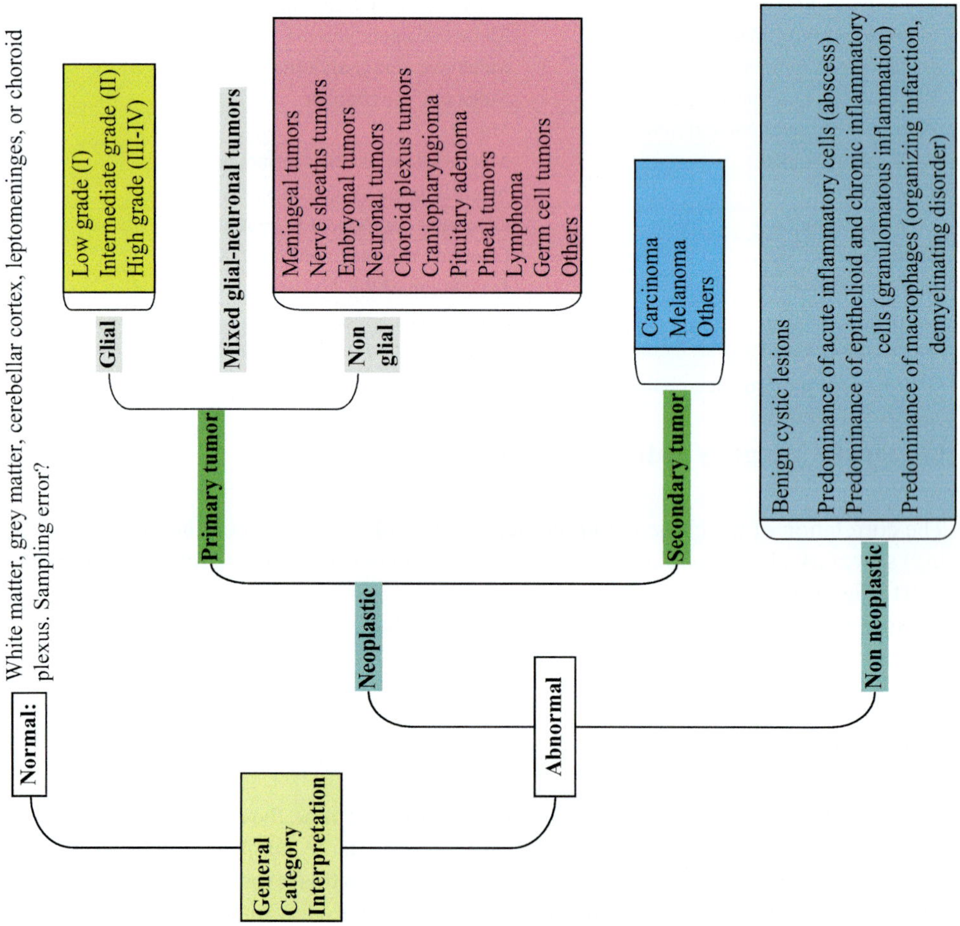

Fig. 4.9 General-category interpretation flow chart

Glial Versus Non-glial

The hallmark for differentiating glial from non-glial tumors is the presence of a fibrillary matrix. All glial tumors, with the exception of oligodendroglioma and some glioblastomas, show a fibrillary background caused by the crisscrossing of the long cytoplasmic processes of glial cells. This important feature becomes manifest more clearly in smears (emphasizes glial processes) than in frozen sections.

Low Versus High Grade

Because, under some circumstances, the neurosurgeon may alter the attempt to aggressively resect a lesion based on the identification of high-grade features, it is advisable to become familiar with the cytomorphologic criteria. With just very few exceptions, the presence of the "AMEN criteria" of **a**typia, **m**itosis, **e**ndothelial hyperplasia, and **n**ecrosis indicates high-grade tumors.

Nonneoplastic

Whenever you see more than few macrophages or inflammatory cells, you have to seriously consider nonneoplastic conditions in the differential. The presence of a large number of inflammatory cells leads the diagnosis in the direction of inflammatory/reactive processes. The few exceptions to this (i.e., lymphoplasmacytic-rich meningioma, some germinomas) do not make this finding less useful. Likewise, the presence of abundant macrophages is unusual in tumors and should suggest a non-neoplastic necrotizing process (i.e., evolving infarction) or a demyelinating disease. Both inflammatory cells and macrophages, usually obscured in frozen sections, are nicely preserved in smears.

Final Recommendations

Perform this algorithm with the necessary prudence and up to the extent possible, keeping in mind three facts: first, that the neurosurgeon's primary interest is to know whether the sample is representative of the lesion and, if that is the case, to know whether it is the lesion he believed was there or, whether he must change the surgical procedure. Second, the scope of the intraoperative diagnosis should be limited to only what is unequivocal. To do that while still providing helpful information, one may use less specific diagnoses that cover two or more potential specific diagnosis. For example, "infiltrating glioma" (diffuse astrocytomas, oligodendroglioma), "metastatic malignant neoplasm" (carcinoma, melanoma), "low-grade neuroepithelial neoplasm" (pilocytic astrocytoma, ganglioglioma, dysembryoplastic neuroepithelial tumor), "high-grade neuroepithelial neoplasm" (glioblastoma, anaplastic astrocytoma, anaplastic oligodendroglioma, medulloblastoma), "macrophage-rich lesion" (demyelinating disorder, infarct). And third, avoiding the over-diagnosis of malignancy during intraoperative consultation is paramount. In this respect, it is advisable to keep in mind those CNS tumors that are most frequently overgraded, such as pleomorphic xanthoastrocytoma, pilocytic astrocytoma, and mixed neuronal-glial tumors; as well as the nonneoplastic lesions that are potentially misinterpreted as neoplasms, like reactive gliosis, evolving infarcts, and demyelinating disorders. Finally, we ought to assume that some cases are simply so difficult that they are not diagnosable at the time of intraoperative consultation. Thus, in such circumstances, major patient management decisions should be deferred until the evaluation of permanent sections. Remember, *no diagnosis is preferable to a wrong diagnosis.*

Suggested Reading

Kepes JJ. Pitfalls and problems in the histopathologic evaluation of stereotactic needle biopsy specimens. Neuropathology. 1994;5:19–33.

Kleinschmidt-DeMasters BK, Prayson RA. An algorithmic approach to the brain biopsy–part I. Arch Pathol Lab Med. 2006;130:1630–8.

Kresak JL, Rivera-Zengotita M, Foss RM, Yachnis AT. CNS intraoperative consultation: a survival guide for non-neuropathologists. Methods Mol Biol. 2014;1180:369–76.

Lacruz CR, Catalina-Fernández I, Bardales RH, Pimentel J, López-Presa D, Sáenz-Santamaría J. Intraoperative consultation on pediatric central nervous system tumors by squash cytology. Cancer Cytopathol. 2015;123:331–46.

Lee HS, Tihan T. The basics of intraoperative diagnosis in neuropathology. Surg Pathol Clin. 2015;8:27–47.

Powell SZ. Intraoperative consultation, cytologic preparations and frozen section in the central nervous system. Arch Pathol Lab Med. 2005;129:1635–52.

Prayson RA, Kleinschmidt-DeMasters BK. An algorithmic approach to the brain biopsy–part II. Arch Pathol Lab Med. 2006;130:1639–48.

Savargaonkar P, Farmer PM. Utility of intraoperative consultations for the diagnosis of central nervous system lesions. Ann Clin Lab Sci. 2001;31:133–9.

Taratuto AL, Sevlever G, Piccardo P. Clues and pitfalls in stereotactic biopsy of the central nervous system. Arch Pat Lab Med. 1991;115:596–602.

Yachnis AT. Intraoperative consultation for nervous system lesions. Semin Diagn Pathol. 2002;19:192–206.

Chapter 5
Normal Brain and Gliosis

Recognition of the abnormal rests on a clear knowledge of the normal.

It is very important to become familiar with the cytologic appearance of normal brain if we want to be able to determine whether a smear is normal or not. A useful exercise is to examine smears from various regions of normal brain made from unfixed necropsy brain tissue with a relatively short postmortem delay. In this way, we will ascertain that the normal appearance varies considerably depending on the region studied – cerebral cortex, white matter, basal nuclei, cerebellar cortex, choroid plexus, leptomeninges, or pineal gland. Therefore, at the time of evaluating a smear, we must keep in mind both this regional variability and the precise site from which a brain biopsy specimen has been taken.

On the other hand, because of intense reactive changes of brain tissue tend to be interpreted as a tumor, becoming familiar with the cytologic appearance of reactive gliosis also is extremely important.

White Matter Pattern

Normal white matter smears easily and produces evenly distributed preparations with a pearly white macroscopic aspect. Shearing forces in the smear rip neuropil (a complex of axons, dendrites, and synapses) into tiny spherules, appearing as a finely granular background with a distinctive feltlike appearance. Scattered in this background, there are small, empty vacuoles representing dissolved myelin and a low cellular population consisting basically of oligodendrocytes and to a lesser extent of astrocytes. Both of them appear to have small, round to oval nuclei with little, if any, recognizable cytoplasm and with no visible cytoplasmic processes (naked nuclei). The cytological discrimination between these two normal glial cells is difficult, but not necessary. However, astrocytes have slightly larger and more oblong (potato-like) nuclei than do oligodendrocytes, which have smaller and round (orange-like)

C. R. Lacruz et al., *Central Nervous System Intraoperative Cytopathology*, Essentials in Cytopathology 13, https://doi.org/10.1007/978-3-319-98491-9_5

nuclei. If the biopsy originates from a region with long interneuronal connection pathways, the presence of very long fine fibers corresponding to axons may be observed, which may extend across several microscopic fields. Vascularization consists of delicate capillaries with elongated endothelial cells arranged parallel to the capillary wall (Fig. 5.1a, b). There may also be arterioles with thicker walls, in which cells are arranged parallel (endothelial cells) or perpendicular (muscle cells) to the lumen (Fig. 5.1c).This bidirectional arrangement is never found in neoplastic vessels, in which cells are arranged more or less parallel to the lumen. We should also keep in mind that in samples of deep normal periventricular white matter, ependymal nests may be found.

When you become familiar with this pattern, it cannot be confused with anything else, even though, on occasion, low-grade astrocytoma has been mentioned as a possible differential diagnosis. However, low-grade astrocytoma shows a clearly fibrillary (no felt-like) background, as well as greater cellular density and variability.

Gray Matter Pattern

Smears from the cerebral cortex, thalamus, and basal ganglia are similar. Tissue tends to smear less evenly than tissue from white matter, accumulating elements of larger size, such as blood vessels and neurons, at the edge of the smear. The background is also eosinophilic and granular (feltlike), but without vacuoles of myelin. On the other hand, cellularity, even though variable in number, shape, and size, depending on which part of the brain the biopsy comes from, is always higher than in white matter. Together with the glial cells described above, we have additionally the presence of numerous neurons of variable appearance, but with characteristic nuclear and cytoplasmic features. Neurons appear as large cells with abundant cytoplasm, distinct cell borders, and round, prominent nucleolated nuclei. Small neurons are less easy to identify with certainty, and when numerous – for example, the neurons of the hippocampus, in the medial temporal lobe – can be misinterpreted as neoplastic cells. Just as for white matter, capillaries are particularly distinctive, but the smears also contain arterioles and small arteries (Fig. 5.2a, b).

As previously mentioned, pathologists should be aware that in smears from the hippocampus, the admixture of small and large neurons may look remarkably like astrocytoma. But, once again, the characteristic eosinophilic and finely granular "feltlike" background of normal neuroglial tissue (Fig. 5.2c) contrasts with the clearly fibrillary background of astrocytoma.

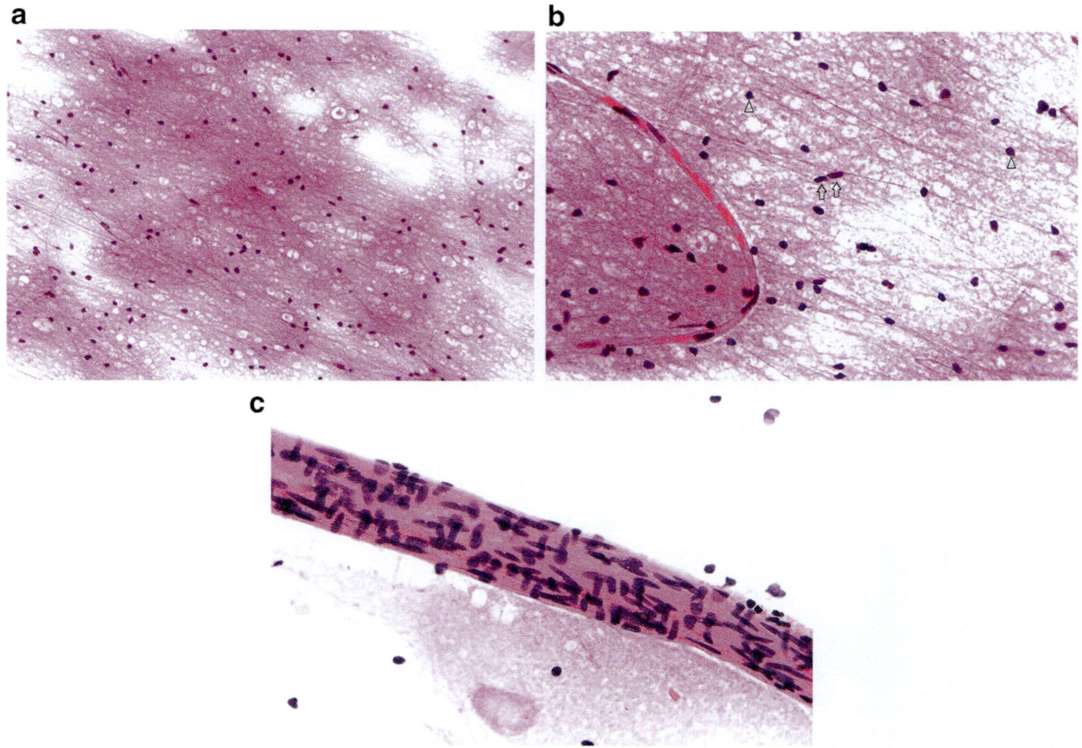

Fig. 5.1 *White matter*. (**a**) Evenly distributed smear displaying a finely granular "feltlike" background, small vacuoles, and sparse isomorphic cellularity. (**b**) High-magnification view demonstrating astrocytes with oblong nuclei (*arrows*), oligodendrocytes with round nuclei (*arrowheads*), and empty vacuoles representing dissolved myelin. Also note the very long axons and a slim capillary lined by endothelial cells. (**c**) Muscular arteriole displaying bidirectional arrangement of the cells in the vessel wall, parallel (endothelial cells) and perpendicular (muscle cells) to the direction of the vessel (**a**–**c**; Smears, H&E)

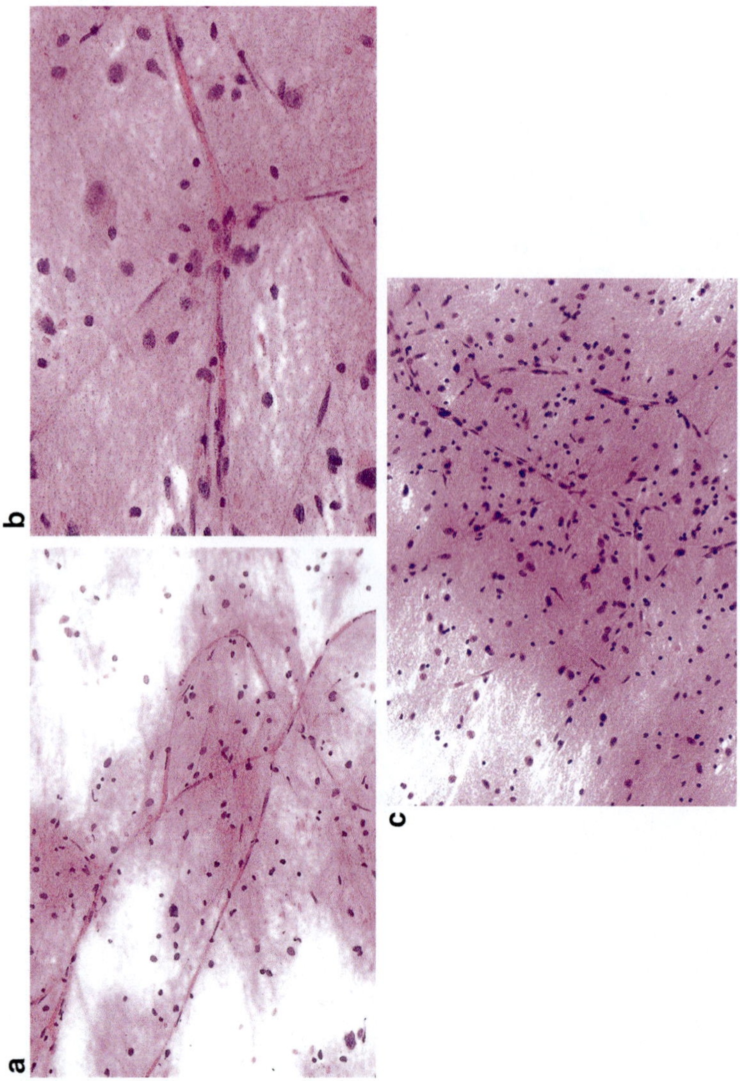

Fig. 5.2 *Gray matter*. (**a**) This preparation shows less evenly distributed cell aggregates and anisocytosis. (**b**) Under high magnification, the larger cells are neurons admixed with small glial cells. Unlike white matter, the fine granular background is devoid of myelin vacuoles. (**c**) In preparations from the hippocampus, the admixture of small and large neurons may look remarkably like astrocytoma. However, the finely granular "feltlike" background is characteristic of normal neuropil (**a–c**; Smears, H&E)

Cerebellar Cortex Pattern

The appearance of this pattern is quite different from the foregoing gray matter pattern, because it is clearly much more cellular. The predominant cells are neurons from the internal granular layer, which look like small, round, hyperchromatic cells without visible cytoplasm. We should remember that this type of neuron is the smallest cell in the human body, its size being smaller even than the mature lymphocyte. In this "sea" of small cells, in an isolated fashion, as if they were islands, voluminous Purkinje's neurons may be observed. These cells show a wide cytoplasm with an expansive dendritic tree and large vesicular nucleus with a visible nucleolus. The background around the exterior of the cellular lakes displays the finely granular neuropil appearance (Fig. 5.3a, b). The rest of the cerebellar subcortical structures have an appearance similar to the patterns of white matter and gray matter described above.

Due to the predominance of internal granular neurons, this type of smear must be differentiated from smears originating from "small round blue cell tumors" –embryonal tumors, small-cell carcinoma, and lymphoma – even though the smaller size and higher uniformity of granular cells give some clues about their benignity (all mentioned tumors are distinctly more anaplastic).

Choroid Plexus Pattern

A normal choroid plexus may be present in biopsy specimens from the ventricles. It is important to recognize this normal pattern to avoid mistakes with choroid plexus tumors. The choroid plexus, because of its vascular-stromal framework, tends to smear poorly and results in a cohesive crush preparation. Its vessels show a complex arched papillary appearance, characteristic of a plexus, lined by a row of cuboidal epithelial cells (Fig. 5.4a). The cells that appear isolated, due to the squash trauma, show a wide polygonal "cobblestone-shaped" cytoplasm and small, round, basally located nuclei. In adults, choroid epithelial cells often bear a single prominent paranuclear cytoplasmic vacuole (Figs. 5.4b).

Smears from choroid plexus papilloma are highly cellular and show papillae, monolayer fragments, tridimensional aggregates, and single cells. On the other hand, the cells in the papillae tend to be arranged in a more piled-up and pseudostratified fashion than in the normal choroid plexus.

Leptomeningeal Pattern

Large cell clusters from the pia-arachnoid may be present in biopsy specimens from the brain surface. The cytoplasm of arachnoid cap cells is wide and delicate, whereas the nuclei are round to ovoid with finely granular dispersed chromatin, often giving

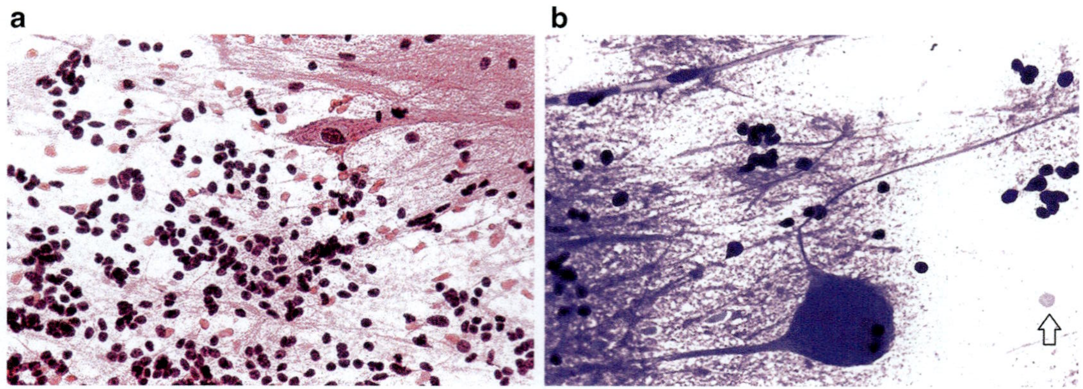

Fig. 5.3 *Cerebellar cortex*. (**a**) Characteristic findings include small internal granular cell neurons and large Purkinje's neurons. Note the homogeneous pink neuropil at the right upper corner (Smear, H&E). (**b**) A rotund Purkinje's neuron exhibits a fine axon and coarser dendritic tree. Compare the erythrocyte size (*arrow*) with that of internal granular cell neurons (Smear, Romanowsky)

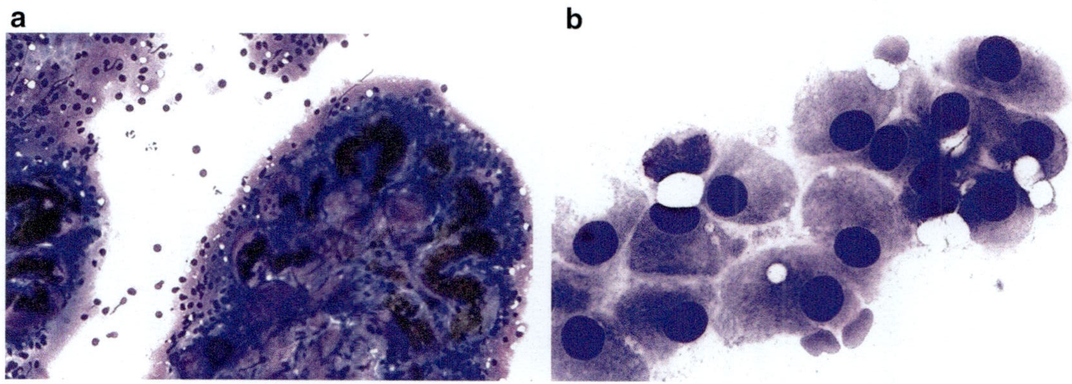

Fig. 5.4 *Choroid plexus.* (**a**) Cohesive tissue fragments with central vascular stroma lined by low-prismatic epithelium. (**b**) A high-magnification view shows normal choroid epithelium with round nuclei and polygonal "cobblestone" cell bodies. Also note large paranuclear cytoplasmic vacuoles (**a**, **b**; Smears, Romanowsky)

the appearance of central clearings. As against cells from the choroid plexus, arachnoidal cells have poorly defined boundaries, giving rise to sheets with a syncytial appearance (Fig. 5.5a, b).

Not infrequently, a tendency is observed in arachnoid cell sheets to have a whorl-like cellular arrangement (particularly arachnoid granulation samples), which is why they may be confused with meningiomas in the absence of clinico-radiologic data.

Pineal Pattern

The cytomorphologic features of the native pineal gland tissue vary with age. *Infant pineal gland* preparations are highly cellular composed of uniform, round, single pinealocytes with indistinct cytoplasm. Nuclei display fine dispersed chromatin and indistinct nucleoli. The background is finely granular (neuropil-like) and calcifications are absent (Fig. 5.6a). Smears from *adult pineal gland* are less cellular, displaying tissue fibrillary fragments and single cells with ill-defined cytoplasm and moderate nuclear pleomorphism; microcalcifications, referred to as *corpora arenacea* or simply "brain sand," also are a common finding (Fig. 5.6b).

In children, the somewhat high cellularity mimics a pineocytoma, whereas in adults, the fibrillary background, nuclear pleomorphism, and calcifications can mimic a low-grade glial neoplasm.

Table 5.1 summarizes the various smears patterns of normal brain tissue and its potential pitfalls.

Gliosis

Reactive astrocytosis or gliosis is a nonspecific response of the brain tissue to a broad variety of neoplastic and nonneoplastic irritating injuries. That is, it is not an isolated disease entity but rather a stereotypic tissue response. Thus, in the presence of a population of astrocytes suggestive of a reactive process, the first thing to do is to find its cause, and if a cause is not found, the next step will be to differentiate reactive glial proliferation from neoplastic glial proliferation. It is worthwhile to spend some time on this latter aspect –*gliosis* versus *low-grade astrocytoma* – because there is no other issue in the field of neuro-intraoperative diagnosis so debated and so widely commented on. In fact, it is believed that the differentiation between these two processes can be very difficult and be the source of wrong diagnoses of malignancy, and it is good to know that in view of this difficult issue, the cytological method can be very useful by providing information and morphologic details in a manner not seen in the corresponding frozen sections.

Starting with the performance of the technique, astrocytoma in smears spreads well, whereas reactive gliosis spreads poorly and tends to remain as cohesive "fluffy" clusters which cannot be smeared out after being squashed. With respect to

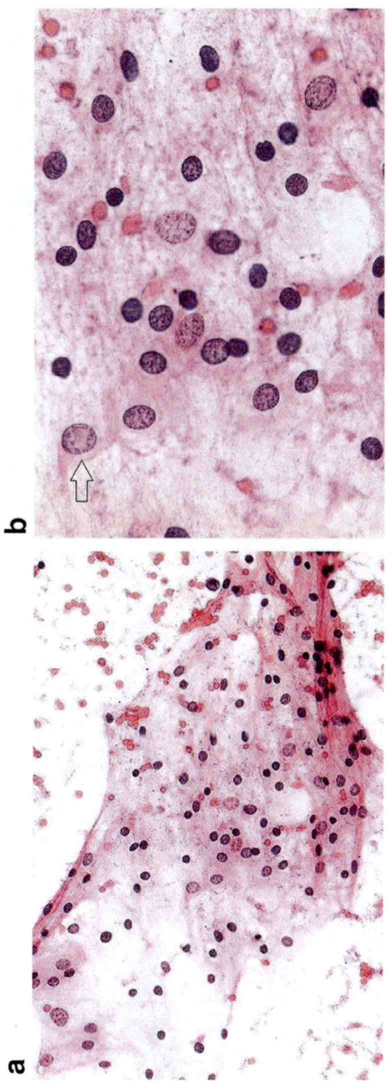

Fig. 5.5 *Leptomeninges*. (**a**) Arachnoid cell sheet with characteristic syncytial appearance. (**b**) High-magnification view showing oval nuclei with finely granular chromatin. Note nuclear clearings giving the appearance of pseudoinclusions (*arrow*; **a**, **b**; Smears, H&E)

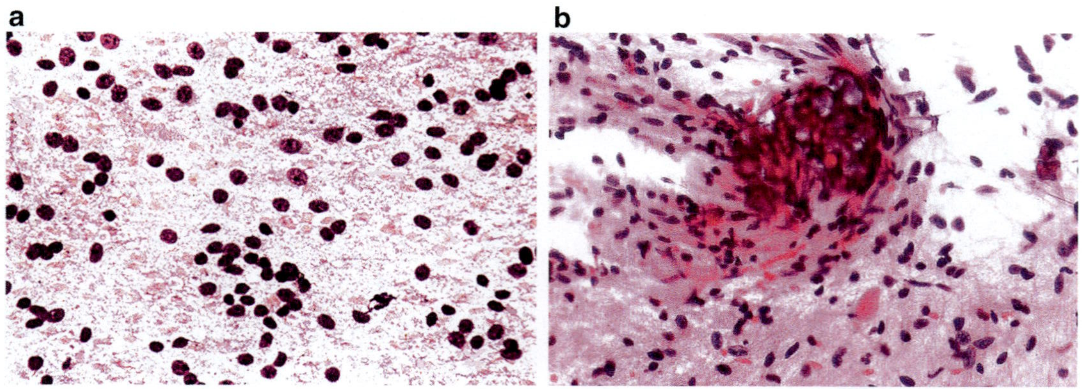

Fig. 5.6 *Native pineal gland*. (**a**) *Children*. Single cell pattern of round cells with indistinct cytoplasm in a loose finely granular background. Note the moderate anisokaryosis of normal pinealocytes. (**b**) *Adults*. In this preparation the nuclear pleomorphism, microcalcifications ("brain sand"), and fibrillary background of the aging pineal gland are well seen (**a**, **b**; Smears, H&E)

Table 5.1 Normal brain tissue patterns and potential misdiagnosis

Tissue type	Misdiagnosis
White matter	Low-grade glioma
Gray matter	Mixed neuronal-glial tumors
	Infiltrating glioma
Cerebellar cortex	Embryonal tumors
	Lymphoma
	Small-cell carcinoma
Choroid plexus	Choroid plexus papilloma
Leptomeninges (arachnoid granulations)	Meningioma
Pineal gland (children)	Pineocytoma
Pineal gland (adults)	Low-grade glioma

purely morphologic data, the background, which is clearly fibrillary in the case of a tumor, in gliosis is variable depending on the nature of the originating process. In most cases, a few thickened fibers travel through the background, although most of the matrix is fine "feltlike" neuropil. Against this variable background, reactive astroctytes and other cells embedded in their gliotic meshwork remain bound together, whereas more distant groups are sheared away in their own clusters. The individual reactive astrocytes appear uncrowded and evenly dispersed, displaying well-defined radial processes and minimal, if any, nuclear atypia (Fig. 5.7a, b). The nuclear changes are more of the reactive type including increase in size, binucleation, or "mirror nuclei" (nuclei that occur in physically contiguous matched pairs) and fairly well-defined nucleolus than those of authentic atypia (hyperchromatism, irregular contours). Colloquially speaking, it may be said that the reactive astrocyte is a cell "too well-made" to be neoplastic. On the other hand, in response to other processes, reactive gliosis is often accompanied by telltale non-glial elements such as inflammatory or neoplastic cells, foamy macrophages, hemosiderin pigment, or necrotic debris, which, combined with radiologic features, should prompt a consideration of other diagnoses (Fig. 5.8a, b). In very difficult cases – no well-sampled lesions and no clinico-radiologic correlation – a generic diagnosis of "hypercellular astroglial tissue, differential includes low-grade astrocytoma vs reactive gliosis; deferred to permanents" is adequate. Table 5.2 summarizes useful features in differentiating gliosis from low-grade astrocytoma in smears.

Piloid Gliosis

The so-called piloid gliosis is an exuberant chronic reactive gliosis with abundant Rosenthal fibers (RFs). It is a common process adjacent to cysts and slow-growing tumors (e.g., pineal cyst, syrinx, craniopharyngioma, hemangioblastoma), particularly in the midline axis (third ventricle, brainstem, cerebellum, and spinal cord), the same areas that tend to be home to pilocytic astrocytoma. To complicate more this

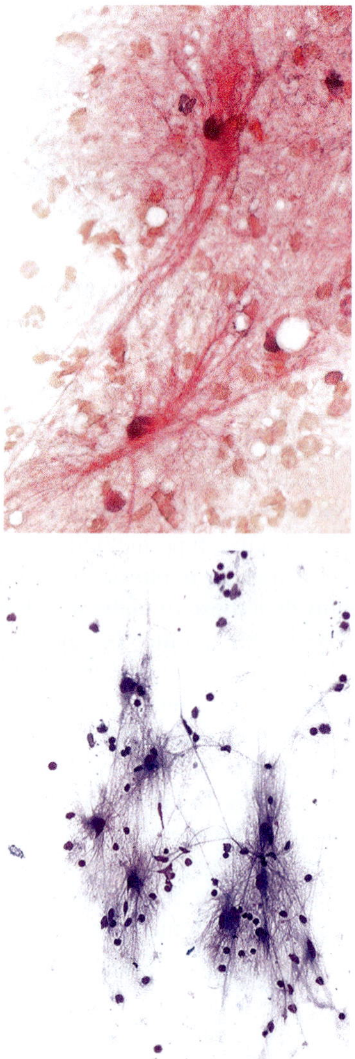

Fig. 5.7 *Reactive gliosis*. (**a**) Clump of evenly spaced reactive astrocytes and some inflammatory cells (Smear, Romanowsky). (**b**) Two stellate-shaped reactive astrocytes with tapering cytoplasmic processes and mild nuclear enlargement (Smear, H&E)

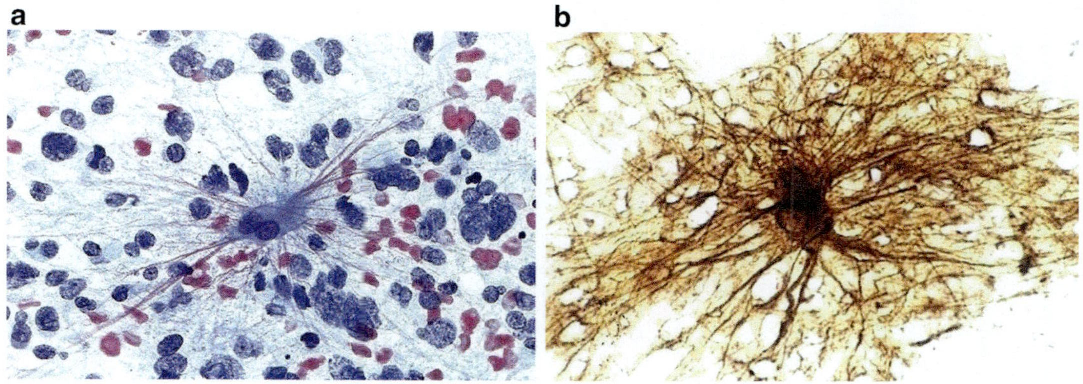

Fig. 5.8 *Reactive gliosis*. (**a**) Binucleation (mirror nuclei) and tapering processes radiating out from all around the cell suggest it is nonneoplastic. Compare this morphology with the surrounding glioblastoma tumor cells (Smear, Papanicolaou). (**b**) Typical hypertrophic reactive astrocyte with extensive radiating processes trapping not stained lymphoma cells (Smear, GFAP immunostain)

Table 5.2 Gliosis versus low-grade astrocytoma

	Gliosis	Astrocytoma
Smearing	Poorly	Easily
Background	Variable	Fibrillary
Cellular distribution	Even/uncrowded	Uneven/overlapped
Nuclear features	Bland/binucleation	Hyperchromatism/angulations
Cell bodies	Stellate-shaped	Non-discernible/eosinophilic
Non-glial elements	Common	Usually absent
Imaging features	Non-glioma appearance	Glioma appearance

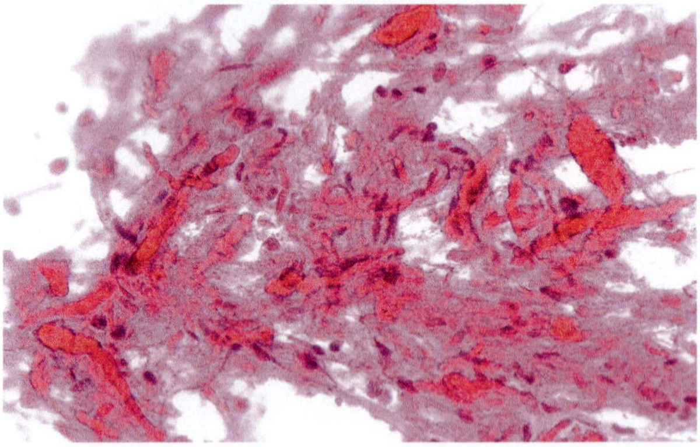

Fig. 5.9 *Pilocytic gliosis*. The long processes forming a compact layer are intermixed with numerous hyaline Rosenthal fibers (Smear, H&E)

scenario, this form of chronic reactive astrocytosis is often more fibrillar in nature, and smears may show numerous long processes forming a compact layer with abundant RFs (Fig. 5.9); therefore, it can easily be misinterpreted as pilocytic astrocytoma. As a general rule, if you find more RFs than cells, you should think of gliosis before tumor. However, in ambiguous cases, the term "piloid astroglial tissue" can be used as the intraoperative diagnosis.

Contaminants

It also behooves us to keep in mind the possibility of the presence of foreign elements such as anucleate squames and glove powder that are unrelated to the process in cytologic smears. The presence of these two contaminants is relatively frequent even with careful handling of slides. The possibility of contamination with anucleate squames must be taken into account in order to avoid confusing them with epidermoid/dermoid cysts or with craniopharyngioma (Fig. 5.10a). On the other hand, the inexperienced may mistake glove powder for psammoma bodies or *cryptococci* (Fig. 5.10b). Also bone fragments (dust), which form during the drilling of a burr hole may contaminate the specimen and can be mistaken for dystrophic calcification as part of the disease process (Fig. 5.10c). Awareness of these possible pitfalls can mitigate the chance of misinterpretation.

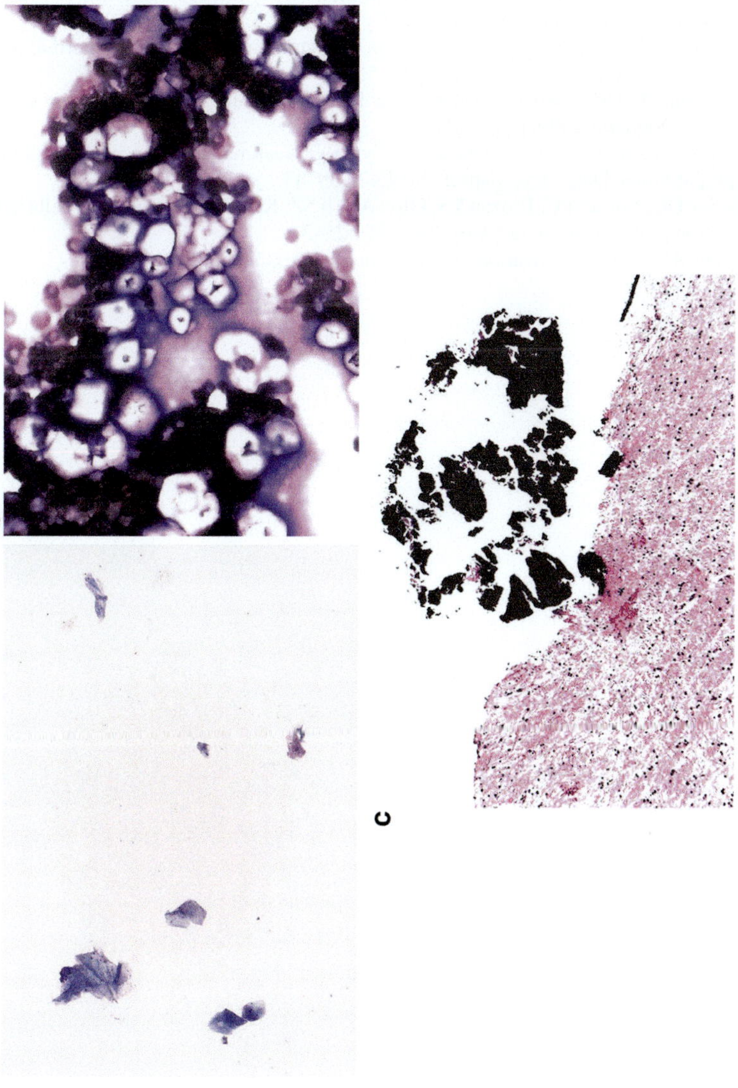

Fig. 5.10 *Contaminants*. (**a**) Anucleate squames seen as a contaminant on a glass slide (Romanowsky). (**b**) Talc crystals of glove powder on a glass slide appear as crystalloid, polygonal structures with a dark striation in the middle (Romanowsky). (**c**) Bone dust from the drill hole as seen in sections. Although this calcified material is obviously artifactual, when intimately associated with tissue fragments in smears can be interpreted to be integral to the process (stereotactic biopsy)

Suggesting Reading

Adams JH, Graham D, Doyle D. Brain Biopsy: The smear technique for neurosurgical biopsies. Philadelphia: JB Lippincott; 1981. p. 15–8.

Chandrasoma PT, Apuzzo MLJ. Stereotactic brain biopsy. New York: Igaku-Shoin; 1989. p. 75–87.

Crain BJ, Bigner SH, Johnston WW. Fine needle aspiration biopsy of deep cerebrum. A comparison of normal and neoplastic morphology. Acta Cytol. 1982;26:772–8.

Jiménez-Heffernan JA, Bárcena C, Agra C, Asunción A. Cytologic features of the normal pineal gland of adults. Diagn Cytopathol. 2015;43:642–5.

Lacruz CR, Escalona J. Diagnóstico citológico de los tumores del sistema nervioso central. Barcelona: César Viguera; 2000. p. 19–23.

Murro D, Alsadi A, Nag S, Arvanitis L, Gattuso P. Cytologic features of the normal pineal gland on squash preparations. Diagn Cytopathol. 2014;42:939–43.

Parwani AV, Taylor DC, Burger PC, Erozan YS, Olivi A, Ali SZ. Keratinized squamous cells in fine needle aspiration of the brain. Acta Cytol. 2003;47:325–31.

Pekny M, Nilsson M. Astrocyte activation and reactive gliosis. Glia. 2005;50:427–34.

Part II
Neoplastic

Chapter 6
Astrocytic Tumors

Astrocytic tumors constitute the most numerous and heterogeneous group of gliomas, with an incidence estimated at 60% of all primary intracranial neoplasms. Because of the variety and complexity of astrocytic tumors, it is advisable to divide the intraoperative study into two important groups: (1) diffuse astrocytic tumors, a group of widely infiltrative neoplasms –considered to be surgically incurable – that includes diffuse astrocytomas (grades II to IV), diffuse midline glioma, and gliomatosis cerebri, and (2) localized "nondiffuse" astrocytic tumors, a group of relatively circumscribed neoplasms – in which attempt of total surgical resection is the treatment of choice – that includes pilocytic astrocytoma, subependymal giant cell astrocytoma, and pleomorphic xanthoastrocytoma. Therefore, distinguishing diffuse astrocytic tumors (any type) from localized "nondiffuse" astrocytic tumors (any type) during surgery remains a main goal to improve treatment planning.

Diffuse Astrocytomas

As a group, diffuse astrocytomas (diffuse astrocytoma, anaplastic astrocytoma, and glioblastoma) represent the largest group (> 90%) of astrocytic tumors. Glioblastoma is the most frequent, with low-grade examples comparatively uncommon, particularly in the elderly. They may be located throughout the neuroaxis spinal cord included, but preferentially involve the cerebral hemispheres in adults and the brainstem in children and adolescents (the cerebellum is a highly unusual site). These tumors are slightly more common in men than women (1.3:1 ratio) and significantly more common in white than black people. Because of their wide infiltration beyond their grossly and radiologically apparent margins, diffuse astrocytomas (any grade) are considered to be surgically incurable. In addition, they have an inherited tendency for malignant transformation.

C. R. Lacruz et al., *Central Nervous System Intraoperative Cytopathology*, Essentials in Cytopathology 13, https://doi.org/10.1007/978-3-319-98491-9_6

The clinical picture is variable, depending on the degree of malignancy and the location of the tumor. Common symptoms in patients with low-grade tumors are new-onset seizures, motor disturbances, difficulties with speech and vision, and changes in behavior, all of these undergoing a progressive development in the course of several months. The evolution of most glioblastomas usually takes a short time (less than 3–4 months), with raised intracranial pressure and mental disturbances. Some patients may present more acutely with seizures or stroke. In low-grade tumors, MRI displays ill-defined or relatively discrete areas of T1 hypointensity and T2/FLAIR hyperintensity (due to tumoral edema) without contrast enhancement, whereas glioblastomas typically have an irregular contrast-enhancing ring around a dark necrotic center. Tumors that cross the corpus callosum are often referred to as "butterfly lesions" because of bilateral involvement of the white matter in the centrum semiovale.

Grossly, diffuse astrocytomas are ill-delimited neoplasms with blurred margins, translucent appearance, gray-pink coloration, and a certain tendency to cystification (micro- or macrocysts). In the more aggressive forms, we additionally find necrotic and hemorrhagic areas that give the tumor a variegated or "geographic" appearance (see Chap. 3, Fig. 3.1a).

From the histologic point of view, they present a broad gradient of malignancy that may be summarized in three progressive grades:

Diffuse astrocytoma (WHO grade II). A slowly growing, infiltrating glioma composed of well-differentiated astrocytes with fibrillary or gemistocytic features and mild nuclear atypia (Fig. 6.1a, b)

Anaplastic astrocytoma (WHO grade III). A malignant infiltrating astrocytoma with increased cellularity, mitoses, and nuclear atypia (Fig. 6.2)

Glioblastoma (WHO grade IV). A highly malignant, infiltrating glioma with predominant astrocytic differentiation and fully developed anaplastic features: marked atypia, microvascular proliferation, atypical mitoses, necrosis, and cellular pleomorphism (Fig. 6.3a, b, c).

These forms usually are not independent entities but instead represent different grades of malignancy of the same oncologic process. Therefore, not infrequently we can find different grades of dedifferentiation/malignancy within the same tumor (intratumoral heterogeneity), or we can see how the grade of malignancy increases with each successive recurrence (tumoral progression). In this respect, the marked tendency of anaplastic astrocytoma to progress to glioblastoma in about 2 years (secondary glioblastoma) is well known. However, most glioblastomas (roughly 90%) occur unassociated with demonstrable precursor lesions (primary glioblastoma).

Currently, diffuse astrocytoma and anaplastic astrocytoma are grouped together on the basis of their *isocitrate dehydrogenase-1 or − 2* (*IDH1/2*) genes mutational status into either IDH-mutant (70–80%) or IDH-wild type (20–30%). Similarly, glioblastomas are grouped into IDH-mutant (5–10%; often corresponds to secondary glioblastoma) or IDH-wild type (90–95%; often corresponds to primary glioblastoma). A single point mutation in codon 132 of *IDH1* converting arginine to histidine accounts for up to 90% of all mutations. Immunostain IDH1 R132H can detect this

a b

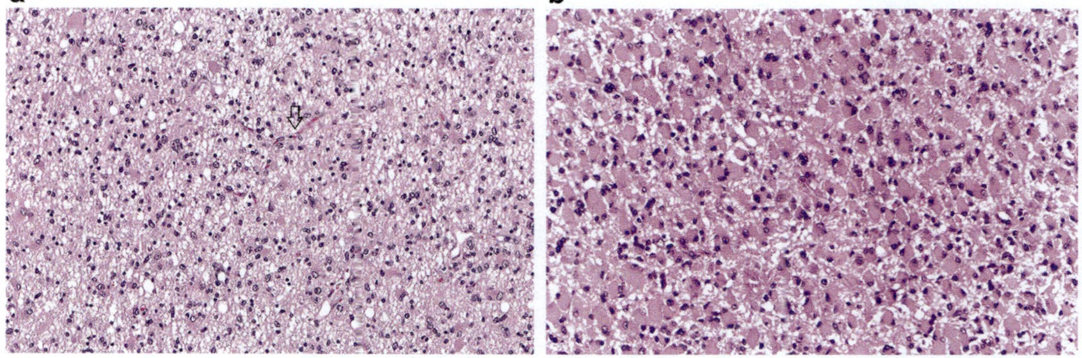

Fig. 6.1 *Diffuse astrocytoma WHO grade II, histology*. (**a**) Fibrillary variant. Hyperchromatic nuclei with irregular contours are embedded in a dense fibrillary matrix. Also note characteristic microcystic changes and a capillary vessel (*arrow*). (**b**) Gemistocytic variant. Pleomorphic astrocytes with plump bellies of eosinophilic cytoplasm and eccentric nuclei predominate

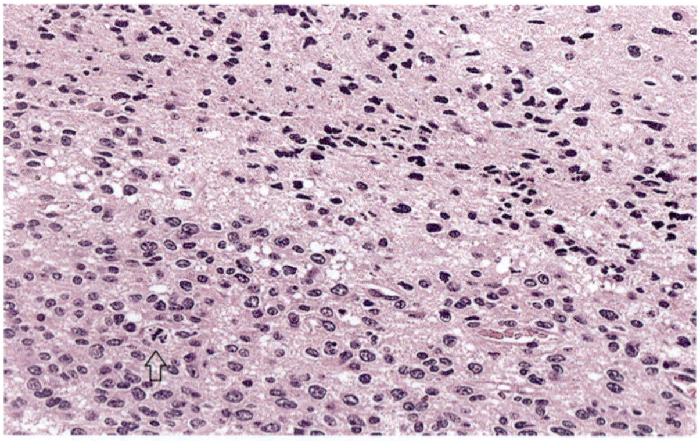

Fig. 6.2 *Anaplastic astrocytoma WHO grade III, histology*. This degree of nuclear pleomorphism and atypia could be present in either astrocytoma grade II or III. Without mitotic activity (*arrow*) the lesion would be grade II

particular mutation, although IDH sequencing of *IDH1* codon 132 and *IDH2* codon 172 is recommended to look for rarer mutations in immunonegative examples, especially if there are reasons to suspect an IDH-mutant glioma (i.e., a previous history of lower-grade – II or III –glioma, an adolescent or young adult patient, loss of ATRX expression by IHC). Overall, *IDH1/2* mutations serve as important biomarkers for diffuse gliomas; the finding of an *IDH* mutation confers a better prognosis regardless of tumor grade and other variables, serving as an independent prognostic factor. The vast majority of IDH-mutant diffuse astrocytomas, as well as the anaplastic astrocytomas and glioblastomas that evolve from them, also harbor class-defining loss of function in *TP53* and *ATRX* genes. Thus, a *typical immunohistochemical staining panel* may include IDH1 R132H protein (cytoplasmic positivity), p53 protein (nuclear positivity), ATRX protein (loss of nuclear immunostaining in tumor cells), and MIB-1 for proliferation index (nuclear positivity). Another form of high-grade astrocytoma that most often occurs in the pediatric population is characterized by histone H3F3 mutations and occurs either in the cerebral hemispheres (G34 codon mutations) or in the midline (K27 codon mutations), the latter leading to the new WHO entity termed diffuse midline glioma, H3 K27 M-mutant (see later).

Regarding therapy, the *most relevant molecular test for patients with high-grade gliomas* is the methylation status of the promoter for O6-methylguanine-DNA methyltransferase (*MGMT*). Epigenetic *MGMT* promoter methylation results in decreased expression of the gene with improved response to alkylating agents (i.e., temozolomide) and with longer survival, regardless of therapy. This epigenetic silencing of *MGMT* occurs in around 75% of IDH-mutant glioblastomas and around 20% of IDH-wildtype glioblastomas and can be assessed by PCR-based tests of genomic tumor DNA.

General Diagnostic Approach

Cytologic preparations of astrocytic neoplasms are invaluable diagnostic aids because they reveal, better than frozen sections, the features of the astrocytic cells. Smears show the presence of well-defined cytoplasmic processes that cross each

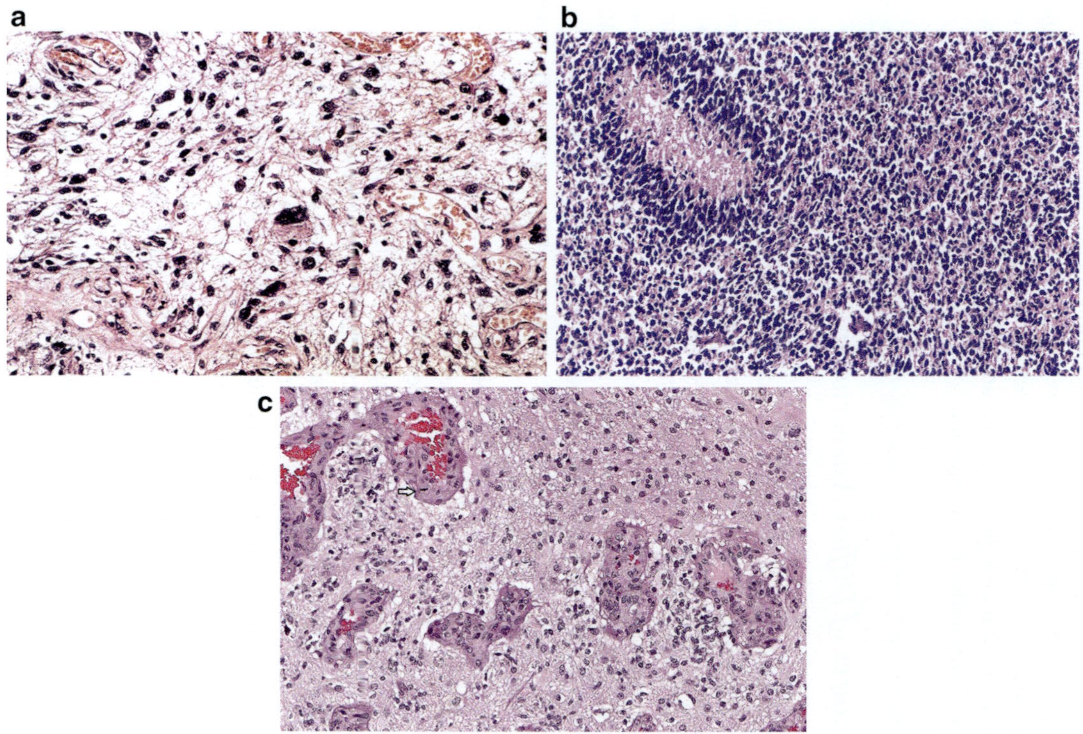

Fig. 6.3 *Glioblastoma WHO grade IV, histology.* (**a**) Pleomorphic astrocytic cells and anomalous vessels are characteristic features. (**b**) Palisading necrosis, the hallmark feature of glioblastoma, appears surrounded by densely packed small tumor cells in this case. (**c**) Typical microvascular hyperplasia characterized by small multilayered vessels with plump, mitotically active (*arrow*) endothelia

other in multiple directions, giving rise to a fibrillary appearance. These processes may be shortened, thickened, or distorted in comparison with normal/reactive astrocytes but, in any event, are able to occupy the intercellular space producing the characteristic fibrillary background. By the contrary, in frozen sections, it is very difficult to evaluate whether the background is composed of astrocytic fibers (fibrillary/thread-like in smears) or neuropil of normal brain (finely granular/felt-like in smears), a matter of great importance in interpretation. The grade of the tumor, low or high, may be inferred from the degree of cell **a**typia and from the presence or absence of **mi**tosis, **e**ndothelial proliferation, and **n**ecrosis ("AMEN" criteria), all characteristics perfectly noticeable in smears.

Cytologic Features of Diffuse Astrocytoma

Smears show fibrillary tissue fragments with a characteristic lumpy appearance, in which there are increased cellularity, mild nuclear atypia, and uneven cellular distribution in comparison with normal brain. The cytoplasm is either eosinophilic or not discernible, and as a result many cells appear as naked nuclei against the fibrillary background. Nuclei are oval to elongate and have mild to moderate hyperchromatism and irregular contours, which is of great value for distinguishing tumor cells from normal and reactive astrocytes. The vessels are of mature capillary type (Fig. 6.4a, b). The *gemistocytic variant* is the one consisting in great part of this type of astrocytes (at least 20% of the tumor cells). Gemistocytes (from the Greek *gemistos* for laden or full) are characterized by abundant glassy pink cytoplasm and eccentrically placed nuclei. The randomly oriented cytoplasmic processes, even though fewer, broader, and shorter than in the previously mentioned diffuse astrocytoma, are very evident in smears forming a coarse network (Fig. 6.5a, b). The pure forms of *protoplasmic astrocytoma* are very infrequent. The tumor is so named because its cells resemble the small "protoplasmic" astrocytes of the cortex. Because of the scarcity of glial filaments, specimens from this variant have a low consistency and spread very easily on the glass slide producing a myxoid background that is poor in fibers. The tumor cells show scant cytoplasm that extends itself in radial processes that are shorter and more ill-defined (coweb-like) than in the other variants. Nuclei are round to oval with finely granular to condensed chromatin and small nucleoli. The background usually displays a metachromatic myxoid appearance with Romanowsky stains (Fig. 6.6a–c).

Features common to the three variants are the absence of mitosis, microvascular proliferation, and necrosis, and the presence of which is not considered to be compatible with the diagnosis of diffuse astrocytoma.

a b

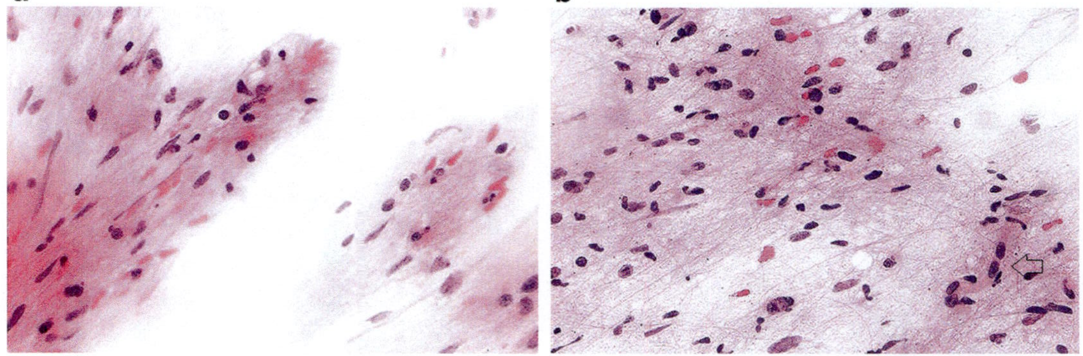

Fig. 6.4 *Diffuse astrocytoma WHO grade II, fibrillary variant*. (**a**) Cellular tissue fragments have a characteristic uneven, lumpy appearance. In contrast to normal brain, there is fibrillary background, increased cellularity and mild nuclear atypia. (**b**) Cytoplasms are not discernible and nuclei show irregular contours and slight hyperchromatism. Vessels are of the capillary type (*arrow*; **a**, **b**; Smears, H&E)

a b

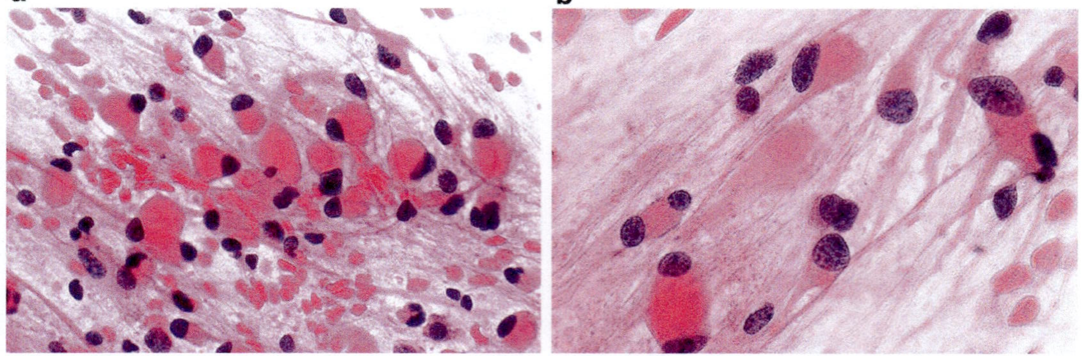

Fig. 6.5 *Diffuse astrocytoma WHO grade II, gemistocytic variant*. (**a**) Characteristic gemistocytic astrocytes with peripherally displaced nuclei and glassy pink cell bodies. (**b**) A high-magnification view shows fewer and coarser cytoplasmic processes contrasting those seen in fibrillary diffuse astrocytoma (**a**, **b**; Smears, H&E)

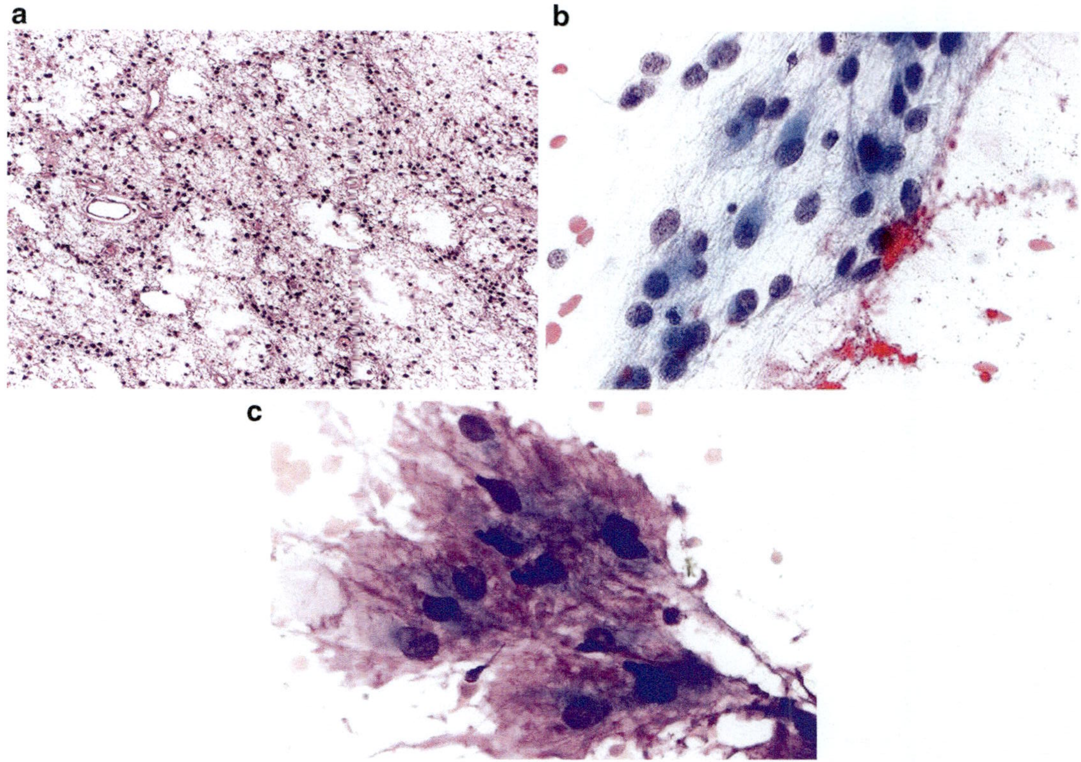

Fig. 6.6 *Diffuse astrocytoma WHO grade II, protoplasmic variant*. (**a**) Histology. Characteristic appearance with numerous microcysts and small tumor cells. (**b**) Evenly distributed preparation with small cells showing round to oval nuclei and sparse cytoplasmic processes (Smear, Papanicolaou). (**c**) Metachromatic myxoid material surrounding the tumor cells (Smear, Romanowsky)

Differential Diagnosis Considerations of Diffuse Astrocytoma

The differential diagnosis includes normal brain tissue, reactive glial proliferation, and other low-grade gliomas (mainly pilocytic astrocytoma). We have already seen the differentiation of the first two processes in the previous chapter, whereas distinguishing diffuse astrocytoma from other low-grade gliomas may be difficult and will depend on the predominant cell type. Thus, pilocytic astrocytoma should be considered in the case of the standard (fibrillary) variant, subependymal giant cell astrocytoma in the case of the gemistocytic variant, and oligodendroglioma and dysembryoplastic neuroepithelial tumor in the case of the protoplasmic variant (these differential diagnoses are covered in the description of each of these tumors) (Table 6.1).

Table 6.1 Characteristics of diffuse astrocytoma

Cytologic features
Lumpy tissue fragments and mature capillary vessels
In comparison with normal brain, smears show:
Fibrillary (no felt-like) background
Increased cellularity with uneven disposition
Mild nuclear atypia
Gemistocytic variant
Large, plump cells with eccentric nuclei predominate
Protoplasmic variant
Small cells with short, cobweb-like processes predominate
Differential diagnosis and pitfalls
Normal brain tissue
Reactive gliosis
Pilocytic astrocytoma
Gemistocytic variant
Subependymal giant cell astrocytoma
Protoplasmic variant
Oligodendroglioma
Dysembryoplastic neuroepithelial tumor

Cytologic Features of Anaplastic Astrocytoma

It may be preferable to use the term "high-grade diffuse astrocytoma" to refer to this tumor, because in the strict sense of the word "anaplasia" means the total absence of differentiation, which is not the case in this neoplasm. Particularly, in smears the astrocytic character is preserved in most cells, keeping the cytoplasmic processes and therefore the fibrillary background. However, the malignant traits, outlined only in the low-grade variant, appear here developed with increased cellularity, atypia, and mitotic activity. Nuclear atypia is evident, with increasing variations in nuclear size, shape, and coarsening of chromatin. The vessels are often more prominent than in the low-grade variant, being frequently associated with tumor cells to form perivascular aggregations. Discrete cells, with well-defined cell boundaries and variable cytoplasmic processes, are more conspicuous than in low-grade, diffuse astrocytoma. By definition, microvascular proliferation and necrosis must be absent (Fig. 6.7a, b).

Differential Diagnosis Considerations of Anaplastic Astrocytoma

Due to the presence of moderate to high cellularity and increased atypia, the distinction from normal white matter and reactive gliosis is not a significant problem, but other gliomas with atypia and cellular pleomorphism, such as pleomorphic xanthoastrocytoma, some pilocytic astrocytomas, anaplastic oligodendroglioma, and undersampled glioblastoma, should be considered. In the latter two cases, a generic diagnosis of "high-grade, diffuse glioma" suffices for the purposes of an intraoperative consultation. With respect to pleomorphic xanthoastrocytoma and pilocytic astrocytoma, their differential diagnosis is covered in the description of each of these tumors (Table 6.2).

Cytologic Features of Glioblastoma

The cytologic appearance of glioblastoma multiforme reflects the adjective that describes it, because it is extremely variable and pleomorphic. Some cases show an appearance essentially similar to that of anaplastic astrocytoma (Fig. 6.8a), whereas in others, it resembles that of a high-grade undifferentiated tumor, somewhat similar to embryonal tumors (Fig. 6.8b). In this spectrum of progressive dedifferentiation, we may find that all intermediate possible aspects, such as cellular anaplastic changes, vascular proliferative changes, and necrotic phenomena add up and combine among each other. We may summarize all of this by saying that they always

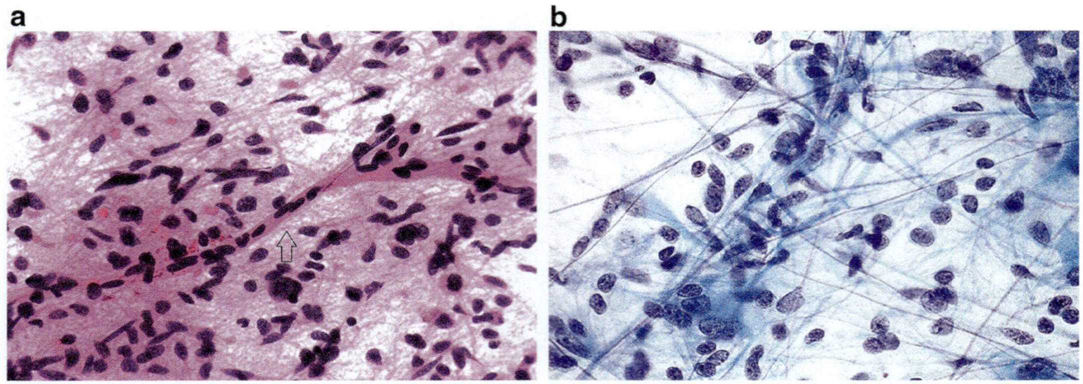

Fig. 6.7 *Anaplastic astrocytoma WHO grade III*. (**a**) Dark, elongated and sometimes angulated nuclei without apparent nucleoli are typical of anaplastic astrocytoma and glioblastoma, but in WHO grade III tumors, the vessels are still of capillary type (*arrow*; Smear, H&E). (**b**) This preparation from a *diffuse midline (pontine) glioma* shows a prominent fibrillary network and well-defined atypical astrocytic cells (Smear, Papanicolaou)

Table 6.2 Characteristics of anaplastic astrocytoma

Cytologic features
Fibrillary background
Increased cellularity and pleomorphism
Distinct nuclear atypia and mitotic activity
Perivascular aggregates
Differential diagnosis and pitfalls
Pleomorphic xanthoastrocytoma
Pilocytic astrocytoma with degenerative-type atypia
Anaplastic oligodendroglioma
Undersampled glioblastoma

form very cellular smears, in which the following background features, vascular changes, and cell types combine in a variable fashion.

Background

It may be fibrillary, necrotic, or necrotic-fibrillary. The presence of necrosis is of great value for the classification of a diffusely growing glial tumor such as a glioblastoma. In smears, necrotic debris often appears amorphous, somewhat granular, and thick acellular (Fig. 6.9a). However, to be diagnostic, necrotic debris needs to display some remaining structures such as faint eosinophilic nuclei, pyknotic nuclei, or cell ghosts (Fig. 6.9b). In some cases, necrosis is so extensive that it constitutes all the material obtained in the biopsy, which creates serious problems for the differential diagnosis. In order to avoid this, it is useful to tell the neurosurgeon to take a new biopsy from the peripheral band of neoplasia surrounding the necrotic center, radiologically identified as a ring-like image.

Vascular Changes

We may find microvascular "glomeruloid" proliferation, abnormal fistulous vessels with intraluminal endothelial proliferation, and vascular thrombosis. Frequently, these atypical vessels appear surrounded by a large number of tumor cells, thus accentuating the pseudopapillary appearance that started in the anaplastic astrocytoma (Fig. 6.10a–c).

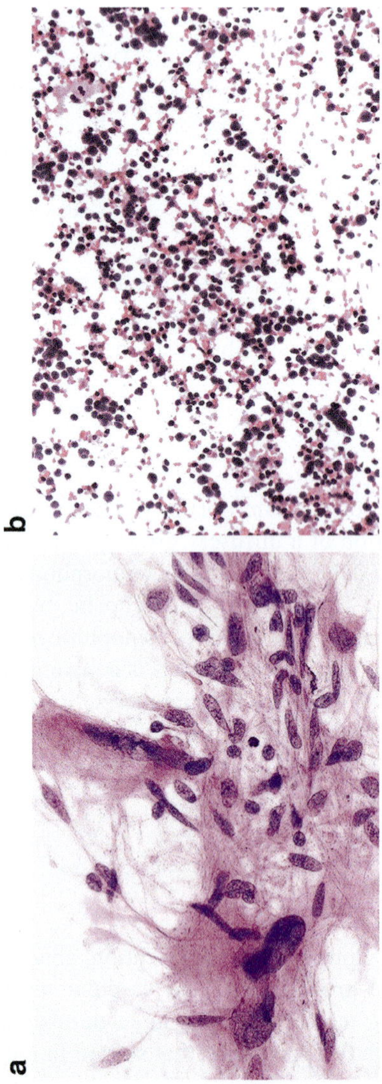

Fig. 6.8 *Glioblastoma, cytology*. (**a**) Preparation from a conventional glioblastoma showing atypical astrocytic cells in a fibrillary background. With the exception of giant cells, the overall appearance is similar to that of anaplastic astrocytoma. (**b**) This preparation from a small-cell glioblastoma shows a discohesive pattern of small cells lacking astrocytic features and granular necrotic debris (**a**, **b**; Smears, H&E)

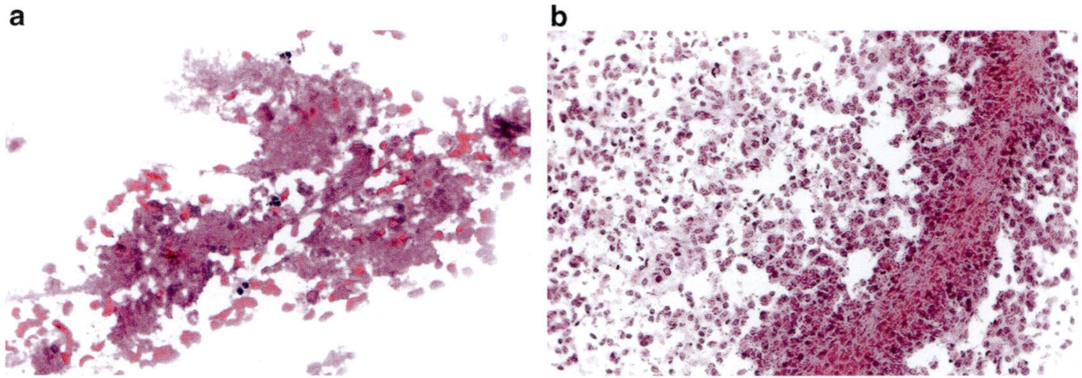

Fig. 6.9 *Glioblastoma, necrosis.* (**a**) Cytological preparations of tissue from the nonenhancing center will show little other than necrosis. Unlike infarcts and demyelinating disease, only smeared granular debris (no macrophages) is the result. (**b**) In this case, necrotic granular debris is intermixed with ghost cells and karyorrhectic nuclei (**a**, **b**; Smears, H&E)

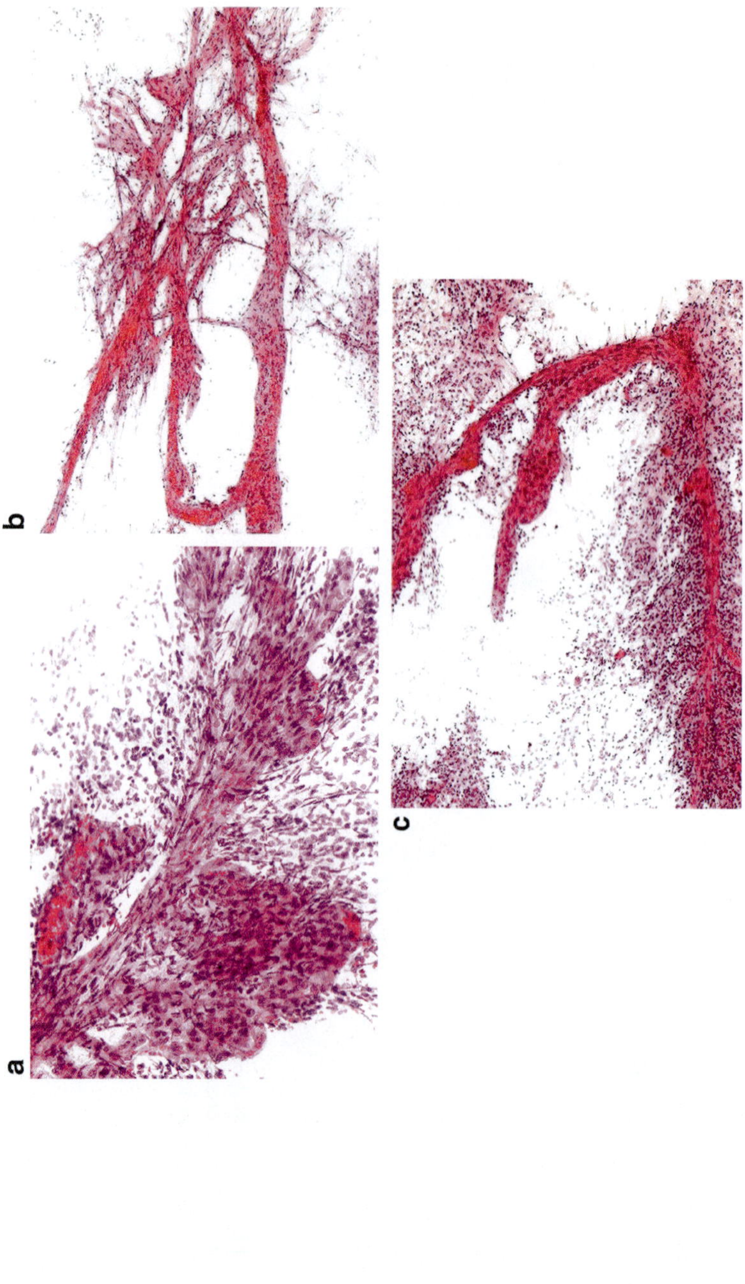

Fig. 6.10 *Glioblastoma, vascular changes.* Microvascular "glomeruloid" proliferation (**a**), fistulous vessels with intraluminal endothelial proliferation (**b**), and thrombosed vessels, known as "black veins" by the surgeon (**c**) are common in glioblastomas. Note that these abnormal vessels are surrounded by abundant tumor cells (**a–c**; Smears, H&E)

Cell Types

We may find, even on the same smear, pleomorphic astrocytic cells (sometimes giant multinucleated) and cells that lack overt astrocytic features, such as bipolar (fusiform) cells, monopolar (tadpole) cells, small undifferentiated cells, and large epithelioid cells. Independently of the cell type, intercellular cohesiveness is very low, and, therefore, tumor cells appear isolated or form, at most, small loose groups. On their part, the nuclei, like the cells, display a sharp variety in size, number, and appearance and may be large or small, single or multiple, with or without nucleolus, etc. The chromatin is coarse and irregular, and the nuclear membrane often shows numerous folds and creases that give the nucleus a multilobed appearance (Fig. 6.11a–c).

Morphologic Variants

The predominance of some of these cell types gives rise to the different morphologic variants of glioblastoma. Thus, in *giant cell glioblastoma*, the smear is primarily composed of very large and bizarre giant cells, with wide irregular cytoplasm expanding into multiple processes (Fig. 6.12a–c). In *gliosarcoma*, a variant in which areas of glioma alternate with areas of conspicuous mesenchymal component, both malignant, a mixed pattern is observed consisting of atypical glial cells and clusters of variably sarcomatous elements. The glial component is astrocytic, often with gemistocytes, whereas the sarcomatous component is usually undifferentiated and spindle shaped but may be rhabdoid, chondroid, or osteoblastic (Fig. 6.13a–c). Lastly, in *epithelioid glioblastoma*, epithelioid cells with plump cytoplasm, sharp cell borders, and round "open" nuclei with nucleoli predominate, making differential diagnosis with metastatic carcinoma/melanoma challenging. Rhabdoid and gemistocytic morphology can also be seen (Fig. 6.14a, b).

Differential Diagnosis Considerations of Glioblastoma

Other high-grade gliomas, non-glial primary tumors, metastatic tumors, and non-neoplastic necrotic processes should be considered. Other high-grade gliomas (anaplastic astrocytoma, anaplastic oligodendroglioma) usually do not exhibit such a variegated picture and so many signs of aggressiveness as glioblastoma does. In any event, as previously mentioned, an intraoperative diagnosis of "high-grade, diffuse glioma" is adequate. Differentiating metastatic carcinoma from glioblastoma may be difficult with frozen sections, but it can be done more easily with smears. Glioblastoma is composed of discohesive cells that often have a glial aspect featuring cytoplasmic processes. In contrast, metastatic carcinomas form cohesive cell groups, and their cells have smooth surfaces without processes. With respect to non-tumoral necrotic lesions, it is as important attempting to recognize their causal agent

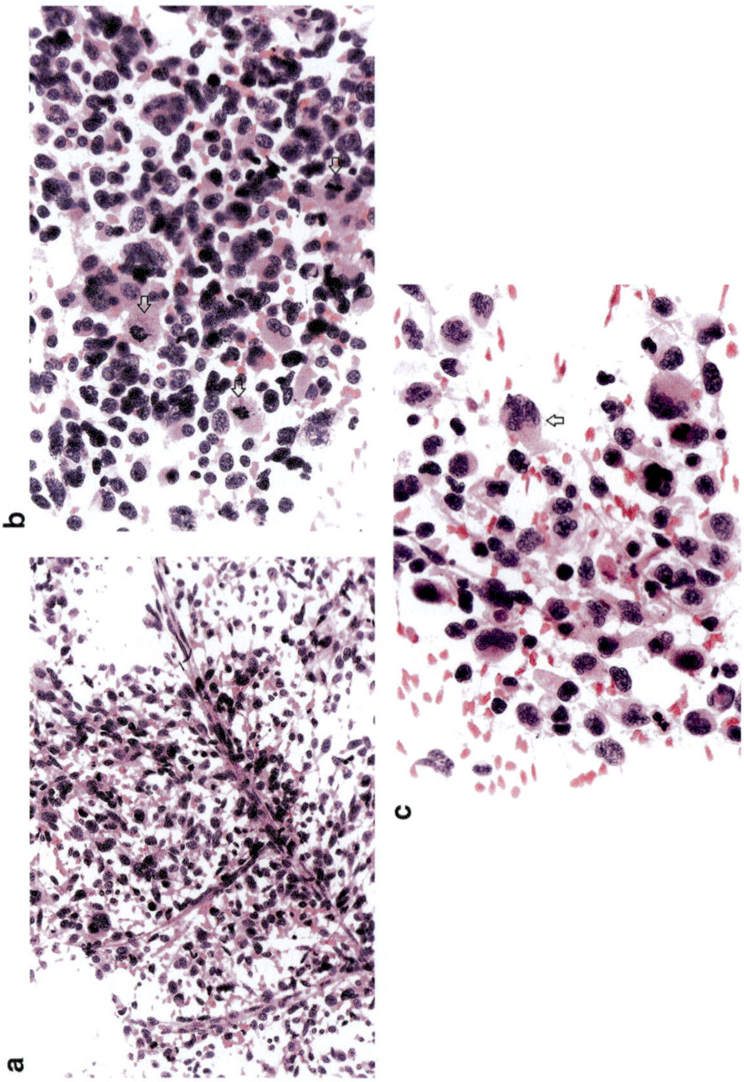

Fig. 6.11 *Glioblastoma, cell types*. (**a**) Tumor cells are pleomorphic and tend to remain close to blood vessels giving a pseudopapillary appearance. (**b**) Predominantly single cell pattern with anaplastic features and frequent atypical mitotic figures (*arrows*). (**c**) Considerable cellular pleomorphism with astrocytic, epithelioid, fusiform, small undifferentiated, and tadpole-shaped (*arrow*) cells on the same preparation. Also note numerous folds and indentations of the nuclear membranes (**a–c**; Smears, H&E)

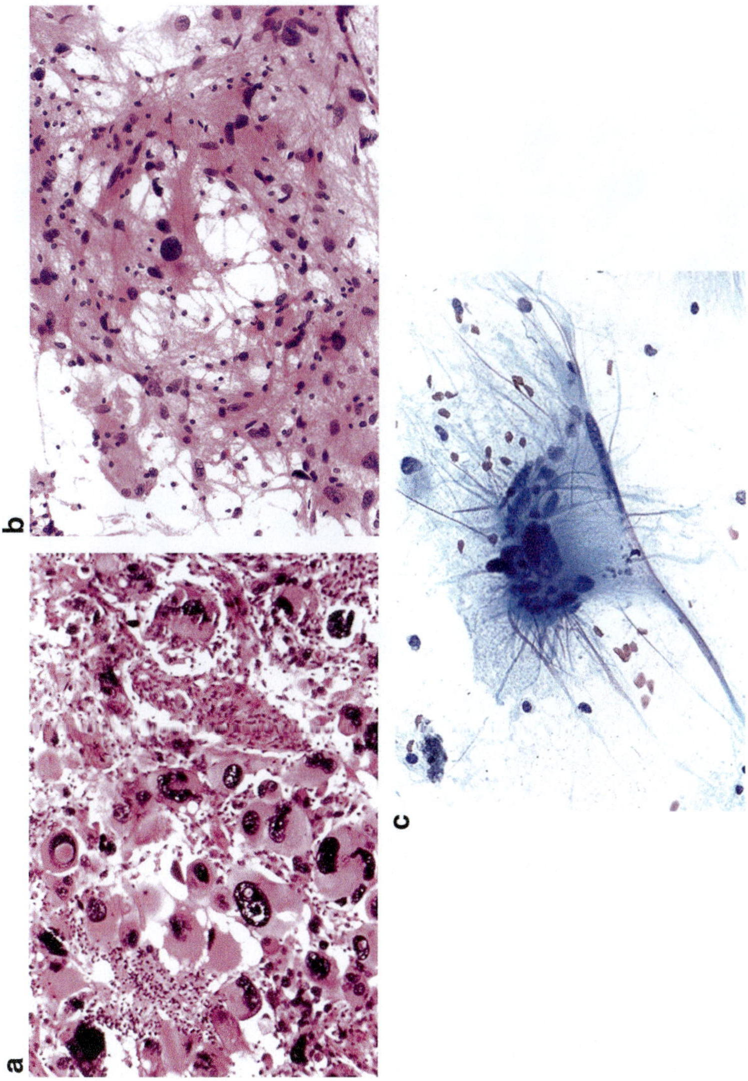

Fig. 6.12 *Giant cell glioblastoma.* (**a**) Histology. The defining feature of this lesion is very large tumor cells with marked pleomorphism and bizarre nuclear features. (**b**) Cytologic preparation showing large bizarre mononucleate and multinucleate tumor cells with intervening smaller astrocytoma cells (Smear, H&E). (**c**) Giant cells are quite large and exhibit numerous multipolar processes, the hallmark of astrocytic cells (Smear, Papanicolaou)

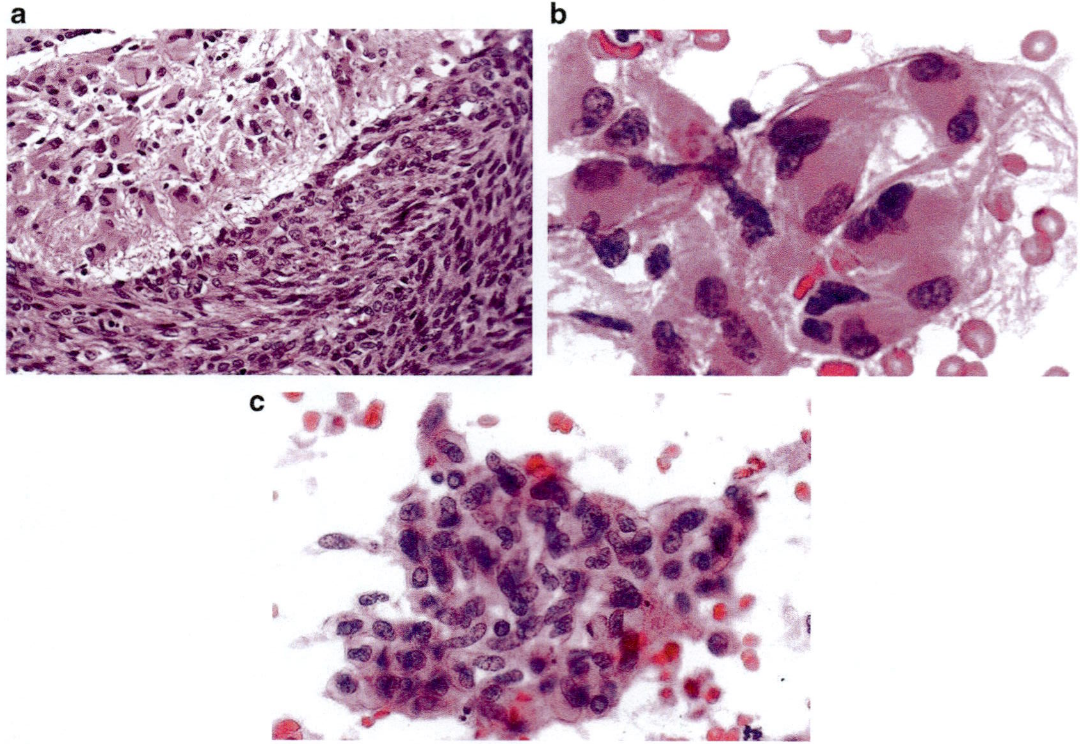

Fig. 6.13 *Gliosarcoma*. (**a**) Histology. A biphasic pattern with areas displaying glial and mesenchymal differentiation characterizes this variant. Alternating areas of astrocytic (**b**) and densely packed sarcomatous cells (**c**) can be seen in cytologic preparations from this tumor (**b**, **c**; Smears, H&E)

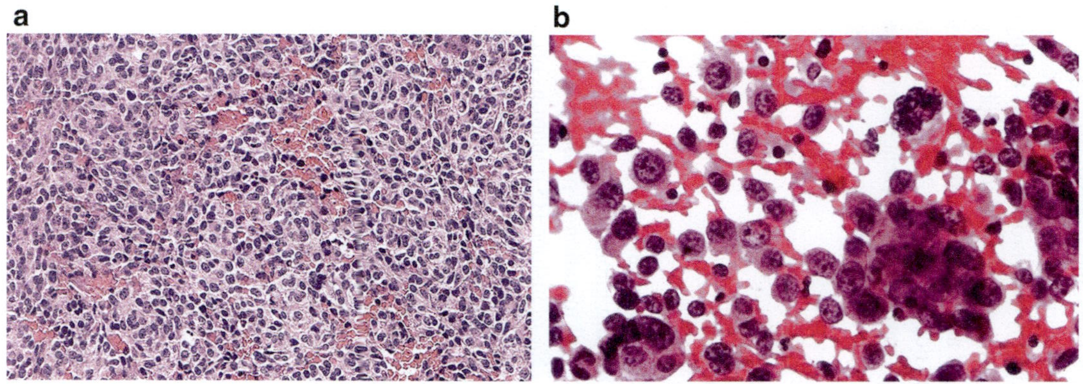

Fig. 6.14 *Epithelioid glioblastoma*. (**a**) Histology. Epithelioid tumor cells and lack of fibrillary background simulate metastatic carcinoma or melanoma. (**b**) Well circumscribed cells with a paucity of cytoplasmic processes, both isolated and in aggregates, more typically associated with metastatic carcinoma or melanoma, predominant in this variant. Also note vesicular nuclei and prominent nucleoli (Smear, H&E)

as to rule out the presence of neoplastic cells, if needed with additional smears. *Radiation necrosis with radiation-induced atypia* presents an especially difficult case. Advanced imaging techniques including PET can suggest a diagnosis of radiation necrosis, but biopsy/resection of questionable lesions is often performed to rule out a recurrent tumor. Radiation-induced atypia may be dramatic and affect numerous cell types including tumor cells and reactive astrocytes, which exhibit bizarre bubbly nuclei and abundant pink cytoplasm. Coagulative necrosis (that is difficult to smear), extensive vasculopathy (fibrinoid necrosis, telangiectasia, and hyaline thickening), dystrophic calcification (amorphous basophilic aggregates), and a minimal inflammatory infiltrate, if any, complete the cytologic picture of this process (Fig. 6.15a, b). However, it is not always possible to distinguish radiation necrosis with radiation-induced atypia from tumor recurrence, being an intraoperative report of "glioma with necrosis and radiation changes, grading deferred" adequate (Table 6.3).

Diffuse Midline Glioma

Diffuse midline glioma, H3 K27 M-mutant, is not a morphologic/architectural variant but represents a diffusely infiltrating glioma (any grade) with predominant astrocytic differentiation and a specific point mutation at position K27 (codon K27) in the histone H3 coding genes. About 75% of histone H3 mutations occur in *H3F3A*, encoding the H3.3 isoform, whereas 20–25% of mutations occur in *HIST1H3B or HIST1H3C*, encoding H3.1. An antibody to the K27 M mutant protein can reliably identify these cases, regardless of whether the protein results from mutations in *H3F3A* or *HIST1H3B/C*. These tumors most often involve the ventral brain stem (histone H3 K27 M mutations are found in up to 70% of *diffuse pontine gliomas*), thalamus, and spinal cord in children and young adults. Most patients present with the classic triad (multiple cranial neuropathies, long tract signs, and ataxia) or CSF obstruction, typically developing over a short period of time (1–2 months). On MRI, diffuse midline gliomas are usually T1-hypointense and T2-hyperintense; contrast enhancement and necrosis may be present. Regardless of histologic grade, the prognosis is poor (WHO grade IV tumor) with <10% of these patients surviving beyond 2 years.

Smears features and differential diagnosis are similar to those diffuse astrocytomas (any grade), with frequent overrepresentation of giant cells (Fig. 6.7b). Therefore, during intraoperative consultation, report as "diffuse glioma."

Gliomatosis Cerebri

This process is now considered as only an unusual growth pattern of any diffuse glioma, rather than a distinct entity. It has a clinicoradiologic pattern of widespread brain invasion involving three or more cerebral lobes. Also bilateral growth and

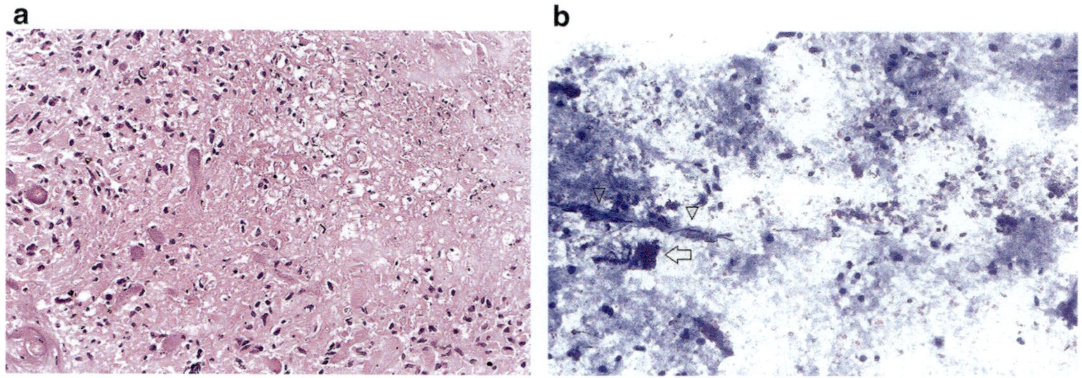

Fig. 6.15 *Radiation necrosis*. (**a**) Tissue section displaying a large focus of coagulative necrosis that lacks the distinctive pseudopalisading of glioblastoma. Also, note hyalinized vessels and large, bizarre glial cells in the adjacent brain parenchyma. (**b**) Cytomorphologic findings include necrotic granular debris, polymorphic gliosis, dystrophic calcification (*arrow*), rigid vessels (*arrowheads*), and some inflammatory cells. Unlike evolving infarcts and demyelinating lesions, macrophages are uncommon (Smear, Papanicolaou)

Table 6.3 Characteristics of glioblastoma

Cytologic features
Fibrillary and/or necrotic background
Anomalous vessels with microvascular proliferation
Very high cellularity with discohesive pattern
Marked cellular pleomorphism with
Distinct nuclear atypia (multilobed appearance, coarse chromatin)
Often tumor cells conserve fibrillary processes (diagnostic clue)
Beware of no diagnostic smears of sampling:
Central necrosis
Gliotic edge
Variants/patterns:
Giant cell (bizarre, multinucleated giant cells predominate)
Small cell (small, undifferentiated cells predominate)
Gliosarcoma (mixed pattern of glial and sarcomatous cells)
Epithelioid (large, epithelioid cells predominate)
Differential diagnosis and pitfalls
Other anaplastic gliomas
Pleomorphic xanthoastrocytoma
Metastatic carcinoma/melanoma
Embryonal tumors
CNS lymphomas
Sarcomas
Nonneoplastic necrotic processes
Necrotizing infections
Ischemic lesions
Radiation necrosis with radiation-induced atypia

regular extension to infratentorial structures are frequently noted. Common symptoms are seizures, aphasia, and changes in personality/mental status, and neuroimaging displays diffuse and sometimes impressive enlargement of the involved structures without tissue destruction (autopsy specimens usually show intact gross anatomy). The histologic pattern is that of an extensive infiltrating process without formation of appreciable tumor nodules and may be encountered in any of the newly defined integrated diffuse glioma diagnoses. Thus, neoplastic cells most commonly display an astrocytic phenotype, but oligodendroglial, mixed oligoastrocytic, and glioblastoma phenotypes may be seen.

Cytologic Features

The predominant pattern is a population of small, immature glial cells that tend to be bipolar, with a dense and often elongated microglia-like nucleus. This cytomorphology is presumably originated by adaptation of the avidly infiltrating tumor cells to the underlying histoarchitecture (white matter tracks). Most of such cells do not have well-defined cytoplasm and cytoplasmic processes and appear isolated or forming small clusters with angiotropic tendency. Additionally, large tumor cells with irregular pleomorphic nuclei can be seen (Fig. 6.16a, b). During intraoperative consultation, report these cases as "diffuse glioma.".

Differential Diagnosis Considerations

Given its infiltrating character with preservation of the underlying histoarchitecture, reactive gliosis may be a differential diagnosis. This distinction is not difficult on the basis of the clear cytomorphologic differences between reactive astrocytes (stellate morphology, minimal nuclear atypia) and the predominant cell type in gliomatosis cerebri (ill-defined cytoplasm and cytoplasmic processes, elongated and hyperchromatic nuclei, marked atypia).

Pilocytic Astrocytoma

Pilocytic astrocytoma (PA) occurs most frequently in children and young adults with a peak incidence in the teens, being the most common pediatric glioma (33% of all gliomas in this age group). A majority of cases arise in the cerebellum (commonest location), optic pathway, hypothalamic/third ventricular region, dorsal aspect of the brain stem and spinal cord, but may be seen in the cerebral hemisphere as well, where most frequently involve the periventricular areas of the frontotemporal lobes (anywhere expected tumor). PA occurs sporadically or in association with *neurofibromatosis type 1* (NF-1). Aberrant activation of the mitogen-activated protein kinase (MAPK) pathway, due to *BRAF-KIAA1549* fusion gene (66–70%) or *BRAF* V600E mutation (8–9%), appears to play a critical role in the pathogenesis of sporadic cases, whereas this is activated in the setting of NF-1 by functional loss of neurofibromin (product of the *NF1* gene and a negative regulator of MAPK pathway signaling). Other than *BRAF* alterations, alterations in *FGFR1*, *KRAS*, *PTPN11*, *NTRK3*, and *NTRK2* have also been reported in sporadic PAs, but at much lower frequencies.

PA is a low-grade neoplasia (WHO grade I), which is why it behaves clinically as a slowly evolving lesion with focal neurologic deficits or ventricular obstruction. In neuroimaging, the majority of PAs appear as circumscribed, round to oval

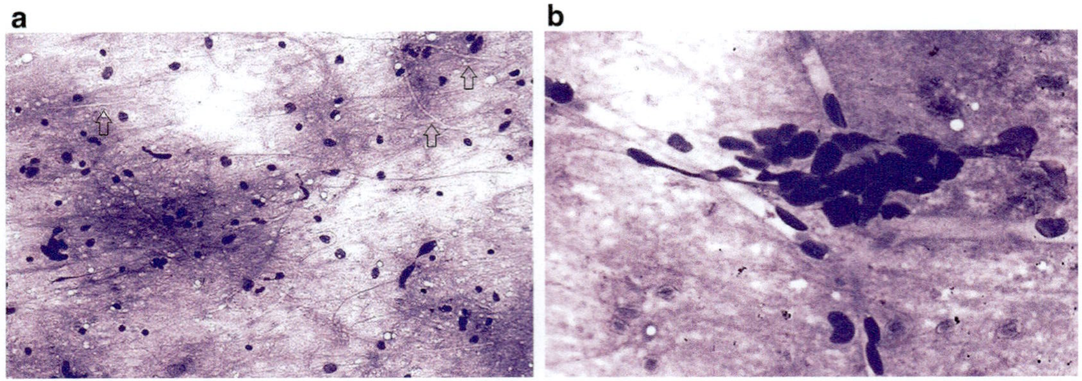

Fig. 6.16 *Gliomatosis pattern*. (**a**) Because many normal or reactive cellular elements will contaminate the available tissue, the monotony of cells in more solid tumors is lost in gliomatosis, but cells with elongated rod-shaped nuclei and indistinct cytoplasm are characteristic. Also note small vacuoles of disintegrated neuropil and long axons as negative images (*arrows*). (**b**) A cluster of hypercromatic tumor cells show angiotropic tendency. Unlike most forms of gliosis, no cytoplasm is apparent (**a**, **b**; Smears, Romanowsky)

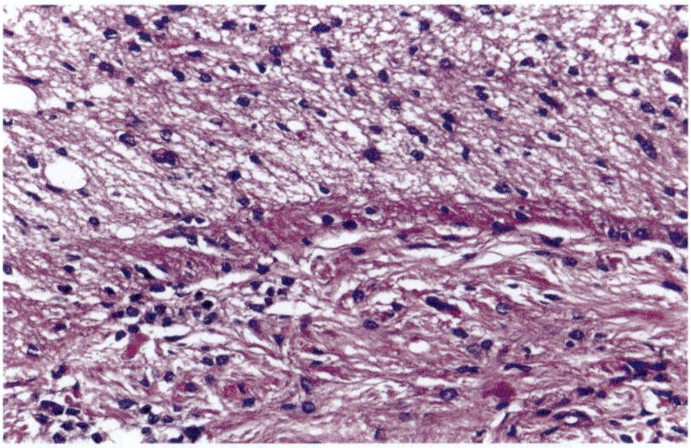

Fig. 6.17 *Pilocytic astrocytomas* often demonstrate biphasic pattern with loose, spongy areas (*above*) admixed with a densely fibrillar element, frequently with Rosenthal fibers (*below*)

enhancing masses with little, if any, perilesional edema. Because of its high tendency to cystification, PA frequently appears as a cystic lesion with an enhancing mural nodule (the classic finding of cerebellar PA). Examples involving the optic nerve typically manifest as a kinked or buckled enlargement of the nerve.

Macroscopically, this tumor is rubbery and relatively well circumscribed with common intra- or para-tumoral cyst formation.

The name *pilocytic astrocytoma* is due to the fact that this neoplasia is composed mostly of bipolar astrocytes with extremely long cytoplasmic processes (piloid/hair cells). Other elements characteristic of this tumor are multipolar "protoplasmic" astrocytic cells, Rosenthal fibers (RFs), and eosinophilic granular bodies (Fig. 6.17).

Pilomyxoid astrocytoma (PMA) is a variant of PA that occurs predominantly in infants and young children and most often involves the hypothalamic/chiasmatic region. The unfavorable location of the majority of PMAs often precludes complete surgical excision, and these tumors have a relatively poor outcome compared with PAs. It is characterized by an abundant myxoid matrix and a monomorphic cell population of spindly, bipolar glial cells.

Malignant transformation of PA occurs only rarely (no more than 1% to 2%), most frequently in the setting of NF1 or in association with irradiation of a previously documented grade I tumor. The so-called anaplastic pilocytic astrocytoma is located most frequently in the brainstem and the spinal cord and is characterized by the presence of anaplastic features, which include brisk mitotic activity (>4 per 10 HPF), moderate to severe nuclear atypia, and hypercellularity, with or without necrosis.

The prognosis of PA is intrinsically favorable, with a roughly 80% 20-year survival rate, and it is worse only when the location prevents radical surgery. Chemotherapy is employed for progressing, unresectable lesions with no evidence of benefit of irradiation on survival. Despite location, the presence of *BRAF-KIAA1549* fusion predicts better clinical outcome (can be detected by FISH assay).

Cytologic Features

Squash preparations show tissue fragments and individual cells in a faint myxoid background. The tumor cells are bipolar with thin, very long hair-like processes (piloid cells) or multipolar with a small cell body and short cobweb-like processes (protoplasmic cells). The nuclei are oval to elongated or round, respectively, with a smooth contoured bland appearance. The characteristic myxoid background, barely discernible with H&E or Papanicolaou stains, is nicely revealed with a metachromatic pink/magenta color in Romanowsky-stained preparations. Scattered here and there, RFs and EGBs may be observed (Fig. 6.18a–c). Both RFs and EGBs are not exclusively found in pilocytic astrocytoma but may be observed in other tumoral and non-tumoral processes; however, their presence, together with the two cell types described above and the myxoid background, completes a cytologic picture of great diagnostic value. Hyalinized and glomeruloid vessels can be prominent features; this, together with the presence of mitotic figures, hyperchromatic nuclei, and degenerative-type atypia including large or giant cells with multiple nuclei circumferentially arranged ("pennies on a plate"), can cause confusion with high-grade astrocytoma, but these features are frequently seen in long-standing lesions and should not prompt tumor overgrading (Fig. 6.19a–c). Preparations from *pilomyxoid astrocytoma* show an enhanced myxoid background and monomorphous spindle cells, with RFs and EGBs typically absent. On the contrary, angiocentric arrangement is an expected feature (Fig. 6.20a–c). The authentic malignant forms (*PA with anaplasia*) manifest themselves through anaplastic cellular changes, mitotic figures, endothelial proliferation, and, sometimes, necrotic debris, which is why the cytologic picture is similar to that of high-grade diffuse astrocytoma.

Differential Diagnosis Considerations

The intraoperative differential diagnoses include other glial neoplasms with fibrillary background, such as diffuse astrocytoma (any grade) and ependymoma, as well as chronic "piloid" gliosis. The main diagnostic problem is to differentiate PA from diffuse astrocytoma, especially in those locations (like the cerebral hemispheres) where PA is not expected. In smear preparations, the presence of "piloid" cells with very long processes and bland nuclei, varicose RFs, globular EGBs, and a variable myxoid background are distinctive features of PA. On the other hand, crowded tissue fragments with a characteristic uneven appearance, angulated nuclei with moderate pleomorphism and hyperchromatism, no discernible or eosinophilic cytoplasm, and a fibrillary, but usually not myxoid background, favor the diagnosis of diffuse astrocytoma. However, if sample is very small and not have all desired characteristics, a report of "astrocytoma with piloid features, grading deferred" is adequate. The presence of perivascular pseudorosettes in smears of PA has been described, resembling in a certain way the cytology of ependymoma, but the cells of

a b c

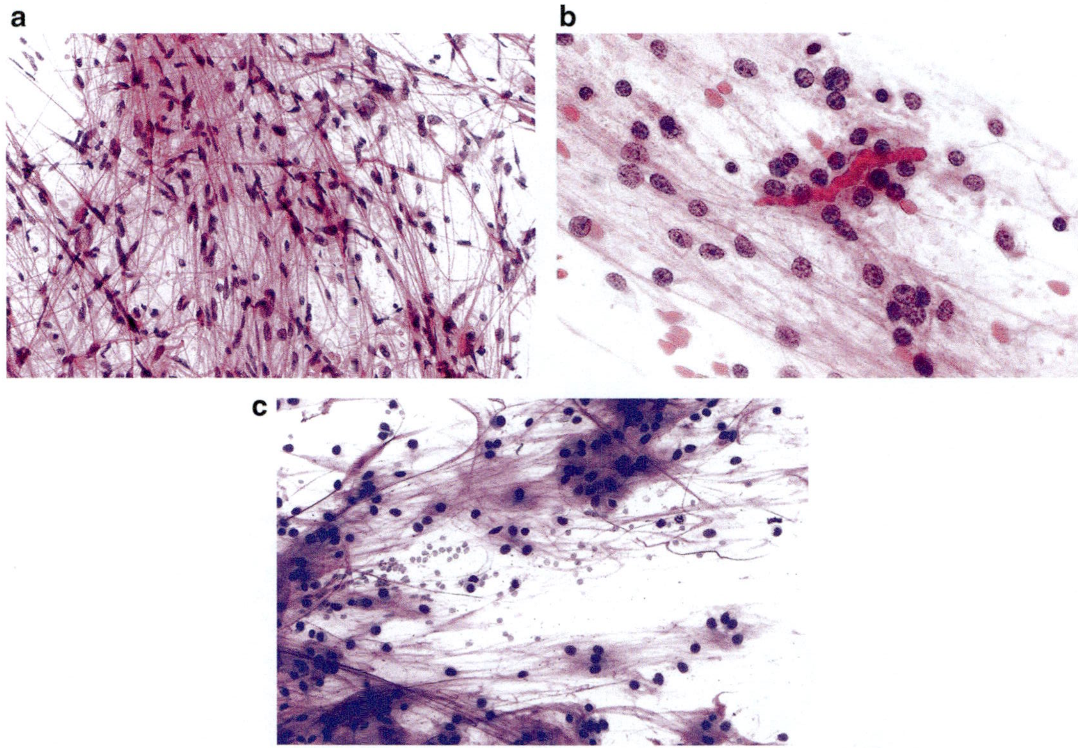

Fig. 6.18 *Pilocytic astrocytoma*. (**a**) Bipolar “piloid” cells exhibiting very long processes. Nuclei are bland with smooth contours (Smear, H&E). (**b**) Brightly eosinophilic Rosenthal fiber with one blunt pole and one tapered end. It is surrounded by “protoplasmic” cells exhibiting round nuclei and short, cobweb-like processes (Smear, H&E). (**c**) The presence of metachromatic myxoid wisps in the background is an additional clue for diagnosis (Smear, Romanowsky)

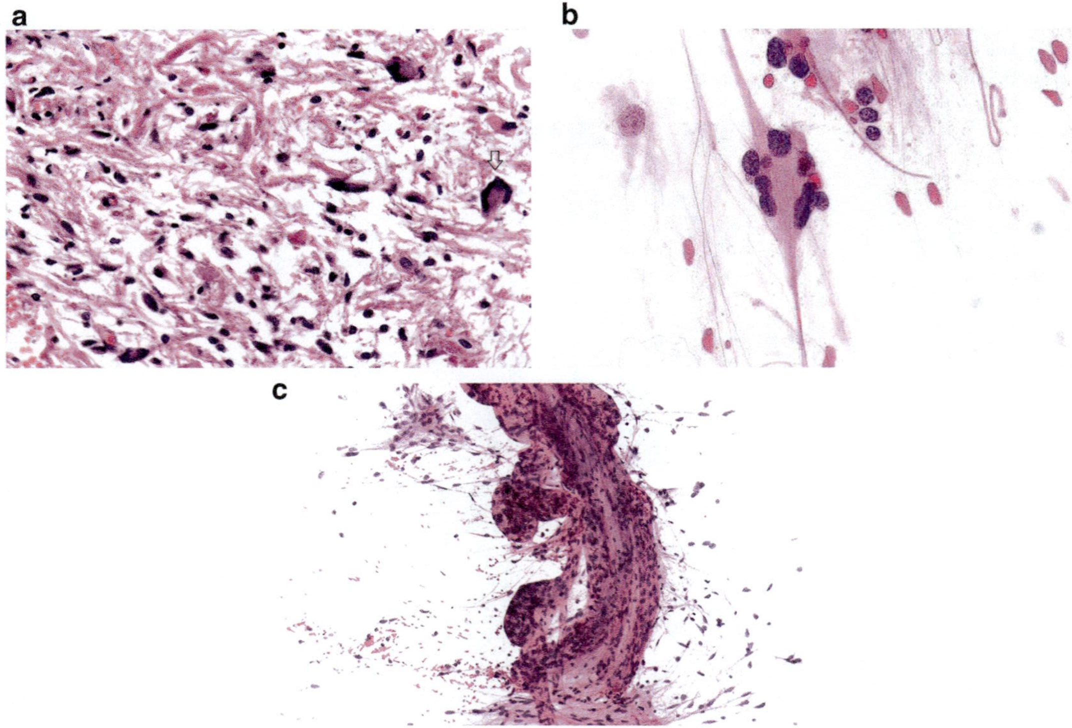

Fig. 6.19 *Pilocytic astrocytoma, atypical (degenerative) changes*. (**a**) Histology. Despite conspicuous cellular atypia, the presence of Rosenthal fibers and eosinophilic granular bodies bespeaks about the indolent behavior of this tumor. Note a characteristic horseshoe or "pennies on a plate" nuclear arrangement (*arrow*). (**b**) A large cell with degenerative-type atypia displays multiple nuclei with peripheral "pennies on a plate" arrangement (as if a stack of pennies was played out peripherally on a plate). (**c**) Angiomatoid vasculature with complex arborization and hyaline mural fibroplasia also is a common finding in long-standing lesions. Note perivascular aggregations of "piloid" tumor cells (**b**, **c**; Smears, H&E)

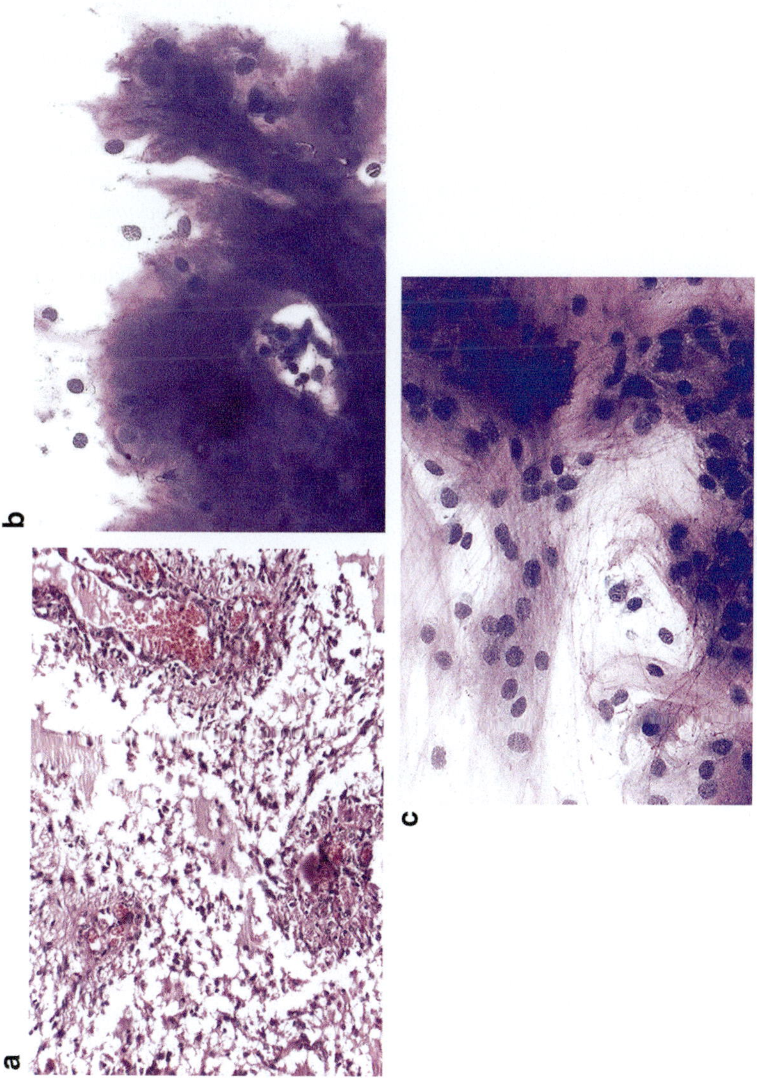

Fig. 6.20 *Pilomyxoid astrocytoma.* (**a**) Histology. This hypothalamic tumor displays a loose myxoid background along with monomorphous bipolar cells arranged in an angiocentric fashion. (**b**) Tissue fragment completely embedded in a dense myxoid matrix. (**c**) High-magnification view showing delicate piloid profiles and bland nuclei as those of pilocytic astrocytoma. The background is clearly myxoid, whereas Rosenthal fibers are absent (**b, c**; Smears, Romanowsky)

Table 6.4 Characteristics of pilocytic astrocytoma

Cytologic features
Fibrillary-myxoid background
Biphasic cellular pattern:
Bipolar “piloid” cells
Multipolar “protoplasmic” cells
Oval to elongate (piloid) or round (protoplasmic) bland nuclei
Rosenthal fibers and eosinophilic granular bodies
Regressive changes
Hyalinized/glomeruloid vessels
Degenerative-type atypia
Pilomyxoid astrocytoma
Enhanced myxoid background
Monomorphous cellular pattern of bipolar cells
Angiocentric arrangements
Differential diagnosis and pitfalls
Diffuse astrocytoma (any grade)
Ependymoma
Piloid gliosis

ependymoma often show a characteristic dual glial-epithelial appearance; additionally, RFs and EGBs are absent. Lastly, piloid gliosis is typically less cellular and does not have protoplasmic cells. Additional sampling and attention to clinical and radiologic features generally allows one to avoid this pitfall (Table. 6.4).

Subependymal Giant Cell Astrocytoma

Subependymal giant cell astrocytomas (SEGAs) are benign (WHO grade I) slow-growing discrete tumors that arise in the walls of the lateral ventricles in children and young adults (mean age at presentation 13 years). Almost always, they occur in the setting of *tuberous sclerosis complex* (TSC), an autosomal dominant syndrome due to mutations in *TSC1* gene on 9q34 (hamartin protein expression) and *TSC2* gene on 16p13.3 (tuberin protein expression). Disruption of the hamartin-tuberin complex causes upregulation of the mTOR pathway and increases proliferation and cell growth. Patients with SEGA usually present with epilepsy, symptoms of increased intracranial pressure (due to obstructive hydrocephalus), or acute hemorrhage. Scans show well-circumscribed, contrast-enhancing masses located in the lateral and/or third ventricles near the foramen of Monro; calcification is an almost constant feature. The SEGA is a sharply delineated, spherical, or multinodular mass of fleshy, gray-pink tissue that is broadly attached to the ventricular wall. The name of the tumor makes reference to its characteristic subependymal location and to its histologic appearance, which is characterized by the presence of large, atypical cells resembling gemistocytes or ganglioid cells (Fig. 6.21a). Because of the mixed glio-neuronal features, some prefer the term "subependymal giant cell tumor" rather than SEGA. Although it is a benign tumor, it represents a possible cause of mortality and morbidity in children with TSC. The standard treatment of symptomatic or enlarging SEGAs is surgical excision, but pharmacological inhibitors of the mTOR pathway (rapamycin and rapalogs, i.e., everolimus) have recently shown to induce involution of SEGAs.

Cytologic Features

Smears show cohesive cell clusters with the intercellular space occupied by fine fibrillary processes. Two predominant cell types are observed: (1) large, plump cells with glassy cytoplasm, resembling gemistocytic astrocytes or ganglioid cells, and (2) smaller spindled elements or "strap" cells. Both cell types have abundant hair-like processes along the cell border giving a "hairy cell" appearance. Nuclei are usually eccentric and neuron-like with open chromatin and prominent nucleoli. Bi- or multinucleated cells and perivascular arrangements (pseudorosettes) may also be present (Fig. 6.21b, c).

Differential Diagnosis Considerations

The differential diagnosis of SEGA includes several tumors containing large astrocytic cells or neurons, particularly gemistocytic astrocytoma, giant cell glioblastoma, and ganglion cell tumors. In gemistocytic astrocytoma, the nucleus has a tendency to protrude from the cytoplasm and does not have a ganglioid appearance, whereas cytoplasmic processes are fewer and broader. Endothelial proliferation, mitosis, and a more polymorphic cellularity distinguish giant cell glioblastoma. Lastly, unlike ganglion cell tumors, SEGA cells exhibit abundant fine processes along the cell borders (Table 6.5).

Pleomorphic Xanthoastrocytoma

Pleomorphic xanthoastrocytoma (PXA) is a relatively rare tumor (less than 1% of all CNS neoplasms) typically presents in later childhood or early adult life, and ignorance of its existence may result in an incorrect diagnosis of malignancy and institution of inappropriate therapy. About 40% of PXAs arise within the temporal lobe, with most of the remainder occurring elsewhere in the cerebral hemispheres. The

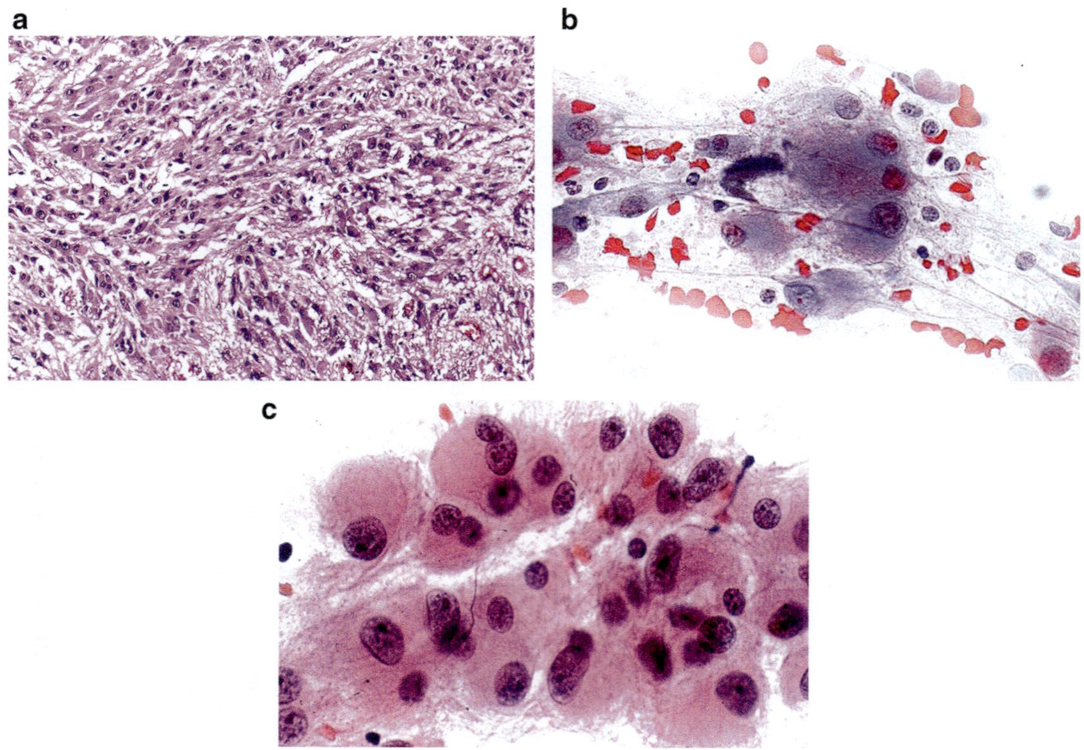

Fig. 6.21 *Subependymal giant cell astrocytoma*. (**a**) Histology. This tumor often displays a "sweeping" pattern with elongated to ganglioid cells. (**b**) Clump of tumor cells with ganglioid and elongated "strap" morphology (Smear, Papanicolaou). (**c**) These tumor cells display a paradoxical appearance: astrocytic-like cytoplasm and ganglion-like nuclei. Note abundant fine processes along the cell border ("hairy cell" appearance) and frequent bi-nucleation (Smear, H&E)

Table 6.5 Characteristics of subependymal giant cell astrocytoma

Cytologic features
Cohesive cell clumps
Large, gemistocyte-like cells
Smaller, strap-like cells
Ganglion-like nuclei
Abundant fine cytoplasmic processes ("hairy cell")
Differential diagnosis and pitfalls
Gemistocytic astrocytoma.
Giant cell glioblastoma
Ganglion cell tumors

tumor maintains a superficial cortical position, often abutting and extending into the overlying pia-arachnoid. Clinically, patients frequently have a chronic seizure disorder (70%) or mass effect symptoms. Neuroimaging demonstration of a well demarcated and partially cystic lesion with a contrast-enhancing mural nodule or plaque is especially suggestive, but they may also be solid or attached to the dura and mimic a meningioma. The term pleomorphic xanthoastrocytoma refers to its histologic appearance, which includes pleomorphic, often bizarre astrocytes with occasional xanthomatous change; EGBs are typical (Fig. 6.22a). The tumor has a relatively favorable prognosis (81% 5-year overall survival) with many cases curable by surgery alone (WHO grade II), but 15% to 20% undergo malignant transformation and patients may die of the disease. Anaplastic PXA (WHO grade III) shows brisk mitotic activity (5 or more mitoses per 10 HPF) and often a "diffuse astrocytoma-like" appearance. PXAs have been shown to harbor the highest frequency of *BRAF* V600E missense mutations within CNS tumors (up two-thirds of cases) that can be detected by immunohistochemistry (BRAF VE 1 antibody staining). The standard treatment of PXAs is surgical excision, but cases harboring *BRAF* V600E mutations may benefit with the use of *BRAF* inhibitors (i.e., vemurafenib).

Cytologic Features

This tumor is less aggressive than its cytomorphologic features would suggest. The characteristic reticulin-glial matrix makes the tissue somewhat difficult to smear. Thus, preparations often show cohesive tissue fragments of markedly pleomorphic cells – gemistocyte-like, spindle, epithelioid, and giant bizarre – with long processes and worrisome, even grotesque, nuclear abnormalities. Hyperchromatism is typical, whereas nuclear pseudoinclusions are often present. Large xanthomatous cells with foamy, lipid filled cytoplasm and globular EGBs are two helpful diagnostic features when present. Lipid droplets may also be seen in the background if a Romanowsky-type stain is utilized. Necrotic debris, significant mitotic activity, and microvascular endothelial proliferation are not common (Fig. 6.22b, c).

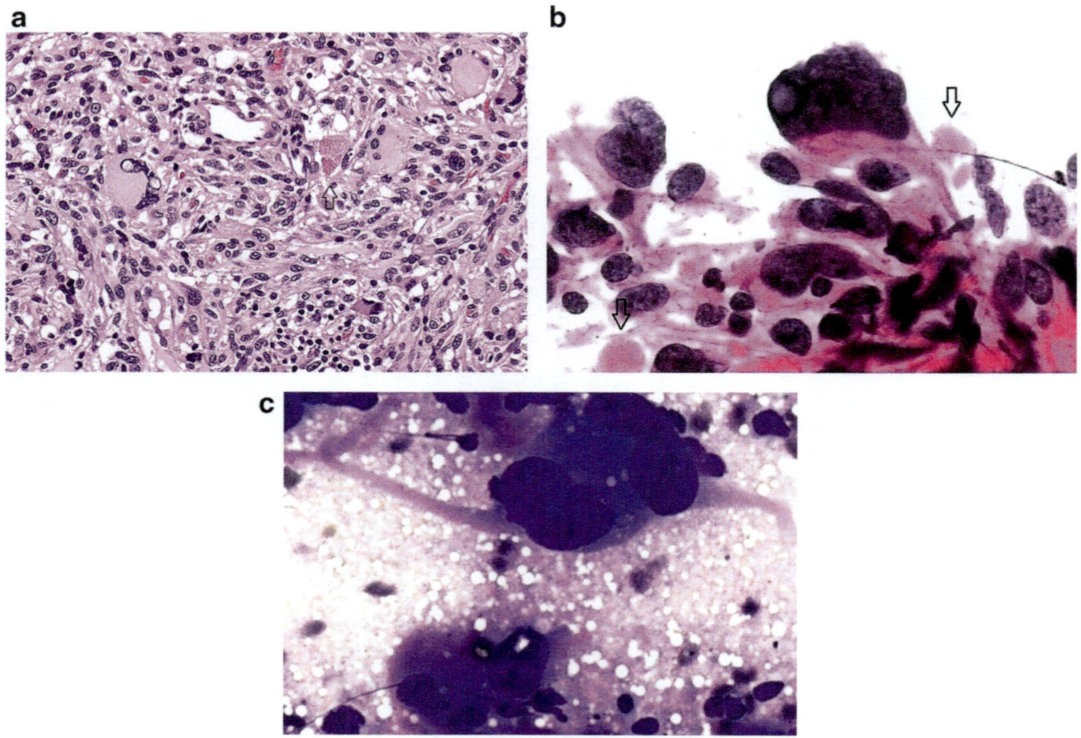

Fig. 6.22 *Pleomorphic xanthoastrocytoma*. (**a**) Histology. Pleomorphism with multinucleated giant cell formation, spindled cells, xanthic astrocytes, perivascular lymphocytic cuffing and eosinophilic granular bodies (*arrow*) characterize this tumor. (**b**) Cellular diversity is the rule in smears. These pleomorphic astrocytic cells exhibit coarse processes and hyperchromatic nuclei. Also note eosinophilic granular bodies (*arrows*; Smear, H&E). (**c**) Pleomorphic multinucleated cells with small cytoplasmic lipidic vacuoles. The background also shows numerous lipid droplets (Smear, Romanowsky)

Table 6.6 Characteristics of pleomorphic xanthoastrocytoma

Cytologic features
Fibrillary tissue fragments
Pleomorphic astrocytic cells with
Bizarre, hyperchromatic nuclei
Glial processes
Xanthomatous change
Fibrillary-lipoid background
Presence of EGBs
Differential diagnosis and pitfalls
Anaplastic astrocytoma
Glioblastoma (particularly giant cell type)
Gliosarcoma.
Pilocytic astrocytoma with degenerative-type atypia
Ganglioglioma

EGBs eosinophilic granular bodies

Differential Diagnosis Considerations

This pleomorphic tumor should be primarily differentiated from high-grade astrocytic tumors, including giant cell glioblastoma and gliosarcoma. The distinction should be based on the absence of necrosis, endothelial proliferation, and brisk mitotic activity, as well as the presence of EGBs and intra–/extracellular lipid droplets. Pilocytic astrocytoma shares several features with PXA (frequent macrocyst formation, presence of EGBs, and the possibility of atypias), but the predominant cellularity of these two tumors is very different – piloid and protoplasmic cells in pilocytic astrocytoma and pleomorphic and xanthomatous cells in PXA. There is also a significant clinical and radiologic overlap between PXA and ganglioglioma, but ganglioglioma is less pleomorphic and has an obvious neuronal component, whereas lipidized "foamy" cells are absent. PXA may be mixed with ganglioglioma in rare cases (Table 6.6).

Suggesting Reading

Ahluwalia CK, Chandrasoma PT. Cytomorphology of subependymal giant cell astrocytoma. A case report. Acta Cytol. 1993;37:197–200.

Altermatt HJ, Scheithauer BW. Cytomorphology of subependymal giant cell astrocytoma. Acta Cytol. 1992;36:171–5.

Bleggi-Torres LF, Gasparetto EL, Faoro LN, Hanel R, et al. Pleomorphic xanthoastrocytoma. Report of a case diagnosed by intraoperative cytophatological examination. Diagn Cytopathol. 2001;24:120–2.

Collins VP, Jones DT, Giannini C. Pilocytic astrocytoma: pathology, molecular mechanisms and markers. Acta Neuropathol. 2015;129:775–88.

Chan JA, Zhang H, Roberts PS, Jozwiak S, et al. Pathogenesis of tuberous sclerosis subependymal giant cell astrocytomas: biallelic inactivation of TSC1 or TSC2 leads to mTOR activation. J Neuropath Exp Neurol. 2004;63:1236–42.

Chen YH, Gutmann DH. The molecular and cell biology of pediatric low-grade gliomas. Oncogene. 2014;33:2019–26.

Chiang JCH, Ellison DW. Molecular pathology of paediatric central nervous system tumours. J Pathol. 2017;241:159–72.

Cloughesy TF, Cavenee WK, Mischel PS. Glioblastoma: from molecular pathology to targeted treatment. Annu Rev. Pathol. 2014;9:1–25.

Eckel-Passow JE, Lachance DH, Molinaro AM, Kyle M, et al. Glioma groups based on 1p/19q, *IDH*, and *TERT* promoter mutations in tumors. N Engl J Med. 2015;372:2499–508.

Finkle HI. Protoplasmic astrocytoma: Cytologic features on tissue imprint preparation. Diagn Cytopathol. 1992;8:430–1.

Franz DN, Agricola K, Mays M, Tudor C, et al. Everolimus for subependymal giant cell astrocytoma: 5-year final analysis. Ann Neurol. 2015;78:929–38.

Gandolfi A, Tedeschi F, Brizzi R. Cytology of giant-cell glioblastoma. Acta Cytol. 1983;27:193–6.

Gielen GH, Gessi M, Hammes J, Kramm CM, Waha A, Pietsch T. H3F3A K27 M mutation in pediatric CNS tumors. A marker of diffuse high-grade astrocytoma. Am J Clin Pathol. 2013;139:345–9.

Hayashi T, Haba R, Kushida Y, Katsuki N, et al. Pilomyxoid astrocytoma of the pineal region: cytopathological features and differential diagnostic considerations by intraoperative smear preparation. Diagn Cytopathol. 2015;43:121–4.

Hawkins C, Walker E, Mohamed N, Zhang C, et al. *BRAF-KIAA1549* fusion predicts better clinical outcome in pediatric low-grade astrocytoma. Clin Cancer Res. 2011;17:4790–8.

Ida CM, Rodriguez FJ, Burger PC, Caron AA, et al. Pleomorphic xanthoastrocytoma: natural history and long-term follow-up. Brain Pathol. 2015;25:575–86.

Jaiswal S, Vij M, Jaiswal AK, Srivastava AK, Behari S. Squash cytology of subependymal giant cell astrocytoma: report of four cases with brief review of literature. Diagn Cytopathol. 2012;40:333–6.

Jiménez-Heffernan JA, Freih Fraih A, Álvarez F, Bárcena C, Corbacho C. Cytologic features of pleomorphic xanthoastrocytoma, WHO grade II. A comparative study with glioblastoma. Diagn Cytopathol. 2017;45:339–44.

Kim SH, Lee KG, Kim TS. Cytologic characteristics of subependymal giant cell astrocytoma in squash smears. Acta Cytol. 2007;51:375–9.

Kim YH, Nobusawa S, Mittelbronn M, Paulus W, et al. Molecular classification of low-grade diffuse gliomas. Am J Pathol. 2010;177:2708–14.

Kobayashi S. Meningioma, neurilemmoma and astrocytoma specimens obtained with the squash method for diagnosis. Acta Cytol. 1993;37:913–2.

Kobayashi S, Hirakawa E, Haba R. Squash cytology of pleomorphic xanthoastrocytoma mimicking glioblastoma. Acta Cytol. 1999;43:652–8.

Korshunov A, Meyer J, Capper D, Christians A, et al. Combined molecular analysis of BRAF and IDH1 distinguishes pilocytic astrocytoma from diffuse astrocytoma. Acta Neuropath. 2009;118:401–5.

Parwani AV, Berman D, Burger PC, Ali SZ. Gliosarcoma: cytopathologic characteristics on fine-needle aspiration and intraoperative touch imprint. Diagn Cytopathol. 2004;30:77–81.

Prayson RA, Estes ML. Protoplasmic astrocytoma: A clinicopathologic study of 16 tumors. Am J Clin Pathol. 1995;103:705–9.

Rodriguez FJ, Scheithauer BW, Burger PC, Giannini C. Anaplasia in pilocytic astrocytoma predicts aggressive behavior. Am J Surg Pathol. 2010;34:147–60.

Roth J, Roach ES, Bartels U, Józwiak S, et al. Subependymal giant cell astrocytoma: diagnosis, screening, and treatment. Recommendations from the international tuberous sclerosis complex consensus conference 2012. Pediatric Neurol. 2013;49:439–44.

Schindler G, Capper D, Meyer J, Janzarik W, et al. Analysis of BRAF V600E mutation in 1320 nervous system tumors reveals high mutation frequencies in pleomorphic xanthoastrocytoma, ganglioglioma and extra-cerebellar pilocytic astrocytoma. Acta Neuropathol. 2011;121:397–405.

Schwartzentruber J, Korshunov A, Liu XY, Jones DT, et al. Driver mutations in histone H3.3 and chromatin remodelling genes in paediatric glioblastoma. Nature. 2012;482:226–31.

Solomon DA, Wood MD, Tihan T, Bollen AW, Gupta W, Phillips JJ, Perry A. Diffuse midline gliomas with histone H3-K27 M mutation: A series of 47 cases assessing the spectrum of morphologic variation and associated genetic alterations. Brain Pathology. 2016;26:569–80.

Takei H, Florez L, Bhattacharjee MB. Cytologic features of subependymal giant cell astrocytoma. A review of 7 cases. Acta Cytol. 2008;52:445–50.

Teo JG, Ng HK. Cytodiagnosis of pilocytic astrocytoma in smear preparations. Acta Cytol. 1998;42:673–8.

Venneti S, Santi M, Felicella MM, Yarilin D, et al. A sensitive and specific histopathologic prognostic marker for *H3F3A* K27 M mutant pediatric glioblastomas. Acta Neuropathol. 2014;128:743–53.

Watanabe T, Nobusawa S, Kleihues P, Ohgaki H. IDH1 mutations are early events in the development of astrocytomas and oligodendrogliomas. Am J Pathol. 2009;174:1149–53.

Weller M, Stupp R, Reifenberger G, Brandes AA, et al. MGMT promoter methylation in malignant gliomas: ready for personalized medicine? Nat Rev. Neurol. 2010;6:39–51.

Wu G, Diaz AK, Paugh BS, et al. The genomic landscape of diffuse intrinsic pontine glioma and pediatric non-brainstem high-grade glioma. Nature Genet. 2014;46:444–50.

Yan H, Parsons DW, Jin G, McLendon R, et al. IDH1 and IDH2 mutations in gliomas. N Engl J Med. 2009;360:765–73.

Yue X, Liu X, Lo S. Diagnosis of astrocytomas in crush preparations. Acta Cytol. 1987;31:83–4.

Chapter 7
Oligodendroglial Tumors

Oligodendroglioma represents the second major category of diffuse gliomas, accounting for 3–4% of all primary brain tumors and approximately 8% of all gliomas. It is a tumor characteristic of young to middle-age adults, with a peak incidence in the 30s and 40s, and is distinctly uncommon in children. These tumors may arise anywhere in the CNS, but most develop in the cerebral hemispheres where they affect the cortex and the subcortical white matter. Their incidence is proportional to the volume of white matter in the region; therefore, the lobe most frequently affected is the frontal lobe, followed by the temporal and parietal lobes, whereas they are rarely found in an occipital or deep location with involvement of the corpus callosum. Brainstem, cerebellum, and spinal cord examples are distinctly unusual.

Clinically, they are slowly progressing neoplasms, with intervals not infrequently of more than 5 years between the onset of symptoms and diagnosis in older studies (before modern neuroimaging). These symptoms include seizures (because of notable corticotropism), headache, focal neurologic deficits, and mental or cognitive disturbances. On scans, they usually appear as well-demarcated, non-enhancing lesions located in the cortex and the subcortical white matter. Conspicuous enhancement and prominent vasogenic edema usually indicate anaplastic change. Calcification is a frequent finding best appreciated on CT and occasionally produces a very characteristic expanded cortical wavy ribbon, the so-called gyriform calcification.

Macroscopically, these tumors are relatively well-defined, soft, pink-grayish masses but with broad zones of infiltration that are not visible to the naked eye. In cases with extensive mucoid degeneration, the tumor may appear gelatinous, whereas the frequent microcalcifications may give it a gritty texture.

There are two WHO histologic grades of oligodendroglioma that have a significant predictor of survival: grade II or well-differentiated tumors and grade III or anaplastic oligodendroglioma.

C. R. Lacruz et al., *Central Nervous System Intraoperative Cytopathology*,
Essentials in Cytopathology 13, https://doi.org/10.1007/978-3-319-98491-9_7

The microscopic image of *WHO grade II oligodendroglioma* is characteristic, consisting of monomorphic cells with round nuclei, perinuclear halos, and a peculiar back-to-back cell disposition that give it a "honeycomb" appearance. The vessels are of the capillary type and form a rich branching network reminiscent of "chicken wire." Though helpful in diagnosis, the characteristic halo (fried egg appearance) is a formalin fixation artifact that is not encountered in rapidly fixed specimens. A small number of cases present a variable image with some cells displaying small bellies of pink cytoplasm (minigemistocytes) (Fig. 7.1a, b).

Anaplastic oligodendroglioma (*WHO grade III*) displays significant mitotic activity, hypercellularity, and microvascular proliferation. Additionally, the anaplastic variant commonly has a more epithelioid cytology with increased cytoplasm, sharper cytoplasmic borders, and prominent nucleoli (Fig. 7.2a, b).

Currently, the diagnosis of oligodendroglioma including anaplastic oligodendroglioma requires the demonstration of both an IDH gene family mutation (the vast majority of oligodendrogliomas are immunoreactive for anti-IDH1 R132H protein) and combined whole arm losses of 1p and 19q (1p/19q codeletion). These 1p and 19q allelic losses are associated with increased response to chemotherapy (e.g., PCV) and with longer survival, regardless of therapy. 1p/19q codeletions and *ATRX/TP53* mutations are relatively exclusive of one another, supporting the argument of two separate lineages of diffuse gliomas that can be identified on a molecular basis to supplement histological diagnosis. In this regard, all infiltrating gliomas should be tested for IDH mutations and 1p/19q codeletion. It is worth noting that there are tumors in the pediatric population histologically similar to adult oligodendrogliomas without the above molecular changes (pediatric-type oligodendroglioma).

Average survival times are 10–15 years for grade II and 5–8 years for grade III. The patient age also is a powerful predictor, with survival inversely proportional to patient age.

Cytologic Features

Frozen sections of oligodendroglioma almost invariably produce misleading cytoplasmic and nuclear artifacts, supporting the fact that cytological technique is preferable for intraoperative consultation. Specimens tend to smear out easily into a sheet of uniform single cells without adhering to blood vessels. In contrast to the rest of gliomas, the background is not fibrillary but finely granular/vacuolated and frequently metachromatic (mucoid) with Romanowsky stains. The characteristic delicate branching "chicken-wire" capillary network is a useful feature preserved in smears (Fig. 7.3a–c). Nuclear morphology is a key microscopic feature – nuclei are uniformly round with a crisp nuclear membrane, delicate "salt-and-pepper" chromatin, and small nucleoli. On the other hand, the cytoplasm is ill-defined and wispy with few glial processes (oligo = few), being the artifactual perinuclear halo seen neither in smear preparations nor in well-fixed specimens. Microcalcifications are observed in a significant number of cases and are more significantly associated with

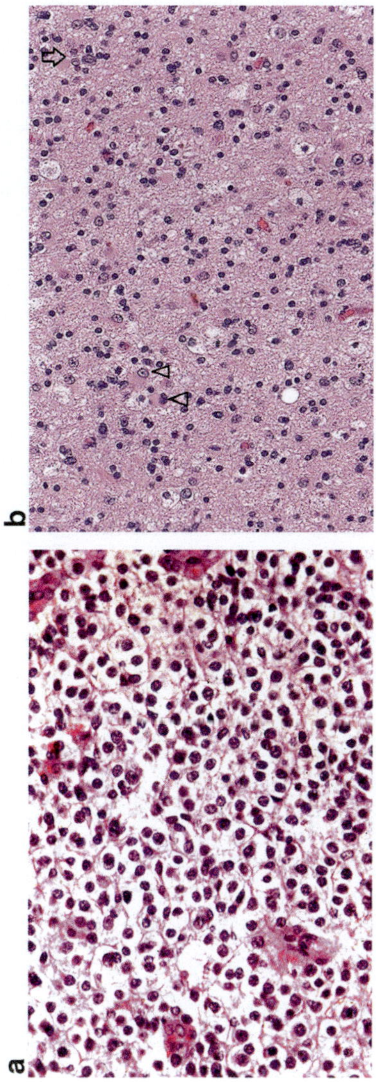

Fig. 7.1 *Oligodendroglioma, histologic features.* (**a**) Delayed formalin-fixed specimen with the characteristic perinuclear halos giving a honeycomb appearance. (**b**) Promptly fixed specimen without the artifactual perinuclear halos. Also note perineuronal satellitosis (*arrow*) and minigemistocytes (*arrowheads*)

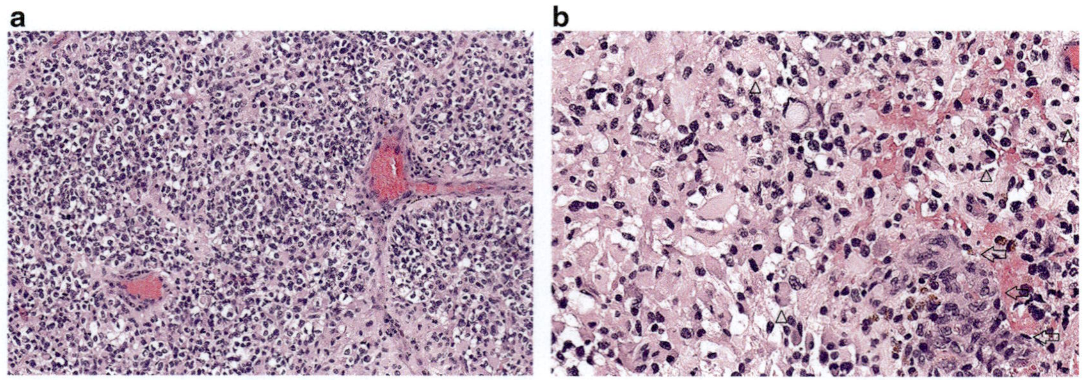

Fig. 7.2 *Anaplastic oligodendroglioma, histologic features*. (**a**) WHO grade III oligodendroglioma can be diagnosed when high cellularity, nuclear pleomorphism, mitosis, and vascular proliferation are observed. Also note artifactual perinuclear halos. (**b**) A high-power view displays microvascular proliferation (*arrows*), minigemistocytes (*arrowheads*), and epithelioid cell morphology. Vascular proliferation is often more linear than the classic "glomeruloid" masses seen in glioblastoma

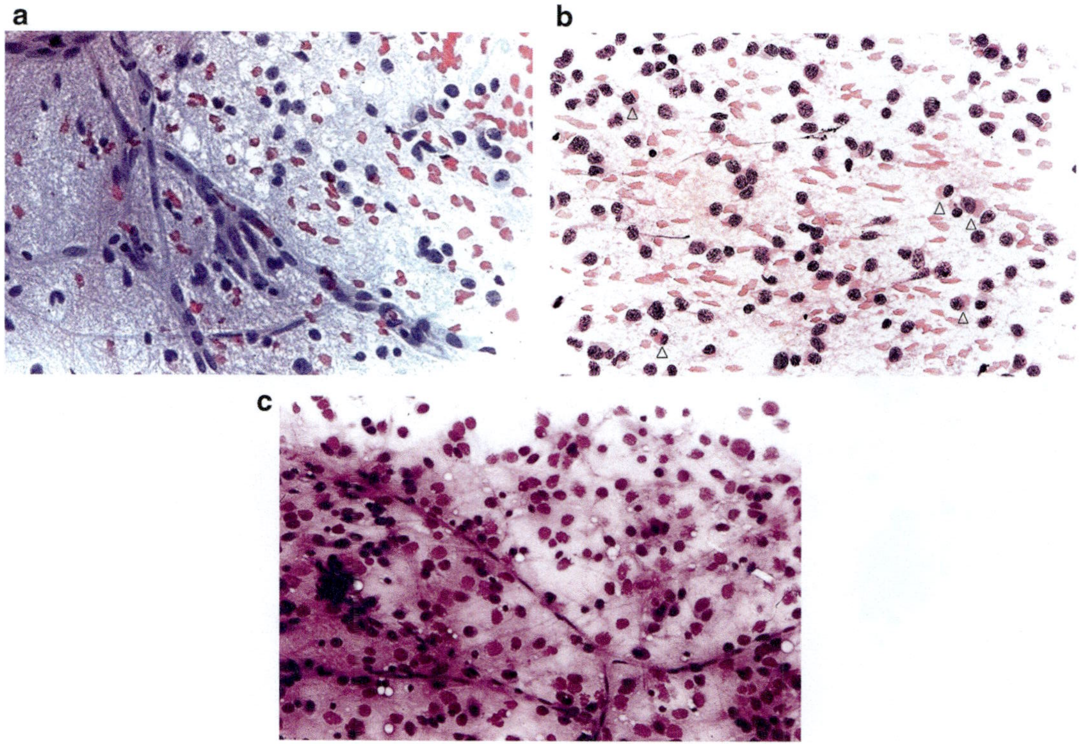

Fig. 7.3 *Oligodendroglioma*. (**a**) Uniform population of small, round cells without perinuclear halos. The background is not fibrillary, but finely granular with slim capillaries and tiny vacuoles (Smear, Papanicolaou). (**b**) Characteristic uniform population of single round nuclei in a clear (no fibrillary) background; some cells display small bellies of pink cytoplasm (*arrowheads*). Also note focal karyomegaly (Smear, H&E). (**c**) This preparation shows mucoid metachromatic background and a "chicken-wire" capillary network (Smear, Romanowsky)

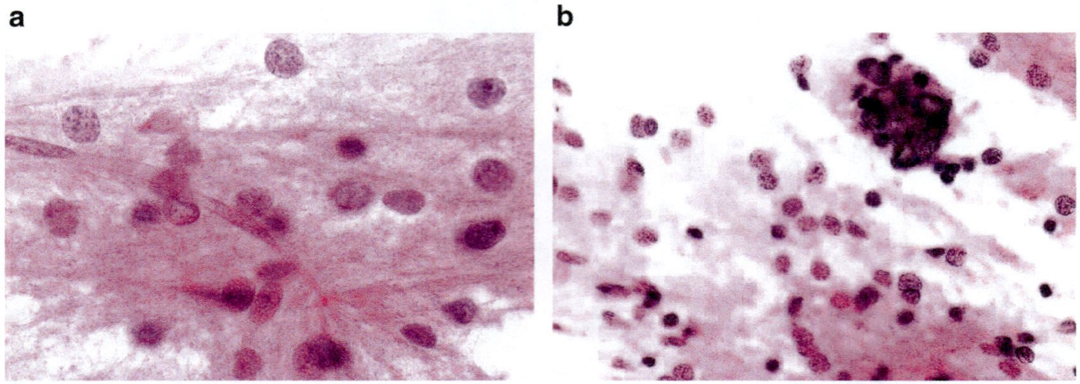

Fig. 7.4 *Oligodendroglioma.* (**a**) Round nuclei with stippled chromatin and small nucleoli in a feltlike (no fibrillary) background with slim capillaries are key features of oligodendroglioma. (**b**) Background microcalcifications also are a frequent finding. Artifactual perinuclear halos are seen neither in smears nor in well-fixed specimens (**a**, **b**; Smears, H&E)

oligodendrogliomas than with other gliomas (Fig. 7.4a, b). Occasionally, it is possible to find, on the same smear, cellular areas with atypical astrocytes together with oligodendroglioma cells as described above, but a diagnosis of *oligoastrocytoma* is strongly discouraged (should only be rendered in the very rare instance of a dual genotype oligoastrocytoma with molecular testing). Moreover, this finding is irrelevant during an intraoperative consultation, since it is sufficient to determine that the pathologic process is a "diffuse glioma" and state that an adequate amount of tissue has been obtained for marker studies that will permit a definitive subclassification. *Anaplastic oligodendroglioma* preserves the general appearance described here but with increased cellularity and pleomorphism (Fig. 7.5a). Nuclei are coarser than they are in grade II counterparts, with accentuated lobulation and mitotic activity (Fig. 7.5b). Within the cellular pleomorphism, multinucleated giant cells (polymorphic variant of Zülch), minigemistocytes, and epithelioid features can be seen. Minigemistocytes have no prognostic significance, but tend to be particularly numerous in these high-grade lesions, displaying small bellies of pink cytoplasm and eccentric nuclei. On their part, tumor cells with epithelioid features have conspicuous eosinophilic cytoplasm with sharper borders and prominent nucleoli (Fig. 7.5c).

Differential Diagnosis Considerations

Since rounded nuclei may be seen in many entities, the differential diagnosis for oligodendroglioma is long. Therefore, we should consider small-cell glial tumors (diffuse astrocytoma, subependymoma), round cell non-glial tumors (dysembryoplastic neuroepithelial tumor, pituitary adenoma, neurocytoma, pineocytoma, lymphoma), and nonneoplastic processes (demyelinating disorders, evolving infarcts). Diffuse astrocytoma shows a dense fibrillary background that is missing in oligodendroglioma. However, given the fact that this distinction is irrelevant during surgery, a prudent pathologist should identify the tumor only as a "diffuse glioma" in either case. A more relevant consideration is the differentiation from subependymoma (WHO grade I tumor), but this neoplasia shows a characteristic prominent fibrillary background that, as we have mentioned, is missing in oligodendroglioma. Dysembryoplastic neuroepithelial tumor (DNT), pituitary adenoma, pineocytoma, and neurocytoma may exhibit a cytologic picture that is practically identical to that of oligodendroglioma. Particularly, on small biopsy specimens, DNT may be indistinguishable from oligodendroglioma (a clue suggesting DNT is the absence of any appreciable cytologic atypia). Pituitary adenoma is easily distinguishable by their location, even if some oligodendrogliomas do extend into the hypothalamic region and aggressive pituitary tumors may extend beyond the sella turcica; therefore, this potential source of error should be kept in mind. In the case of neurocytoma and pineocytoma, the fine neuropil background and the presence of the neurocytic/pineocytomatous rosettes help in distinguishing it. With respect to lymphoid neoplasms, the characteristic finely granular nuclear pattern of oligodendroglioma contrasts with the nuclear features of most CNS lymphomas. Concerning nonneoplastic

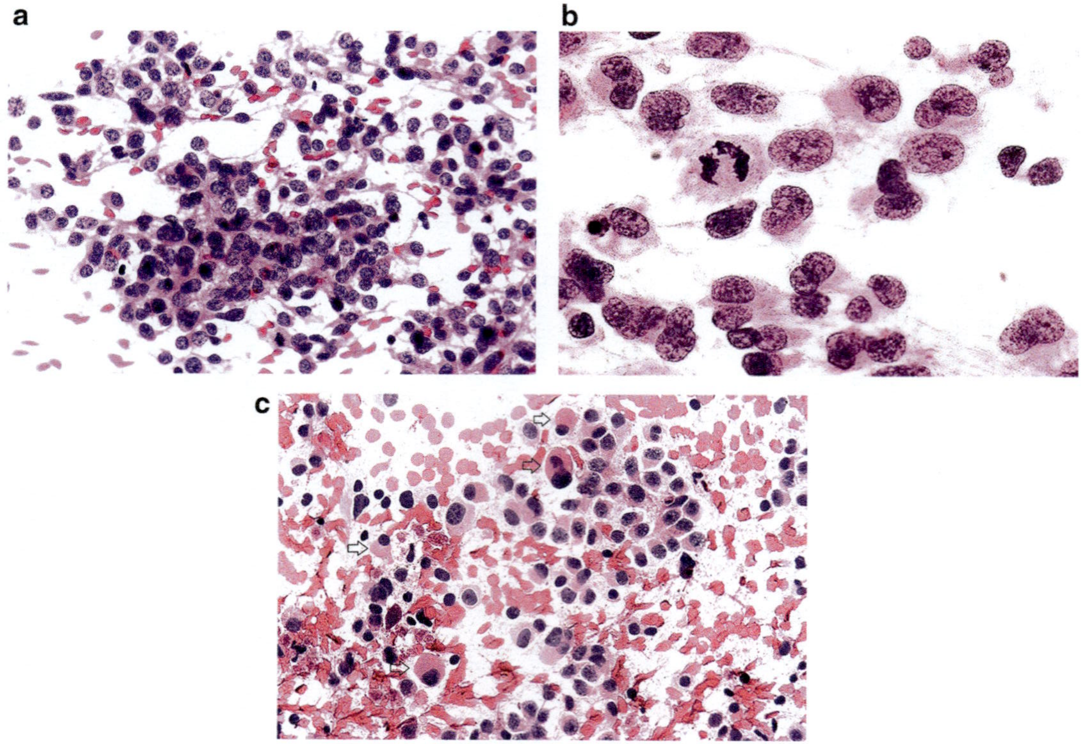

Fig. 7.5 *Anaplastic oligodendroglioma, cytologic features*. Increased cellular density with coarse chromatin and nuclear atypia (**a**), mitotic figures (**b**), and cellular pleomorphism including minigemistocytes (*arrows*) and epithelioid features (**c**) are characteristic attributes of anaplastic oligodendroglioma in cytologic preparations (**a–c**; Smears, H&E)

disorders, oligodendroglioma needs to be distinguished from macrophage-rich processes, such as demyelinating lesions or evolving infarcts, but, in smears, macrophages display abundant foamy cytoplasm and distinct cytoplasmic borders that are missing in oligodendroglioma. *Anaplastic oligodendroglioma* may share cytologic features with anaplastic astrocytoma, glioblastoma, and metastatic carcinoma/melanoma. As we have seen, oligodendroglioma cells lack the characteristic cytoplasmic processes of anaplastic astrocytoma and most glioblastomas, but, in any event, an intraoperative report of "high-grade, diffuse glioma" is adequate for all these tumors, whereas in metastatic carcinoma/melanoma, we should look for the presence of cohesive cell groups and specific differentiation (keratin, neuroendocrine features, melanin, etc.), as well as the absence of minigemistocytes and other cytomorphologic features of oligodendroglioma elsewhere in smears (Table 7.1).

Table 7.1 Characteristics of oligodendroglioma

Cytologic features
Single cell pattern of uniform cells
Round nuclei with finely granular chromatin and small nucleoli
Ill-defined, wispy cytoplasm (no perinuclear halos)
Finely granular or mucoid (no fibrillary) background
Capillary branching network
Anaplastic oligodendroglioma
Increased cellularity and pleomorphism
Coarser chromatin
Prominent mitotic activity
Epithelioid features and minigemistocytes
Microvascular proliferation
Differential diagnosis and pitfalls
Diffuse astrocytoma
Subependymoma
Dysembryoplastic neuroepithelial tumor
Pituitary adenoma
Neurocytoma
Pineocytoma
Lymphoma
Macrophage-rich processes
Anaplastic oligodendroglioma
Anaplastic astrocytoma
Glioblastoma
Metastatic carcinoma/melanoma

Suggested Reading

Eckel-Passow JE, Lachance DH, Molinaro AM, Kyle M, et al. Glioma groups based on 1p/19q, *IDH*, and *TERT* promoter mutations in tumors. N Engl J Med. 2015;372:2499–508.

Goh SGN, Chuah KL. Role of intraoperative smear cytology in the diagnosis of anaplastic oligodendroglioma. Acta Cytol. 2003;47:293–8.

Kim YH, Nobusawa S, Mittelbronn M, Paulus W, et al. Molecular classification of low-grade diffuse gliomas. Am J Pathol. 2010;177:2708–14.

Klysik M, Gavito J, Boman D, Miranda RN, Hanbali F, De Las Casas LE. Intraoperative imprint cytology of central neurocytoma: The great oligodendroglioma mimicker. Diagn Cytopathol. 2010;38:202–7.

Koeller KK, Rushing EJ. From the archives of the AFIP: Oligodendroglioma and its variants: radiologic-pathologic correlations. Radiographics. 2005;25:1669–88.

Kreiger PA, Okada Y, Simon S, Rorke LB, Louis DN, Golden JA. Losses of chromosomes 1p and 19q are rare in pediatric oligodendrogliomas. Acta Neuropathol (Berl). 2005;109:387–92.

Mitsuhashi T, Shimizu Y, Ban S, Ogawa F, Matsutani M, Shimizu M, Hirose T. Anaplastic oligodendroglioma. A case report with characteristic cytologic features including minigemistocytes. Acta Cytol. 2007;51:657–60.

Monabati A, Kumar PV, Roozbehi H, Torabinezhad S. Cytologic findings in metastatic oligodendroglioma. Acta Cytol. 2003;47:702–4.

Nguyen GK, Jonson ES, Mielke BW. Comparative cytomorphology of pituitary adenomas and oligodendrogliomas in intraoperative crush preparations. Acta Cytol. 1992;36:661–7.

Park J-Y, Suh Y-L, Han J. Disembryoplastic neuroepithelial tumor. Features distinguishing it from oligodendroglioma on cytologic squash preparations. Acta Cytol. 2003;47:624–9.

Sahm F, Reuss D, Koelsche C, Capper D, et al. Farewell to oligoastrocytoma: in situ molecular genetics favor classification as either oligodendroglioma or astrocytoma. Acta Neuropath. 2014;128:551–9.

Watanabe T, Nobusawa S, Kleihues P, Ohgaki H. IDH1 mutations are early events in the development of astrocytomas and oligodendrogliomas. Am J Pathol. 2009;174:1149–53.

Wesseling P, van den Bent M, Perry A. Oligodendroglioma: pathology, molecular mechanisms and markers. Acta Neuropathol. 2015;129:809–27.

Yan H, Parsons DW, Jin G, McLendon R, et al. IDH1 and IDH2 mutations in gliomas. N Engl J Med. 2009;360:765–73.

Chapter 8
Ependymal Tumors

Ependymal tumors are considered to originate from radial glial-like stem cells or precursors thereof lining the wall of the ventricles or the wall of the spinal canal, which is why they can occur along the entire neuroaxis. Ependymoma and its variants account for 5–9% of all primary brain tumors in adults, 6–12% in children, and 30% in infants, being the third most common pediatric CNS tumor. Thought most are sporadic, they may also be seen as a part of *neurofibromatosis type 2*, nearly all of which are spinal and tend to present with multiple masses.

Ependymal tumors are traditionally divided into four histologic types, ependymoma, anaplastic ependymoma, subependymoma, and myxopapillary ependymoma, which correspond to different grades of malignancy. *Ependymoma* corresponds to WHO grade II, and *anaplastic ependymoma* corresponds to WHO grade III, whereas *subependymoma* and *myxopapillary ependymoma* are slowly growing neoplasms and correspond to WHO grade I. However, no association between histological grade and biological behavior or survival has been definitively established. Moreover, given that specific genetic alterations and molecular groups have recently been proposed as prognostic/predictive factors, the practice of histologically grading ependymoma may soon become obsolete altogether (Table 8.1).

Two molecular groups, ST-EPN-*RELA* and PF-EPN-A (together comprising two-third of all cases), have the worst outcome. In contrast, patients in the other subgroups have an excellent prognosis with 5-year overall survival rates close to 100%. ST-EPN-*RELA* accounts for 70% of pediatric supratentorial ependymomas and is characterized by the *C11orf95-RELA* fusion gene (testing may be performed by PCR or FISH for break-apart probes). PF-EPN-A is characterized by a balanced genome with the CpG island methylator phenotype (CIMP) and primarily occurs in infants and young children. In general, ependymomas in children fare far worse.

C. R. Lacruz et al., *Central Nervous System Intraoperative Cytopathology*, Essentials in Cytopathology 13, https://doi.org/10.1007/978-3-319-98491-9_8

Table 8.1 Key characteristics of nine molecular subgroups of ependymoma

Group	Genetic characteristic	Dominant histology	Age at presentation	Outcome
ST-EPN-*RELA*	*RELA* fusion gene	CL/AN	All age groups	Poor
ST-EPN-*YAP1*	*YAP1* fusion gene	CL/AN	Infants/children	Good
ST-SE	Balanced genome	SE	Adults	Good
PF-EPN-A	Balanced genome	CL/AN	Infants	Poor
PF-EPN-B	Wide polyploidy	CL/AN	Children/adults	Good
PF-SE	Balanced genome	SE	Adults	Good
SP-EPN	*NF2* mutation	CL/AN	Children/adults	Good
SP-MPE	Wide polyploidy	MPE	Adults	Good
SP-SE	6q deletion	SE	Adults	Good

Based on data from: Pajtler KW, et al. *Cancer Cell.* 2015;27:728–43
ST supratentorial, *PF* posterior fossa, *SP* spinal, *EPN* ependymoma, *SE* subependymoma, *MPE* myxopapillary ependymoma, *CL/AN* classic/anaplastic

Ependymoma

There is a clear correlation among the locations of ependymomas, the age of the patient, and symptomatology. Thus, *ependymoma of the fourth ventricle* (about 60%) predominates in the pediatric age and may present with hydrocephalus, symptoms of increased intracranial pressure, and cerebellar ataxia; *those in the spinal cord* (about 10%) have a peak incidence between 40 and 50 years of age, usually arise within cervicothoracic segments, and present with neck/back pain, numbness and paresthesias of the distal extremities, and atrophy of hand musculature, whereas *supratentorial ependymomas* (approx. 30%) affect pediatric as well as adult patients and may present with seizures, focal neurologic deficits, and symptoms of intracranial hypertension. In neuroimaging, ependymomas most often appear as well-circumscribed, variably enhancing, intraventricular masses that partially or completely fill the ventricle. Parenchymal masses are usually discrete and tend to abut or at least extend to a ventricle; however, tumors with no apparent ventricular relationship do occur occasionally. Spinal examples are intraaxial, sausage-shaped lesions. Cystic change and *syrinx* (a cavitated, gliotic-lined defect) are common in supratentorial and spinal locations, respectively.

Macroscopically, they are soft, tan to cherry-red masses with well-demarcated "placenta-like" borders, which facilitate their complete resection. (See Chap. 3, Fig. 3.1b) Tumors arising in the caudal fourth ventricle often flow through the foramina of Luschka and Magendie to grow into the cerebellopontine cistern surrounding the brainstem, as well as down through the foramen magnum – like a "tongue" of tumor – into the upper cervical spine (*plastic ependymomas*).

Histologically, *classic ependymoma* is a tumor composed of monomorphic glial cells with a round to oval nuclei arranged against a fibrillary background. Key histologic features are perivascular pseudorosettes and ependymal rosettes (Fig. 8.1a–c).

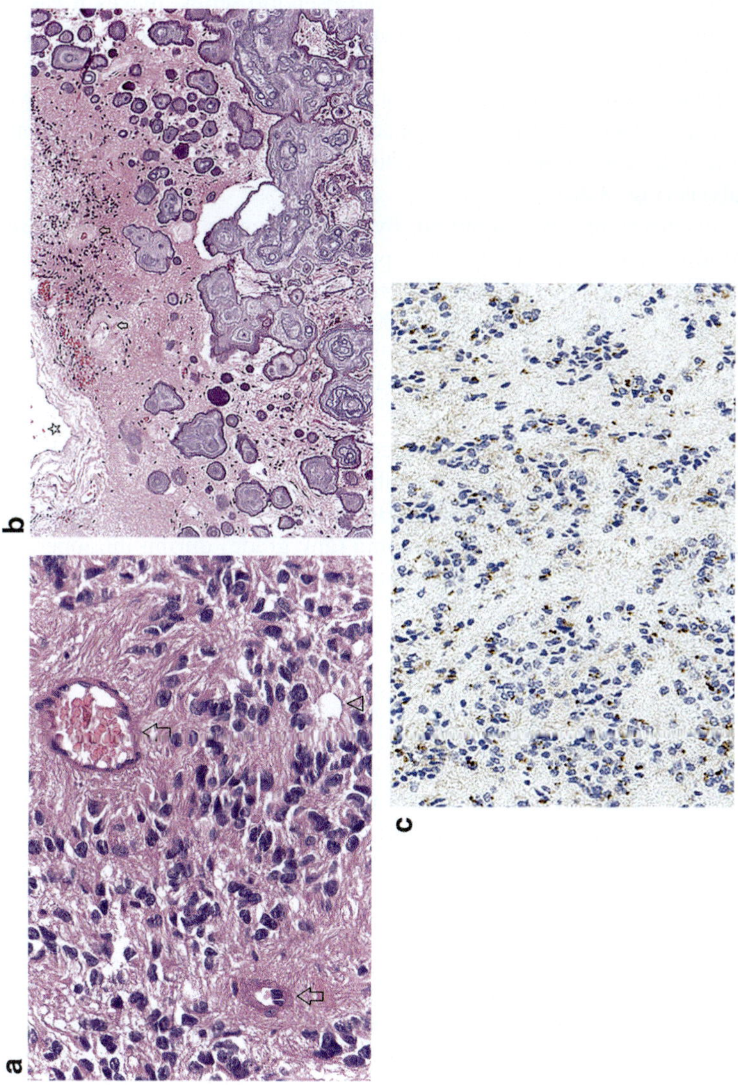

Fig. 8.1 *Classic ependymoma WHO grade II*. (**a**) Typical histologic features include small glial cells, perivascular pseudorosettes (*arrows*), and true, lumen-containing rosettes (*arrowhead*). (**b**) This example is heavily calcified indicating chronicity. Note some perivascular pseudorosettes at the periphery (*arrows*) near the ventricular lumen (*star*). (**c**) An epithelial membrane antigen (EMA) immunostain demonstrates a dot-like pattern of cytoplasmic positivity consistent with ependymoma

Papillary ependymoma, an uncommon variant, shows a predominance of epithelioid cells lining papillae, ependymal channels, and fingerlike projections, which may be confused with choroid plexus papilloma (Fig. 8.2a).

Tanycytic ependymoma consists of elongated spindle bipolar cells resembling tanycytes (from the Greek *tanyos*, meaning to stretch). This feature, together with the common absence of ependymal rosettes and pseudorosettes, makes it easy to confuse it with pilocytic astrocytoma or schwannoma. Most cases are located in the spinal cord (Fig. 8.2b).

Clear cell ependymoma is characterized by cells with clear, glycogen-rich cytoplasm (perinuclear halos) that mimic oligodendroglioma. Most often is supratentorial, cystic, in a child, and show prognostically unfavorable *RELA* gene fusion by molecular analysis (Fig. 8.2c).

Anaplastic ependymoma is diagnosed by the presence of hypercellularity, increased mitotic activity, and microvascular proliferation (Fig. 8.3).

With few exceptions, the *immunohistochemical staining pattern* shared by ependymal tumors is the expression of GFAP, S-100, and vimentin, whereas EMA often shows a characteristic punctuate, dot-like pattern of cytoplasmic positivity (Fig. 8.1c). L1CAM expression is evident in supratentorial ependymomas with the *C11orf95-RELA* fusion gene.

As previously noted, no association between histological grade and biological behavior or survival has been definitively established, being the extent of resection the dominant factor influencing the outcome. Because of this reason, the pathologist needs to consider the diagnosis of ependymoma (any grade) during intraoperative consultation, especially for tumors in ventricular, periventricular, and spinal locations.

Cytologic Features

Ependymomas are cellular tumors that smear in fibrillar tissue fragments, with discohesive sheets of relatively small and uniform cells. Just as in histology, perivascular pseudorosettes and ependymal rosettes are key diagnostic features. Perivascular pseudorosettes, with the characteristic fibrillary zone separating tumor cell nuclei from vessels walls, are responsible for the "arboreal" or "caterpillar" appearance seen in the smears of many cases. These tumor-coated vascular tubes are best preserved at the thicker, less traumatized end of the smear. Tumor cells typically have round to oval nuclei with granular "salt and pepper" chromatin, inconspicuous to small nucleoli, and long tapering processes (Fig. 8.4a, b). *Papillary ependymoma* has an epithelial appearance, with well-defined cytoplasmic borders and broad processes, but shares nuclear features with the more common classic variant. Tumor cells are usually arranged around multilayered papillary fronds and may be little fibrillar tissue (Fig. 8.5a). In *tanycytic ependymoma*, elongated, slender cells with polar glial processes and oval to elongated nuclei are predominant, whereas pseudorosettes may be absent (Fig. 8.5b). *Clear cell ependymoma* resembles classic

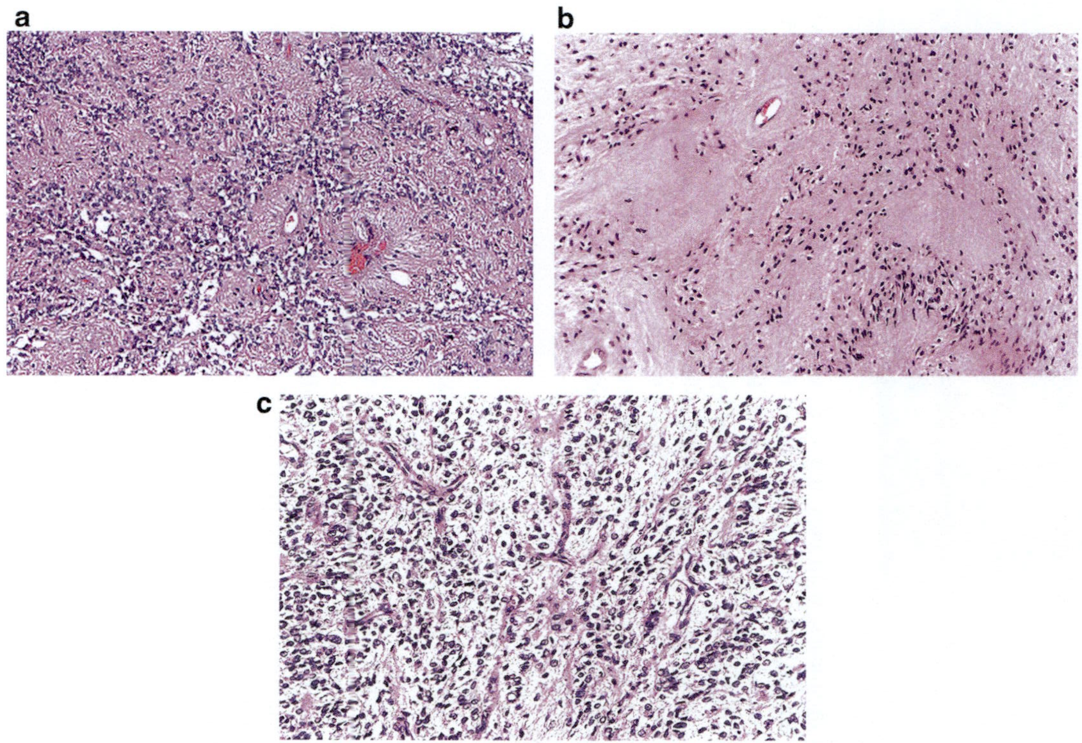

Fig. 8.2 *Ependymoma variants WHO grade II, histologic features*. (**a**) *Papillary ependymoma*. Papillary structures with gliofibrillary "stroma" characterize this variant. The tumor cells are epithelioid and display loss of cohesion between the perivascular aggregates. (**b**) *Tanycytic ependymoma*. A fascicular pattern of elongated spindle cells with less conspicuous pseudorosettes characterize this variant. (**c**) *Clear cell ependymoma*. This tissue section shows sheets of clear cells interrupted by branching "chicken-wire" capillaries resembling oligodendroglioma

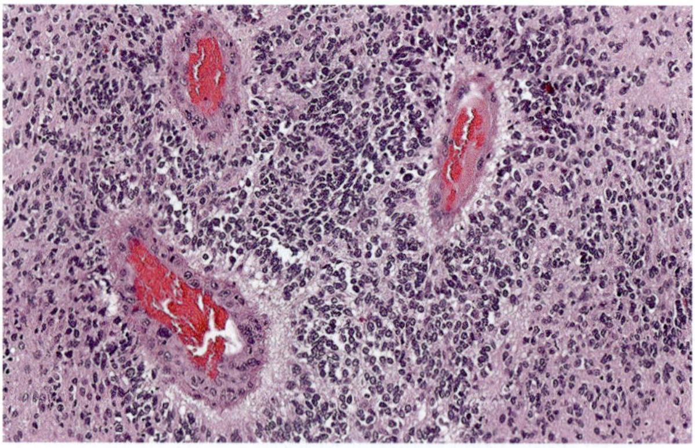

Fig. 8.3 *Anaplastic ependymoma WHO grade III*. (**a**) Increased cellularity, hyperchromatism, brisk mitotic activity, and vascular hyperplasia are characteristic histologic features

ependymoma in smears, with only few cells displaying clear or vacuolated cytoplasm. However, larger grooved and clefted nuclei are characteristic (Fig. 8.5c). *Anaplastic ependymoma* is somewhat similar to ependymoma but shows hypercellular smears with frequent mitosis, vascular hyperplasia, and, sometimes, necrosis. Nuclei are hyperchromatic and frequently clefted or grooved (Fig. 8.6a, b). In summary, it is the very nature of the ependymal cell that conditions the smear appearance of these tumors: on the one hand, their peculiar dual glial-epithelial properties and, on the other, their tendency to group together radially around a central lumen or vessel (Fig. 8.7).

Differential Diagnosis Considerations

The dual character of the ependymal cell gives rise to the paradoxical fact that in the differential diagnosis, both gliomas (particularly pilocytic astrocytoma) and some epithelial tumors, such as choroid plexus papilloma and metastatic papillary carcinoma, should be considered. The presence of specific cell groups (pseudorosettes and rosettes) makes it possible to differentiate it from other low-grade gliomas. An especially difficult case arises with tanycytic ependymoma, which may does not show these characteristics mimicking pilocytic astrocytoma. In this case, we should look for features of pilocytic astrocytoma such as RFs, EGBs, or protoplasmic cells. On their part, choroid plexus papilloma lacks the characteristic fibrillary background of ependymoma, whereas in its papillary structures, the tumor cells are arranged directly along the fibrovascular core, without an interposed fibrillary crown. With respect to papillary metastatic carcinoma, the cytologic benignity of ependymoma and the presence of fibrillary background are major differentiating features. In the case of *anaplastic ependymoma*, poorly differentiated examples may be difficult to identify as ependymal, making distinction from medulloblastoma or other embryonal tumors – particularly ependymoblastoma – challenging. A useful piece of information in differentiating them is that all these tumors are

a b

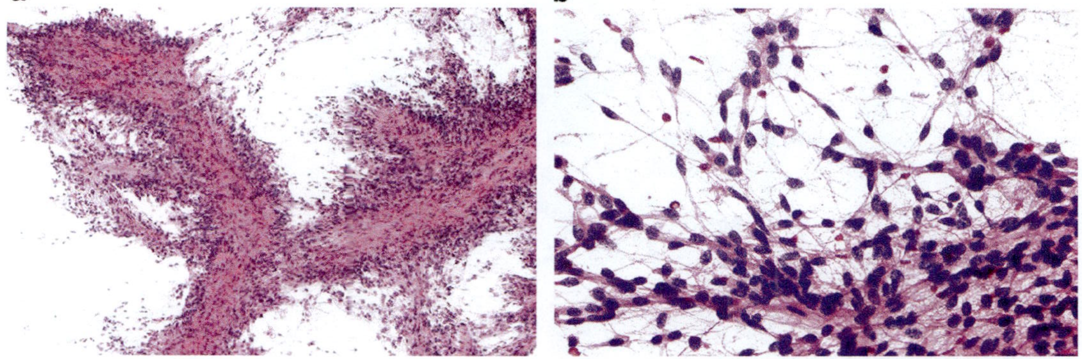

Fig. 8.4 *Classic ependymoma WHO grade II, cytologic features.* (**a**) The characteristic branching "arboreal" appearance of pseudorosettes can be seen well in smears. Tumor cells remain tethered to the vessel wall by their glial tails. (**b**) High-magnification view showing unevenly distributed glial cells in a fibrillary background. Nuclei are small, oval, and uniform (**a**, **b**; Smears, H&E)

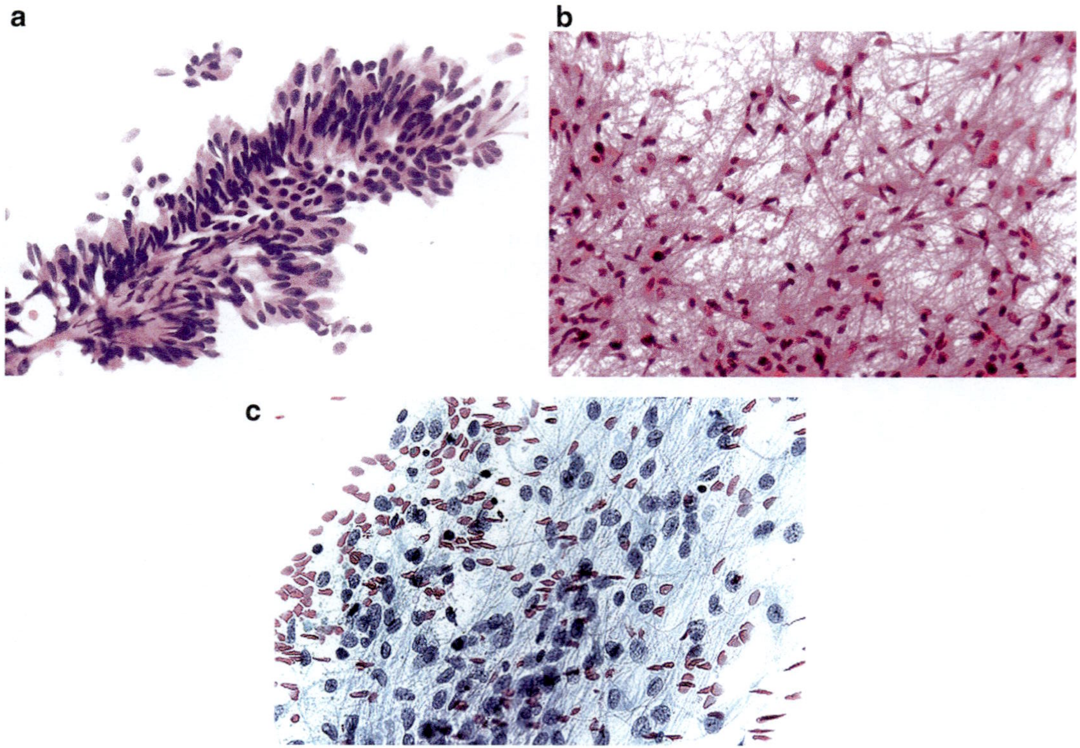

Fig. 8.5 *Ependymoma variants WHO grade II, cytologic features.* (**a**) Papillary ependymoma. Cytologic preparation displaying a papilla with elongated epithelioid cells that have ependymal nuclear features (Smear, H&E). (**b**) Tanycytic ependymoma. The tumor cells are typically spindle-shaped with bipolar or unipolar processes resembling pilocytic astrocytoma (Smear, H&E). (**c**) Clear cell ependymoma. In contrast to oligodendroglioma, this tumor displays characteristic ependymoma features, including ovoid nuclei and fibrillary background. Nuclei of clear cell ependymoma are often larger and more clefted and grooved than those of other variants (Smear, Papanicolaou)

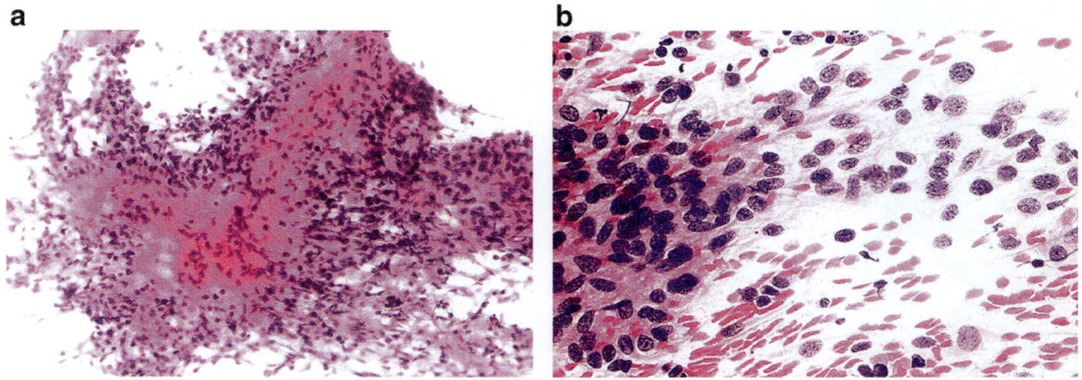

Fig. 8.6 *Anaplastic ependymoma WHO grade III, cytologic features*. (**a**) Crowded tissue fragment with small, hyperchromatic cells. Despite anaplasia, the ependymal cells tend to be arranged around a fibrillary core. (**b**) Nuclei in grade III ependymomas are typically darker and with more irregular contours than those of the grade II counterpart (**a**, **b**; Smears, H&E)

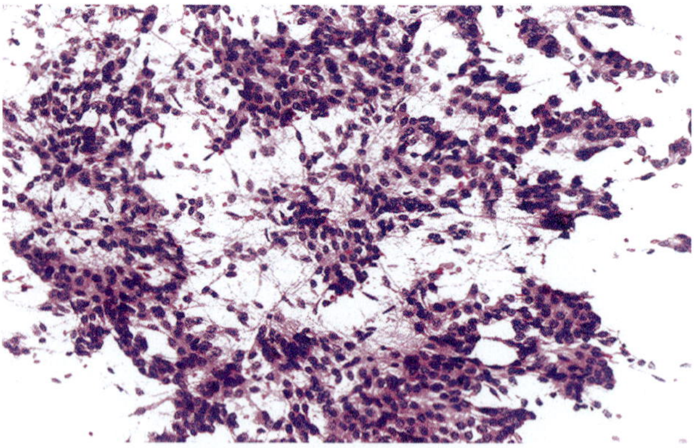

Fig. 8.7 *Ependymoma, dual cell morphology*. Not uncommonly distinct dual glial and epithelial cell populations can be seen in the same preparation. Note that both cell types share the same nuclear features (Smear, H&E)

Table 8.2 Characteristics of ependymoma

Cytologic features
Moderately cellular smears
Fibrillary background
Dual (glial-epithelial) cellular properties
Small oval nuclei with stippled chromatin
Key diagnostic clues
Perivascular pseudorosettes
Ependymal rosettes
Anaplastic ependymoma
Increased cellularity and coarser chromatin
Nuclear grooves and indentations
Mitotic figures and vascular hyperplasia
Useful features usually retained
Perivascular pseudorosettes
Fibrillary background
Differential diagnosis and pitfalls
Pilocytic astrocytoma
Diffuse astrocytoma
Papillary variant
Choroid plexus papilloma
Metastatic papillary carcinoma
Anaplastic ependymoma
Medulloblastoma
Other embryonal tumors

composed of undifferentiated cells with an embryonal (primitive) appearance, whereas conspicuous fibrillary background and perivascular pseudorosettes are lacking (Table 8.2).

Subependymoma

Subependymomas are slow-growing, benign tumors whose preferential location is attached to the wall of fourth (most commonly) or lateral ventricles, although some cases in the septum pellucidum and the spinal cord may be seen. These tumors occur more frequently (about 90%) in middle-age and elderly patients. Usually asymptomatic and incidentally detected, they may produce symptoms through the obstruction of CSF flow or undergo extensive intratumoral or subarachnoid hemorrhage. Radiologically, they are nonenhancing, nodular, and often calcified masses within the ventricles. Histologically, subependymomas are characterized by clusters of ependymal-like nuclei embedded in a dense fibrillary matrix. Microcystic degeneration is common, especially when near the foramen of Monro (Fig. 8.8a). Subependymomas can be cured by surgical excision but may recur if incompletely resected.

Cytologic Features

This neoplasia is difficult to smear because of its firm consistency. This assumes that touch smears are essentially acellular, whereas squash specimens often resist disaggregation and remain as tissue fragments. Under the microscope, they appear as dense fibrillary tissue fragments with clusters of ependymoma-like nuclei, which are arranged in a very similar manner to that observed in histology. Overall, the cellular density is less than in other ependymomas with patches of slightly cellular islands (Fig. 8.8b). In Romanowsky stained preparations, small mucinous blebs from the microcystic content may be observed within the fibrillary background (Fig. 8.8c). Occasionally, large pleomorphic nuclei may be encountered, particularly in multicystic tumors.

Differential Diagnosis Considerations

Due to its particular anatomic location, subependymoma should be differentiated from other ventricular-related tumors such as ependymoma, subependymal giant cell astrocytoma, central neurocytoma, and choroid plexus papilloma and, on the basis of its cytomorphology, from diffuse astrocytoma and oligodendroglioma. Detailed clinicoradiologic information and the characteristic cytologic picture described above readily distinguish subependymoma from these other tumors (Table 8.3).

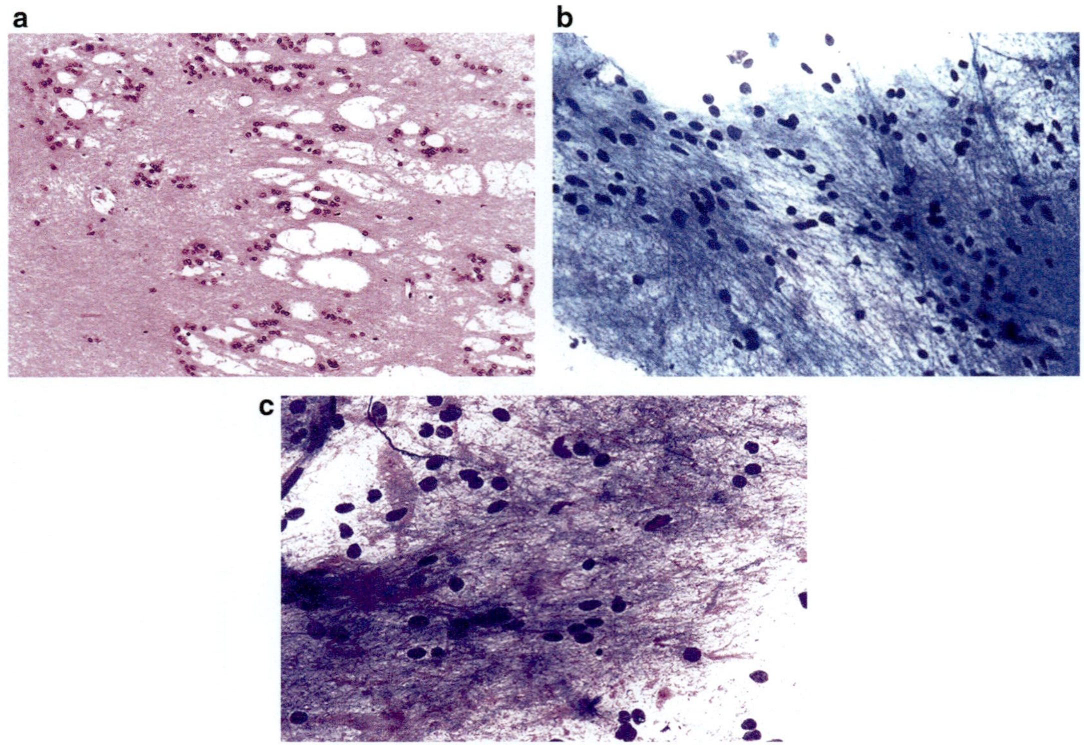

Fig. 8.8 *Subependymoma*. (**a**) Characteristic histologic features include dense fibrillary background, clustered small nuclei, and microcysts. (**b**) Also in cytologic preparations, subependymomas display a dense glial matrix mosaic having either patches of embedded cells or paucicellular fields with few cells (Smear, Papanicolaou). (**c**) This stain reveals metachromatic mucinous blebs from the microcystic content (Smear, Romanowsky)

Table 8.3 Characteristics of subependymoma

Cytologic features
Specimens difficult to smear
Dense fibrillary tissue fragments
Clustered ependymoma-like nuclei
Occasionally
Large, pleomorphic nuclei
Blebs of mucinous material
Differential diagnosis and pitfalls
Ependymoma
Central neurocytoma
Subependymal giant cell astrocytoma
Choroid plexus papilloma
Diffuse astrocytoma
Oligodendroglioma

Myxopapillary Ependymoma

Myxopapillary ependymoma is seen in young to middle-age adults and located almost exclusively in the distal regions of the spinal cord (conus medullaris, filum terminale, and cauda equina). Less frequently, tumors may arise in the upper levels of the spinal cord or may occur extradural, arising in the sacrum or subcutaneous tissues around the sacrococcyx. Clinically, they are associated with chronic low back pain, and scans usually show a sharply circumscribed, contrast-enhancing spinal mass. Grossly, they are soft, sometimes myxoid "bags" that may be invested by a fibrous pseudocapsule derived from the stroma of the filum. Myxopapillary ependymoma histology is characteristic, showing a radial arrangement of cuboidal to spindle glial cells around vascularized myxoid stromal cores or rounded microcysts (Fig. 8.9a). Gross total resection may be curative, but incomplete removal may cause local or widespread dissemination and, even, distant metastases. Therefore, rendering an intraoperative diagnosis of myxopapillary ependymoma is important, since the neurosurgeon should remove the tumor en bloc to prevent recurrence and dissemination.

Cytologic Features

This tumor usually yields highly cellular smears. Aggregates of epithelioid cells are arranged around vascularized stromal cores and globules of myxoid material. This myxoid material is barely discernible with H&E or Papanicolaou stains but is clearly revealed with an intense metachromatic color when Romanowsky-type stains are utilized. Tumor cells are loosely overlapped, displaying cuboidal to elongated appearance with occasional tapering processes and nuclear features of ependymal derivation, namely, ovoid nuclei with finely stippled chromatin and small nucleoli. Sometimes the cells are noticeably elongated and may show delicate processes, similar to tanycytic ependymoma (Fig. 8.9b, c).

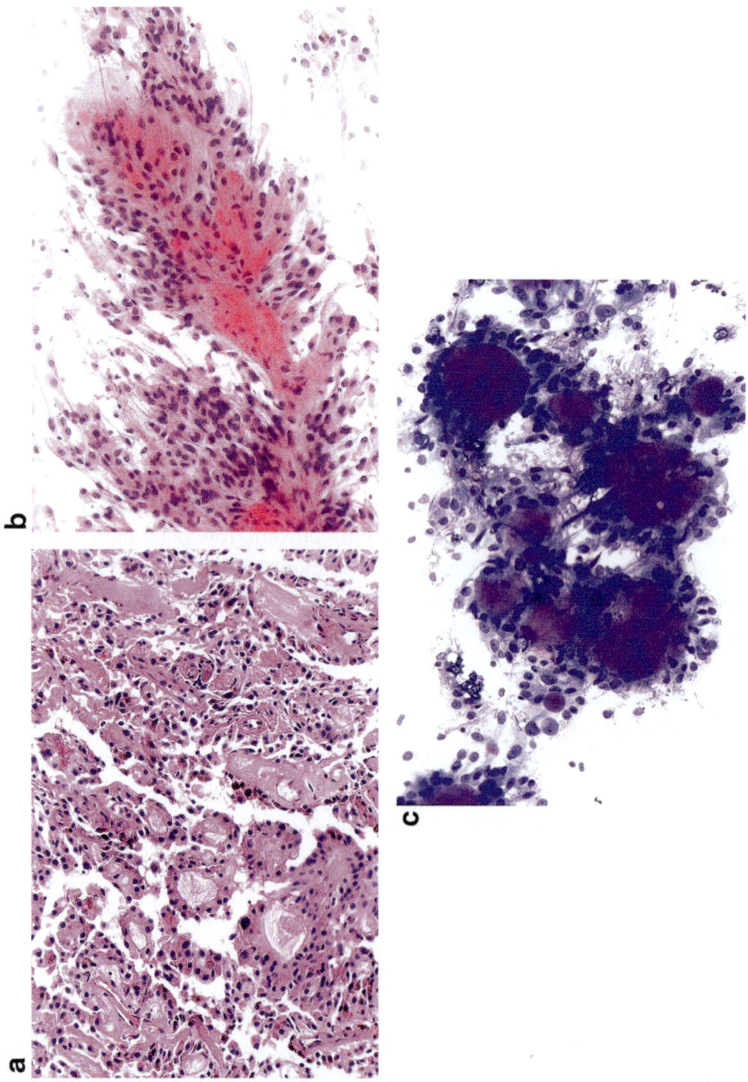

Fig. 8.9 *Myxopapillary ependymoma*. (**a**) Typical histology includes epithelioid cells arranged around hyalinized vascular core papillary structures and rounded mucinous microcysts. (**b**) Highly cellular preparation with slim columnar cells anchored to vascular stromal cores via glial processes (Smear, H&E). (**c**) Balls of epithelioid cells with myxoid cores giving an "adenoid cystic-like" appearance are distinctive features (Smear, Romanowsky)

Table 8.4 Characteristics of myxopapillary ependymoma

Cytologic features
Cellular arrangements around
Vascularized stromal cores
Globules of myxoid material
Cuboidal to slim columnar cell morphology with
Bland nuclei with small nucleoli
Polar tapering processes
Differential diagnosis and pitfalls
Chordoma
Extraskeletal chondrosarcoma
Metastatic mucinous carcinoma
Myxoid liposarcoma

Differential Diagnosis Considerations

Because of its location and the presence of myxoid matrix, the differential diagnosis should be made with chordoma, extraskeletal chondrosarcoma, and metastatic mucinous carcinoma. Extracellular metachromatic material is observed in the smears of these three tumors, but the glial morphology of the ependymal cell (tapering processes) facilitates its distinction from the physaliphorous cell of chordoma, from the small cells of extraskeletal chondrosarcoma, and from the unequivocal epithelial cells of metastatic mucinous carcinoma. In sacral locations, we should also keep in mind the retroperitoneal myxoid liposarcoma due to the presence of a myxoid metachromatic background; however, the characteristic cytomorphology of lipoblasts is very different from that of the ependymal cell. It should be pointed out that, in all these tumors, the extracellular myxoid material is arranged in an amorphous fashion and that we do not observe the characteristic "adenoid cystic-like" globules of the myxopapillary ependymoma (Table 8.4).

Suggested Reading

Azarpira N, Rakei M, Mokhtari M. Cytologic findings in malignant ependymoma. A case report. Acta Cytol. 2010;54:1023–6.

Dvoracek MA, Kirby PA. Intraoperative diagnosis of tanycytic ependymoma. Pitfalls and differential diagnosis. Diagn Cytopathol. 2006;34:289–92.

Inayama Y, Nishio Y, Ishii M, Mita K, et al. Crush and imprint cytology of subependymoma. A case report. Acta Cytol. 2001;45:636–40.

Jimenéz-Heffernan JA, Sanz E, López-Ferrer P. Cytologic features of subependymoma. Acta Cytol. 2003;47:319–20.

Khatua S, Ramaswamy V, Bouffet E. Current therapy and the evolving molecular landscape of paediatric ependymoma. Eur J Cancer. 2017;70:34–41.

Kulesza P, Tihan T, Ali SZ. Myxopapillary ependymoma: Cytomorphologic characteristics and differential diagnosis. Diagn Cytopathol. 2002;26:247–50.
Layfield LJ. Cytologic differential diagnosis of myxoid and mucinous neoplasias of the sacrum and parasacral soft tissues. Diagn Cytopathol. 2003;37:607–12.
Mack SC, Witt H, Piro RM, et al. Epigenomic alterations define lethal CIMP-positive ependymomas of infancy. Nature. 2014;506:445–50.
Manasa PL, Uppin MS, Sundaram C. Analysis of squash smear cytology of ependymomas. Acta Cytol. 2012;56:183–8.
Ng HK. Cytologic features of ependymomas in smears reparations. Acta Cytol. 1994;38:331–4.
Ortega L, Jiménez-Heffernan JA, Sanz E, Ortega P. Squash cytology of intradural myxopapillary ependymoma. Acta Cytol. 2002;46:428–30.
Pajtler KW, Mack SC, Ramaswamy V, Smith CA, et al. The current consensus on the clinical management of intracranial ependymoma and its distinct molecular variants. Acta Neuropathol. 2017;133:5–12.
Pajtler KW, Witt H, Sill M, Jones DTW, et al. Molecular classification of ependymal tumors across all CNS compartments, histopathological grades, and age groups. Cancer Cell. 2015;27:728–43.
Parker M, Mohankumar KM, Punchihewa C, Weinlich R, et al. *C11orf95-RELA* fusions drive oncogenic NF-κB signaling in ependymoma. Nature. 2014;506:451–5.
Raisanen J, Burns DK, White CL. Cytology of subependymoma. Acta Cytol. 2003;47:518–20.
Rushing EJ, Cooper PB, Quezado M, Begnami M, et al. Subependymoma revisited: clinicopathological evaluation of 83 cases. J Neurooncol. 2007;85:297–305.
Shim KW, Kim DS, Choi JU. The history of ependymoma management. Childs Nerv Syst. 2009;25:1167–83.
Takei H, Kosarac O, Powell SZ. Cytomorphologic features of myxopapillary ependymoma. A review of 13 cases. Acta Cytol. 2009;53:297–302.
Tejerina E, Jiménez-Heffernan JA, Ley L, Corbacho C, Sanz E. Intraoperative cytology of subependymoma. Acta Cytol. 2010;54:105–7.

Chapter 9
Other Gliomas

This category of CNS tumors covers a group of three rare glial neoplasms of uncertain histogenesis: astroblastoma, angiocentric glioma, and chordoid glioma. Although the ultrastructural studies suggest a derivation from specialized ependymal cells, these neoplasms also show features that are distinct from ependymomas; therefore, they have not been placed into a definitive category as yet.

Astroblastoma

Astroblastomas are rare intra-axial tumors of children, adolescents, and young adults (average age, 14 years). The vast majority of cases are well-circumscribed, peripheral, cerebral hemispheric masses, with rare examples arising elsewhere. Patients typically present with seizures or expression of mass effect. MRI shows a well demarcated contrast-enhancing mass, which often has a "bubbly" appearance created by multiple intratumoral cysts. Grossly, astroblastomas appear well demarcated and may be cystic. The term astroblastoma is due to its distinctive histologic pattern: perivascular glial cells, with broad or slightly tapered cytoplasmic processes, radiating toward a central blood vessel that often demonstrates sclerosis (astroblastic pseudorosette). In other areas the tumor cells may be detached from the vessel walls, being larger and plumper than in ependymoma (Fig. 9.1a). Although WHO classification does not recommend a specific grading for these tumors, two histologic groups of astroblastomas have been proposed: low grade and high grade. Increased cellularity, cellular atypia, multilayered pseudorosettes, high mitotic activity (greaterthan5 per 10 HPF), and microvascular proliferation are indicative of high-grade lesions. The prognosis is also further complicated by the potential of the astroblastoma to convert into a more malignant type of glioma. However, complete resection typically results in long-term survival, being the treatment of choice for this disease. About 70% of astroblastomas may harbor an *MN1* alteration, including

C. R. Lacruz et al., *Central Nervous System Intraoperative Cytopathology*,
Essentials in Cytopathology 13, https://doi.org/10.1007/978-3-319-98491-9_9

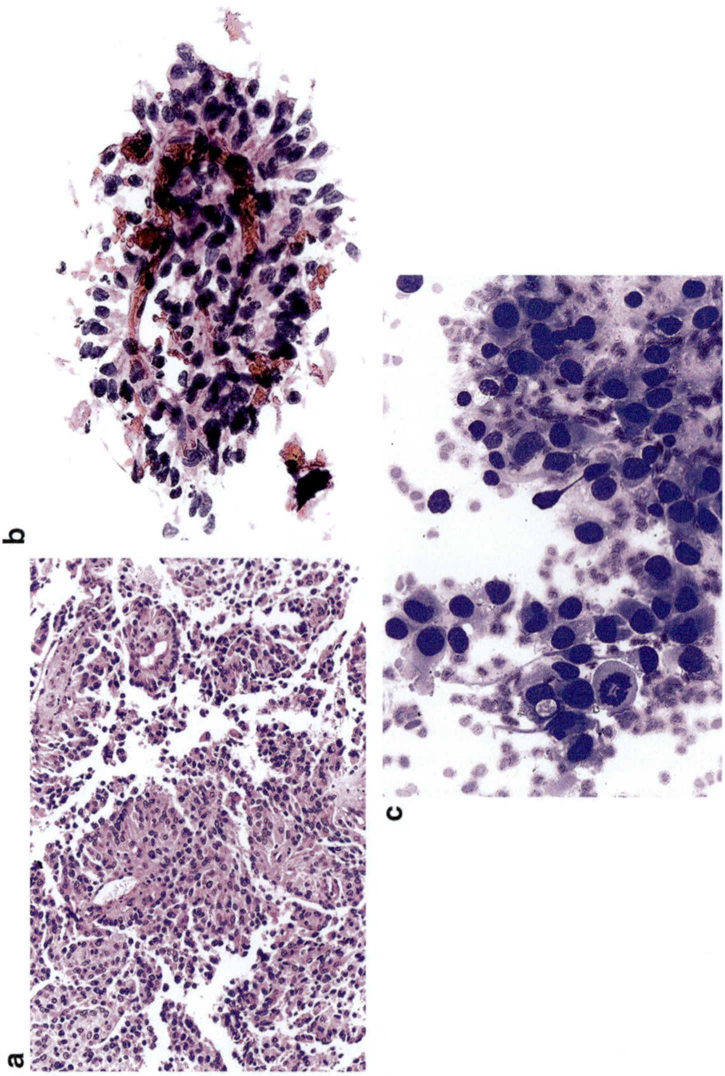

Fig. 9.1 *Astroblastoma.* (**a**) The histologic hallmark is the astroblastic pseudorosette, composed of elongated cells with broad processes radiating toward a central vessel. Unlike ependymoma, a fibrillary background is lacking. (**b**) Characteristic astroblastic pseudorosette showing tumor cells with broad processes radiating toward a central vessel (Smear, H&E). (**c**) Cellular preparation with discohesive cell groups and single cells. The mildly pleomorphic epithelioid cells are typical. Also note monopolar cytoplasmic processes and clear (no fibrillary) background (Smear, Romanowsky)

fusions with *BEND2* or *CXXC5*. Interestingly, the presence of *BRAF* V600E mutations in a subset of astroblastomas (38%) suggests potential clinical utility of targeted anti-BRAF therapy (i.e., vemurafenib).

Cytologic Features

Smears are cellular with perivascular pseudorosettes, discohesive cell groups, and single cells. Astroblastic pseudorosettes are formed by a single layer of tumor cells with stout or slightly tapering processes radiating toward a central vessel. When separate, cells display an epithelioid morphology with occasional monopolar processes, whereas nuclei are somewhat larger and rounder than in ependymoma. The background may look clear or bloody, but no fibrillary (Fig. 9.1b, c).

Differential Diagnosis Considerations

Astroblastoma should be differentiated from other tumors with pseudorosette formation such as ependymoma, subependymal giant cell astrocytoma (SEGA), pilomyxoid astrocytoma, and papillary meningioma. All three glial tumors have abundant processes and therefore a fibrillary background that is missing in astroblastoma. Likewise, cell processes of ependymoma are fibrillary; SEGA cells display abundant fine processes along the cell border ("hairy cells"), whereas pilomyxoid astrocytoma has fibrillary-myxoid background and bipolar spindle cells. However, the intraoperative differentiation from papillary meningioma may be challenging, although the presence of nuclear pseudoinclusions and other features of meningioma (whorls, syncytial aggregates) can aid for identifying the meningothelial nature of the process (Table 9.1).

Angiocentric Glioma

Angiocentric glioma is a low-grade (WHO grade I) distinctive supratentorial epileptogenic neoplasm, which most commonly occurs in children and young adults (mean age, 16 years). They are cortically based masses that behave as slowly evolving lesions with a long-standing history of intractable seizures. MRI shows a superficial, cortical area of T2/FLAIR hyperintensity with frequent stalklike extension toward the subjacent lateral ventricle; lesions generally lack contrast enhancement. Gross findings are not well described (cortical enlargement). The defining histologic feature is a proliferation of remarkably monomorphic spindle-shaped cells with frequent circumferential, parallel, or radial arrangements around vessels of the involved cortex and the subcortical white matter. Subpial aggregation of cells may

Table 9.1 Characteristics of astroblastoma

Cytologic features	
	Cellular smears with:
	Perivascular pseudorosettes
	Discohesive cell groups and single cells
	Epithelioid cells with:
	Large, plump nuclei
	Monopolar, stout, or slightly tapering processes
	Clear or bloody (no fibrillary) background
Differential diagnosis and pitfalls	
	Ependymoma
	Subependymal giant cell astrocytoma
	Pilomyxoid astrocytoma
	Papillary meningioma

also be evident (Fig. 9.2a). Surgical excision, even partial, is usually curative without adjunctive therapy. *MYB-QKI* fusions appear to be a highly specific and sensitive genetic alteration in angiocentric glioma.

Cytologic Features

Smears display loose tissue fragments of bipolar spindled cells, which have a tendency to form perivascular streaming arrays with either single or multilayered cells. Nuclei are slender (more elongated than ependymoma) and remarkable uniform with a stippled chromatin distribution. The tumor cells are often embedded in a homogeneous myxoid background (Fig. 9.2b, c).

Differential Diagnosis Considerations

Angiocentric glioma should be differentiated from ependymoma, subependymoma, and pilocytic astrocytoma. Detailed radiologic information and the characteristic cytologic features described above readily distinguish angiocentric glioma from these other tumors, for example, ependymoma (usually circumscribed enhancing mass, round to oval nuclei), subependymoma (attached to the ventricular wall, clustered dark nuclei), and pilocytic astrocytoma (circumscribed enhancing mass, long "piloid" cells, and small "protoplasmic" cells). Table 9.2 summarizes the characteristics of angiocentric glioma.

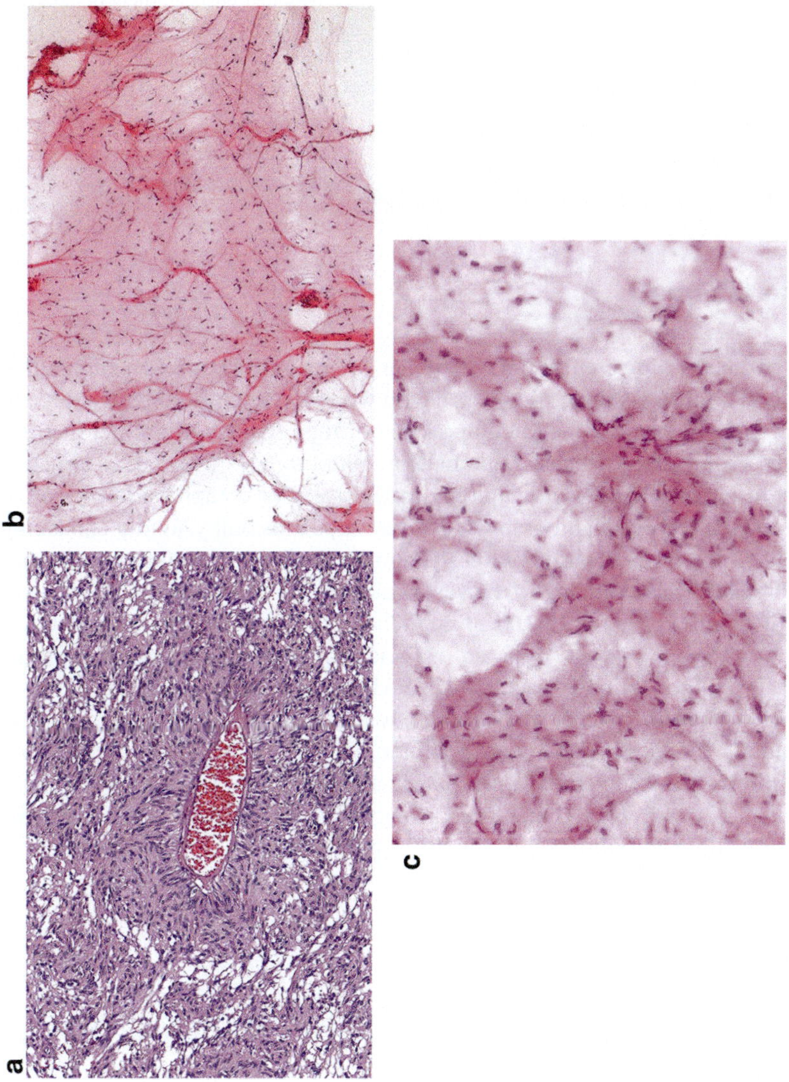

Fig. 9.2 *Angiocentric glioma.* (**a**) Histology. Predominant angiocentric pattern with monomorphous spindle cells often oriented parallel or radial to the vessels. Also note myxoid background. (**b**) This preparation d splays a tissue fragment composed of monomorphous spindle cells embedded in a homogeneous myxoid matrix. Note the tendency of tumor cells to form perivascular linear ensheathments. (**c**) Cytologic bipolarity, angiocentricity, and monomorphism are seen well in cytologic preparations (**b**, **c**; Smears, H&E)

Table 9.2 Characteristics of angiocentric glioma

Cytologic features
Tissue fragments and few single cells
Monomorphic, spindle-shaped cells
Slender nuclei with speckled chromatin
Perivascular ensheathment of cells or radiating
Myxoid background
Differential diagnosis and pitfalls
Ependymoma
Subependymoma
Pilocytic astrocytoma

Chordoid Glioma

Chordoid glioma is a discrete third ventricular tumor with chordoid features that usually affects adults (mean age 46 years), with women outnumbering men three to one. Symptoms are usually due to compression of the regional adjacent structures and include visual disturbances, hypothalamic/pituitary dysfunction, obstructive hydrocephalus, and psychiatric symptoms (possibly from compression of medial temporal lobe structures). Radiographically, they appear as bulky, avidly enhancing masses that fill the third ventricle. Grossly, chordoid gliomas are firm, sometimes mucoid masses densely adherent to the ventricular wall. Histologically, it is characterized by irregular cords or clusters of epithelioid cells embedded within a basophilic myxoid matrix, often with an associated lymphoplasmacytic infiltrate (Fig. 9.3a). The tumor cells are reactive for GFAP and also express nuclear TTF-1 in a similar way to pituicytes and other infundibular region lineage tumors (pituicytoma, spindle cell oncocytoma, and granular cell tumor of the sellar region). Chordoid glioma is a WHO grade II neoplasm, and gross total resection is the optimal treatment. In cases where local circumstances preclude radical surgery, partial resection with adjuvant radiosurgery should be performed.

Cytologic Features

Smears show dispersed or clumps of epithelioid cells, either polygonal or elongated, embedded in a myxoid background. Nuclei are relatively uniform, round to oval, with finely dispersed chromatin and inconspicuous nucleoli. Binucleation and scattered mature lymphocytes may also be seen. The characteristic myxoid matrix, clearly enhanced in Romanowsky-stained preparations, is arranged in the form of bands among the tumor cells, whereas the fibrillary background typical of astrocytomas and ependymonas is not seen (Fig. 9.3b, c).

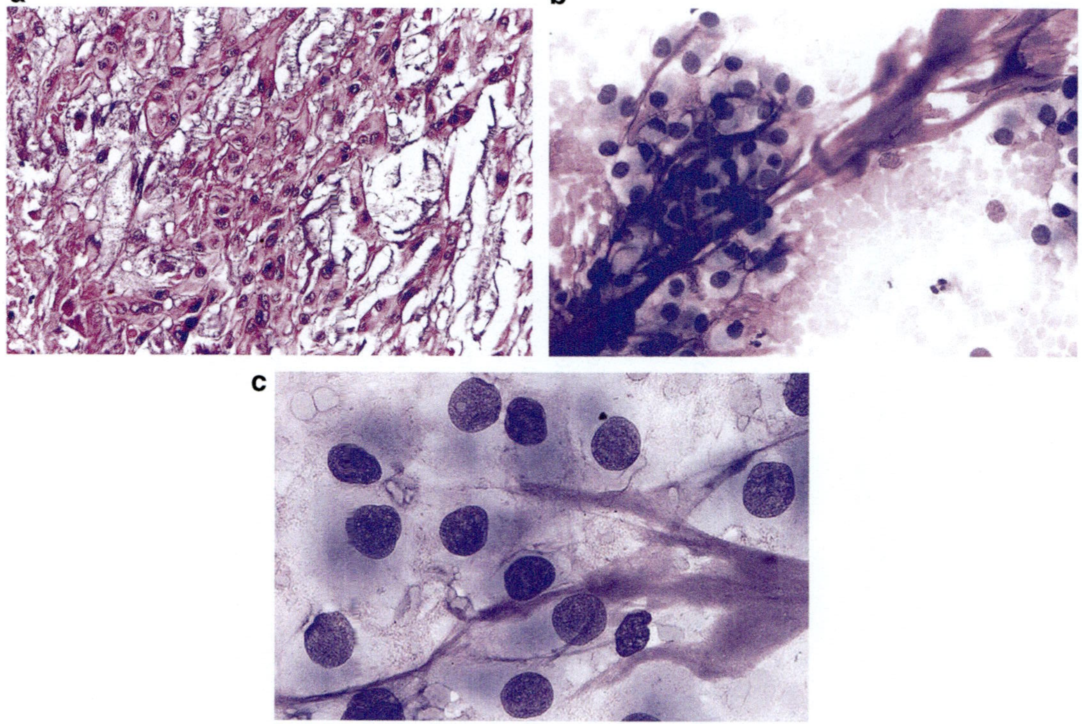

Fig. 9.3 *Chordoid glioma.* (**a**) Histology. Nests and anastomosing cords of epithelioid tumor cells in a bubbly, bluish, myxoid background typify this lesion. (**b**) Cytologic preparations show clustered or single epithelioid cells in a metachromatic myxoid background. In contrast to chordoma, the tumor cells have no cytoplasmic vacuolation. (**c**) Neoplastic nuclei are moderate in size, ovoid, and relatively uniform. Also note the homogeneous cytoplasm (without vacuoles) with uniform sky-blue coloration (**b**, **c**; Smears, Romanowsky)

Table 9.3 Characteristic of chordoid glioma

Cytologic features	
	Clusters and single cells
	Epithelioid or elongated cell morphology
	Plump nuclei with dispersed chromatin
	Homogeneous cytoplasm without vacuoles
	Myxoid (no fibrillary) background
Differential diagnosis and pitfalls	
	Pilocytic/pilomyxoid astrocytoma
	Ependymoma
	Germinoma
	Chordoma
	Chordoid meningioma

Differential Diagnosis Considerations

Due to its particular anatomic location in third ventricle, chordoid glioma should be differentiated from pilocytic/pilomyxoid astrocytoma, ependymoma, and germinoma; whereas on the basis of its myxoid matrix, from the other chordoid tumors, i.e., chordoma and chordoid meningioma. Unlike chordoid glioma, pilocytic/pilomyxoid astrocytomas have long bipolar cells, ependymoma has perivascular pseudorosettes and fibrillary background, germinoma shows a biphasic cellular pattern of large round cells and small lymphocytes in a striped "tigroid" background, whereas chordoma usually displays physaliphorous (bubbly) cells with more conspicuous nucleoli. However, intraoperative differentiation from chordoid meningioma may be challenging. The presence of worlds and nuclear pseudoinclusions favors meningioma, but a preliminary report of epithelioid tumor with chordoid features, with a suggestion of the differential, is adequate. After all, attempt of gross total resection is the recommended procedure for both WHO grade II tumors. Table 9.3 summarizes the characteristics of chordoid glioma.

Suggested Reading

Ahmed KA, Allen PK, Mahajan A, Brown PD, Ghia AJ. Astroblastomas: a surveillance, epidemiology, and end results (SEER)-based patterns of care analysis. World Neurosurg. 2014;82:e291–7.

Ampie L, Choy W, DiDomenico JD, Lamano JB, et al. Clinical attributes and surgical outcomes of angiocentric gliomas. J Clin Neurosci. 2016;28:117–22.

Bandopadhayay P, Ramkissoon LA, Jain P, Bergthold G, et al. MYB-QKI rearrangements in angiocentric glioma drive tumorigenicity through a tripartite mechanism. Nat Genet. 2016;48:273–82.

Bielle F, Villa C, Giry M, Bergemer-Fouquet AM, et al. Chordoid gliomas of the third ventricle share TTF-1 expression with organum vasculosum of the lamina terminalis. Am J Surg Pathol. 2015;39:948–56.

Bonnin JM, Rubinstein LJ. Astroblastomas: a pathological study of 23 tumors, with a postoperative follow-up in 13 patients. Neurosurgery. 1989;25:6–13.

Brat DJ, Scheithauer BW, Staugaitis SM, Cortez SC, et al. Third ventricular chordoid glioma: a distinct clinicopathologic entity. J Neuropathol Exp Neurol. 1998;57:283–90.

Brat DJ, Hirose Y, Cohen KJ, Feuerstein BG, Burger PC. Astroblastoma: clinicopathologic features and chromosomal abnormalities defined by comparative genomic hybridization. Brain Pathol. 2000;10:342–52.

Can B. Cytology of chordoid glioma of the third ventricle. Diagn Cytopathol. 2012;40:185–7.

DeSouza RM, Bodi I, Thomas N, Marsh H, Crocker M. Chordoid glioma: ten years of a low-grade tumor with high morbidity. Skull Base. 2010;20:125–38.

Lehman NL, Hattab EM, Mobley BC, Usubalieva A, et al. Morphological and molecular features of astroblastoma, including BRAFV600E mutations, suggest an ontological relationship to other cortical-based gliomas of children and young adults. Neuro Oncol. 2017;19:31–42.

Lellouch-Tubiana A, Boddaert N, Bourgeois M, Fohlen M, et al. Angiocentric neuroepithelial tumor (ANET): a new epilepsy-related clinicopathological entity with distinctive MRI. Brain Pathol. 2005;15:281–6.

Mott RT, Ellis TL, Geisinger KR. Angiocentric glioma: a case report and review of the literature. Diagn Cytopathol. 2010;38:452–6.

Ni HC, Chen SY, Chen L, Lu DH, Fu YJ, Piao YS. Angiocentric glioma: a report of nine new cases, including four with atypical histological features. Neuropathol Appl Neurobiol. 2015;41:333–46.

Patil M, Karandikar M, Garde S. A rare glial tumor entity: astroblastoma. Indian J Basic Appl Med Res. 2013;3:242–5.

Preusser M, Hoischen A, Novak K, Czech T, et al. Angiocentric glioma report of clinico-pathologic and genetic findings in 8 cases. Am J Surg Pathol. 2007;31:1709–18.

Qaddoumi I, Orisme W, Wen J, Santiago T, et al. Genetic alterations in uncommon low-grade neuroepithelial tumors: BRAF, FGFR1, and MYB mutations occur at high frequency and align with morphology. Acta Neuropathol (Berl). 2016;13:833–45.

Sturm D, Orr BA, Toprak UH, Hovestadt V, et al. New brain tumor entities emerge from molecular classification of CNS-PNETs. Cell. 2016;164:1060–72.

Takei H, Bhattacharjee MB, Adesina AM. Chordoid glioma of the third ventricle: report of a case with cytologic features and utility during intraoperative consultation. Acta Cytol. 2006;50:691–6.

Wang M, Tihan T, Rojiani AM, Bodhireddy SR, et al. Monomorphous angiocentric glioma: a distinctive epileptogenic neoplasm with features of infiltrating astrocytoma and ependymoma. J Neuropathol Exp Neurol. 2005;64:875–81.

Chapter 10
Choroid Plexus Tumors

Choroid plexus tumors (CPTs) account for less than 1% of all intracranial tumors, with papillomas more frequent than carcinomas. Because they commonly affect children, this percentage increases to 2–4% in those younger than 15 years and to 10–20% in those less than 1 year old. Also rare fetal and congenital examples have been described. Without predilection for either sex, they are located preferentially in the lateral ventricles (mainly in the left), followed by the fourth and third ventricles, whereas they are rarely found in the cerebellopontine angles. Tumors also may involve more than one ventricle simultaneously. Supratentorial cases usually appear in children, whereas those located in the posterior fossa are found preferentially in adults. The vast majority of CPTs are sporadic. In a small number of cases, choroid plexus papillomas are components of *Aicardi syndrome*, an X-linked dominant sporadic syndrome occurring almost exclusively in females, with affected patients showing corpus callosum agenesis, chorioretinal abnormalities, and infantile spasms. On the other hand, choroid plexus carcinoma may be a component of the *Li-Fraumeni syndrome*, and approximately 50% of the cases have *TP53* mutations. Recent comparative genomic studies have also identified putative oncogenes (*TAF12*, *NFYC*, *RAD54L*) to be gained in choroid plexus carcinoma, which may become prognostic/diagnostic markers in the future.

Choroid plexus neoplasms either increase the production of cerebrospinal fluid or obstruct its flow, so they usually present with signs of increased intracranial pressure (headache, visual disturbances, nausea/vomiting, papilledema) and hydrocephalus (patients before 2 years of age). In neuroimaging, they appear as solid and strongly enhancing intraventricular masses, often accompanied by diffuse ventricular enlargement. Evidence of brain invasion and heterogeneous enhancement raise concern for choroid plexus carcinoma.

Macroscopically, papillomas are well-demarcated and frequently calcified masses, with a conspicuous papillary or cauliflower-like appearance. They are adhering to the ventricular wall, although well-delimited by the nervous parenchyma. On

C. R. Lacruz et al., *Central Nervous System Intraoperative Cytopathology*, Essentials in Cytopathology 13, https://doi.org/10.1007/978-3-319-98491-9_10

their part, carcinomas are invasive tumors in which solid, necrotic, and hemorrhagic areas may be observed.

Microscopically, three types of choroid plexus tumors are recognized:

Papilloma (WHO grade I) is composed of fibrovascular fronds covered by a single layer of cuboidal to columnar epithelium. The cells have monomorphic round or oval nuclei with a basal location. In contrast to the normal choroid plexus, these cells tend to be more crowded and piled up, displaying a flat rather than cobblestone surface. Mitotic activity is extremely low, whereas calcifications are common (Fig. 10.1a, b).

Atypical papilloma (WHO grade II) is defined as a papilloma with increased mitotic activity (two or more mitosis per ten HPFs is the suggested threshold) without evidence of invasion. Complex architecture, increased cellularity, areas of solid growth, and necrosis may also be present but only one or two of those and not together in constellation.

Carcinoma (WHO grade III) shows clear signs of malignancy, such as frequent mitoses, increased cellular density, blurring of the papillary pattern, nuclear pleomorphism, necrosis, and diffuse brain invasion (Fig. 10.2a, b). Most of these rare malignancies are pediatric, mainly situated in the lateral ventricles, and arise de novo (evolution from papilloma is rarely evident).

An unusual feature of CPTs is that even WHO grade I and WHO grade II tumors have the potential to CSF spread, more often to the spine.

Surgical resection is the optimal treatment for choroid plexus tumors; even gross total resection is the current treatment strategy for choroid plexus carcinoma. Papillomas and well-differentiated carcinomas are curable by surgery, whereas anaplastic carcinomas and with p53 diffuse staining/mutation have a poor outcome despite total resection and adjuvant chemo−/radiotherapy.

Cytologic Features

The smears from *choroid plexus papillomas* (CPPs) are characteristically very cellular and have an epithelial appearance. They display branching papillae with fibrovascular cores, large sheets or monolayer fragments with smooth epithelial surfaces, and isolated columnar to cuboidal (nonciliated) cells arranged in a clear background, the joint presence of all of these components in a single smear being of great diagnostic value. When separate from the vascular core, tumor cells exhibit round to oval nuclei with evenly dispersed chromatin and a moderate amount of cytoplasm (Fig. 10.3a–c). *Atypical papillomas* often have a crowded and tall columnar epithelium with the additional presence of mitoses (Fig. 10.4). The isolated finding of mitotic figures should alert suspicion that the lesion may be a more aggressive tumor and not a simple papilloma. In *choroid plexus carcinomas* (CPCs), the cytomorphologic findings resemble those of either a papilloma or an undifferentiated epithelial tumor, with papillary tissue fragments and individual atypical epithelial cells. Nuclei are voluminous with frequent membrane irregularities and lobulations.

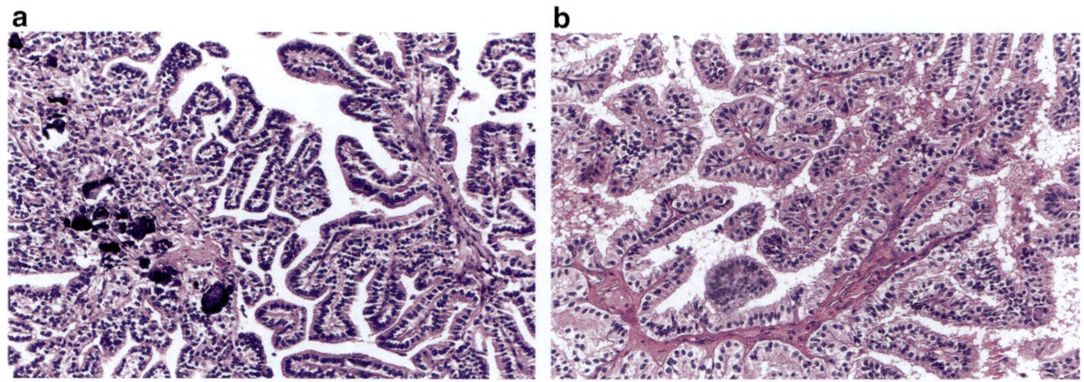

Fig. 10.1 *Choroid plexus papilloma*. (**a**) Typical histologic features include fibrovascular papillary fronds lined by cuboidal to columnar epithelial cells. Also note characteristic calcifications. (**b**) In this case the tumor cells tend to be more crowded and piled up

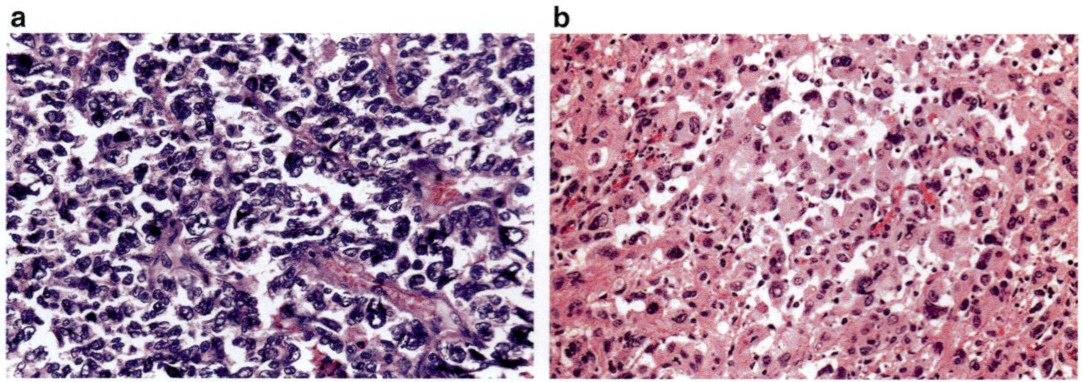

Fig. 10.2 *Choroid plexus carcinoma*. (**a**) Histologic features include papillary structures lined by crowded atypical epithelium. (**b**) In this case crude papillae and sheets of pleomorphic epithelial cells with increased eosinophilic cytoplasm are predominant. Note that both examples are united in their nuclear features

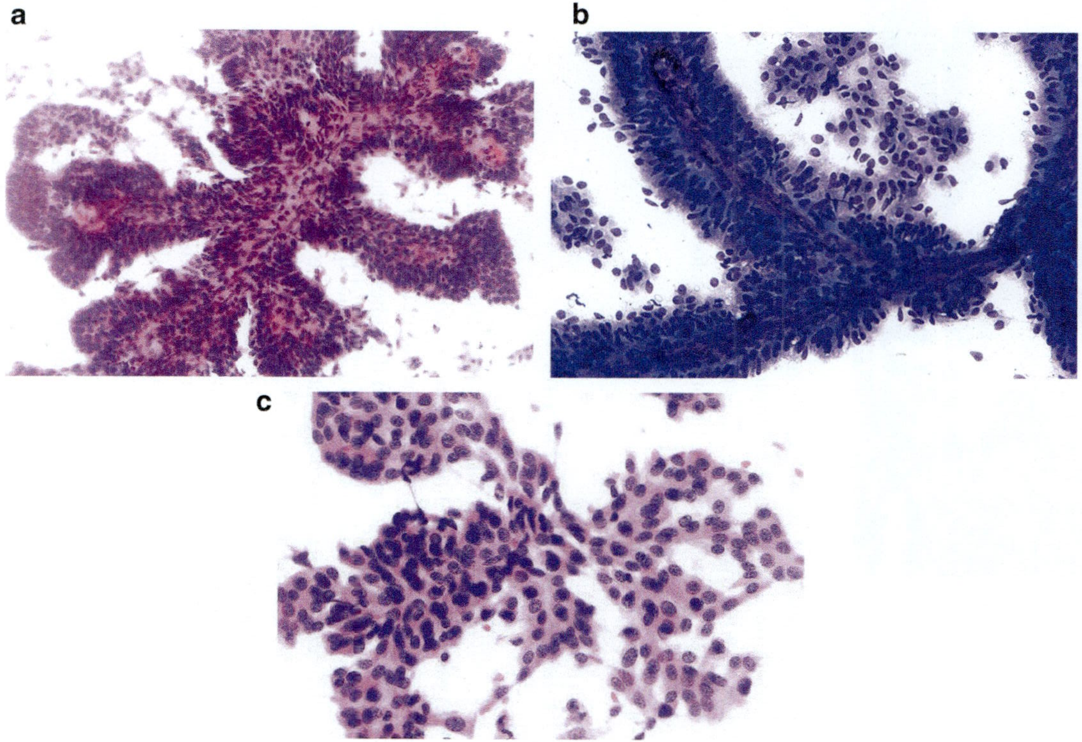

Fig. 10.3 *Choroid plexus papilloma, cytologic features.* (**a**) This highly cellular preparation has branching papillae, small cell clusters, and isolated epithelial cells (Smear, H&E). (**b**) Papilla with a central vascular core. Many cells have a blunt pole that contains the nucleus (Smear, Romanowsky). (**c**) A high-magnification view shows cell sheets with smooth epithelial surfaces. Nuclei have slightly coarser chromatin than their normal counterparts but still lack significant pleomorphism (Smear, H&E)

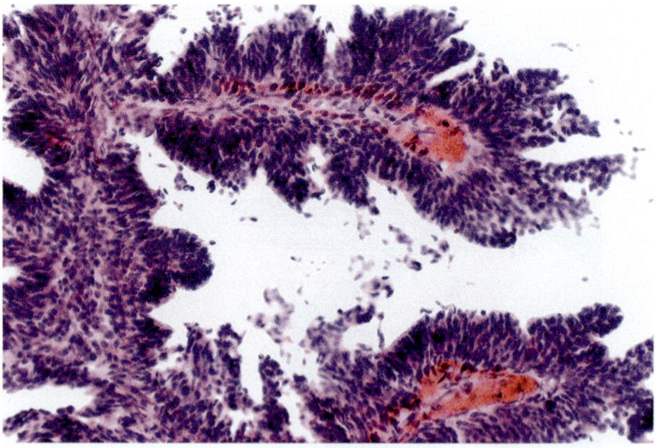

Fig. 10.4 *Atypical choroid plexus papillomas* often have a crowded and tall columnar epithelium (Smear, H&E)

Nucleoli, practically nonexistent in CPP, appear especially prominent here (Fig. 10.5a, b). Solid, undifferentiated examples of CPC display a discohesive pattern of atypical cells with overt malignant features. Mitosis and cell-to-cell wrapping can also be seen, whereas the background often looks granular due to the presence of necrotic debris (Fig. 10.6a, b).

Differential Diagnosis Considerations

Choroid plexus papilloma must be differentiated from normal choroid plexus and from papillary ependymoma. The high degree of cellularity in papilloma smears, together with the presence of the different types of cell clusters described above, is not observed in the normal choroid plexus. On the other hand, the absence of fibrillary background and perivascular pseudorosettes (radial fibrillary processes around blood vessels) differentiate it from ependymoma. These criteria are useful especially for tumors located in the fourth ventricle, because the papillomas of the lateral ventricles and the third ventricle show a clinical-radiologic picture so characteristic that a morphologic diagnosis is virtually not necessary. With respect to the *choroid plexus carcinoma*, the differential diagnosis must be made with metastatic adenocarcinoma, especially if it is of the papillary type (lung, thyroid, digestive tract, or ovaries), because the images may be almost identical. The presence of transitional zones between papilloma and carcinoma, in the same smear, is of great value for identifying the choroid nature of the process. Moreover, in children, the scant likelihood of metastatic carcinoma favors the diagnosis of CPC. By the contrary, the extremely low frequency of this rare tumor in adults favors the likelihood of metastatic adenocarcinoma. Nevertheless, a preliminary diagnosis of malignant epithelial neoplasm with a suggestion of the differential is adequate. Other processes that must be taken into account are melanoma, non-germinomatous germ cell tumors (NGGCTs), and atypical teratoid/rhabdoid tumor (AT/RT). Melanomas are usually

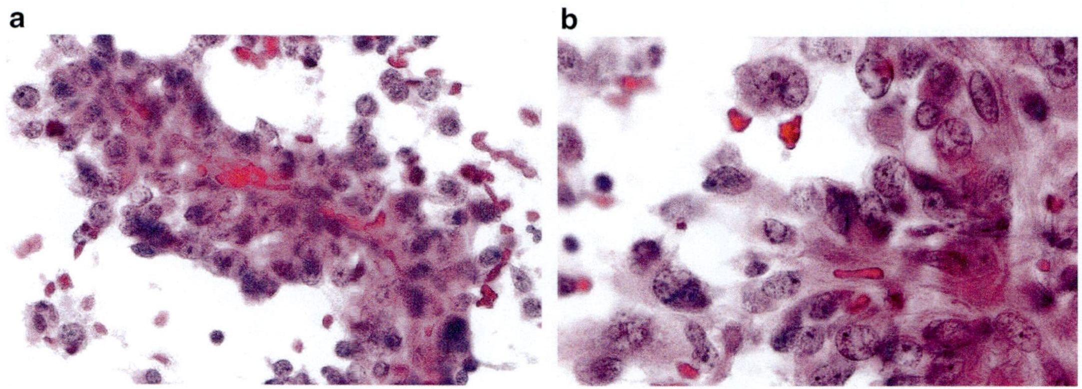

Fig. 10.5 *Choroid plexus carcinoma, cytologic features*. (**a**) Papillary tissue fragments composed of cells with little cytoplasm are consistent with choroid plexus carcinoma. (**b**) This high-power view shows characteristic vesicular nuclei with prominent nucleoli and frequent lobulations (**a**, **b**; Smears, H&E)

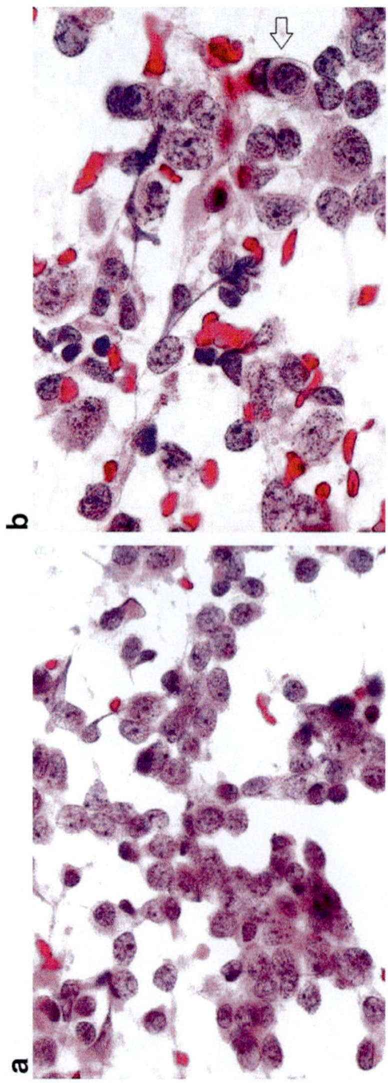

Fig. 10.6 *Choroid plexus carcinoma, cytologic features*. (**a**) Anaplastic example displaying discohesive cells with overt malignant features mimicking poorly differentiated metastatic adenocarcinoma. (**b**) Also note a "cannibalistic" cell engulfing (*arrow*), which is characteristic of malignancy (**a, b**; Smears, H&E)

Table 10.1 Characteristics of choroid plexus tumors

Cytologic features
Cellular smears with the joint presence of:
Papillae with fibrovascular cores
Monolayer fragments
Single cells
Columnar to cuboidal cells with:
Smooth (nonciliated) epithelial surfaces
Round to oval bland nuclei
Clean background
Choroid plexus carcinoma
Malignant cellular characteristics
Areas of transition papilloma-carcinoma
Hemorrhagic or granular (necrotic) background
Differential diagnosis and pitfalls
Normal choroid plexus
Papillary ependymoma
Choroid plexus carcinoma
Metastatic carcinoma
Melanoma
Non-germinomatous (malignant) germ cell tumors
Atypical teratoid/rhabdoid tumor

pleomorphic tumors with epithelioid, fusiform, and bizarre giant cells, whereas melanin can be identified in about 50% of cases. In NGGCTs is advisable the correlation with clinical data, particularly the levels of α-fetoprotein and β-human chorionic gonadotropin in plasma/CSF, usually elevated in these tumors. AT/RT contains rhabdoid cells and also primitive neuroectodermal cells with divergent differentiation along epithelial, mesenchymal, or glial lines. However, solid, undifferentiated examples of CPC and AT/RT (both can exhibit rhabdoid features) may be misdiagnosed even on permanent sections, and making a definitive intraoperative diagnosis of these uncommon entities may be unreliable. In such cases, a descriptive report of "high-grade, malignant anaplastic tumor" is recommended. The distinction can be made in permanent sections by recognition of retained nuclear INI1 (BAF47) expression in CPCs, including in those with rhabdoid morphology (Table 10.1).

Suggested Reading

Barreto AS, Vassallo J, Queiroz LS. Papillomas and carcinomas of the choroid plexus: histological and immunohistochemical studies and comparison with normal fetal choroid plexus. Arq Neuropsiquiatr. 2004;62:600–7.

Buchino JJ, Mason KG. Choroid plexus papilloma. Report of a case with cytologic differential diagnosis. Acta Cytol. 1992;36:95–7.

Cannon DM, Mohindra P, Gondi V, Kruser TJ, Kozak KR. Choroid plexus tumor epidemiology and outcomes: implications for surgical and radiotherapeutic management. J Neuro-Oncol. 2015;121:151–7.

Due-Tønnessen B, Helseth E, Skullerud K, Lundar T. Choroid plexus tumors in children and young adults: report of 16 consecutive cases. Childs Nerv Syst. 2001;17:252–6.

Jeibmann A, Hasselblatt M, Gerss J, Wrede B, et al. Prognostic implications of atypical histologic features in choroid plexus papilloma. J Neuropathol Exp Neurol. 2006;65:1069–73.

Judkins AR, Burger PC, Hamilton RL, Kleinschmidt-DeMasters B, et al. INI 1 protein expression distinguishes atypical teratoid/rhabdoid tumor from choroid plexus carcinoma. J Neuropathol Exp Neurol. 2005;64:391–7.

Kim K, Greenblatt SH, Robinson MG. Choroid plexus carcinoma. Report of a case with cytopathologic differential diagnosis. Acta Cytol. 1985;29:846–9.

Lam S, Lin Y, Cherian J, Qadri U, et al. Choroid plexus tumors in children: a population-based study. Pediatr Neurosurg. 2013;49:331–8.

Ogiwara H, Dipatri AJ Jr, Alden TD, Bowman RM, Tomita T. Choroid plexus tumors in pediatric patients. Br J Neurosurg. 2012;26:32–7.

Pai RR, Kini H, Rao VS, Naik R. Choroid plexus papilloma diagnosed by crush cytology. Diagn Cytopathol. 2001;25:165–7.

Pant I, Chaturvedi S, Suri V, Dua R. Choroid plexus papilloma with cytologic differential diagnosis. A case report. J Cytol. 2007;24:89–91.

Rickert CH, Paulus N. Tumors of the choroid plexus. Microsc Res Tech. 2001;52:104–11.

Savage NM, Crosby JH, Reid-Nicholson MD. The cytologic findings in choroid plexus carcinoma: report of a case with differential diagnosis. Diagn Cytopathol. 2012;40:1–6.

Strojan P, Popović M, Surlan K, Jereb B. Choroid plexus tumors: a review of 28-year experience. Neoplasma. 2004;51:306–12.

Tabori U, Shlien A, Baskin B, Levitt S, et al. TP53 alterations determine clinical subgroups and survival of patients with choroid plexus tumors. J Clin Oncol. 2010;28:1995–2001.

Tena-Suck ML, Gomez-Amador JL, Ortiz-Plata A, Salina-Lara C, Rembao-Bojorquez D, Vega-Orozco R. Rhabdoid choroid plexus carcinoma. A rare histological type. Arq Neuropsiquiatr. 2007;65:705–9.

Tong Y, Merino D, Nimmervoll B, Gupta K, et al. Cross-species genomics identifies *TAF12, NFYC* and *RAD54L* as choroid plexus carcinoma oncogenes. Cancer Cell. 2015;27:712–27.

Wolf JE, Sajedi M, Brant R, Coppes MJ, Egeler RM. Choroid plexus tumours. Br J Cancer. 2002;87:1086–91.

Zaky W, Dhall G, Khatua S, Brown RJ, et al. Choroid plexus carcinoma in children: the head start experience. Pediatr Blood Cancer. 2015;62:784–9.

Chapter 11
Neuronal and Mixed Neuronal-Glial Tumors

This category covers a heterogeneous group of tumors that have the common feature of consisting, in whole or in part, of cells with different degrees of neuronal differentiation (large ganglion cells or small neurocytes). In the mixed neuronal-glial tumors, another component of glial nature (most often astrocytic) is added to this neuronal component. Both are rare neoplasms, which taken as a whole hardly exceed 2–3% of all intracranial tumors. Aside from this low frequency, other common features of neuronal/neuronal-glial tumors are an early age of presentation (most cases are diagnosed in patients less than 25 years old) and a mildly aggressive behavior. With exception of the rare anaplastic ganglioglioma, they are well-circumscribed and slow-growing tumors, which is why their prognosis is intrinsically favorable after gross total resection. In spite of these common features, the locations and histologic pictures vary quite a bit, giving rise to different anatomo-clinical entities. Similarly, the cytologic picture and the differential diagnosis are different and particular for each type, the reason why it behooves us to study them separately.

Dysembryoplastic Neuroepithelial Tumor

Dysembryoplastic neuroepithelial tumors (DNTs) are intracortical, typically multinodular neoplasms that usually become symptomatic during the first two decades of life with chronic, medically intractable partial complex seizures. The temporal lobe (particularly mesial zones) is the most common location for DNTs, although histologically similar tumors have been described in rarer sites such as the basal ganglia, thalamus, lateral ventricle, septum pellucidum, and brain stem. Neuroimaging demonstrates T2-hyperintense nodule(s) limited to cerebral cortex. Grossly, DNTs are mucin-rich intracortical expansions, sometimes with a discernibly nodular growth pattern. The histologic hallmark is the so-called *specific glioneural element*; this is

C. R. Lacruz et al., *Central Nervous System Intraoperative Cytopathology*,
Essentials in Cytopathology 13, https://doi.org/10.1007/978-3-319-98491-9_11

characterized by an alveolar or columnar pattern formed by bundles of axons ensheathed with oligodendrocyte-like cells. Between these elements, normal-looking neurons appear to float in small pools of faintly basophilic matrix (Fig. 11.1a, b). Most DNTs harbor an alteration in *FGFR1*, either TKD duplication or a single nucleotide variation, whereas the presence of an IDH mutation or 1p/19q codeletion excludes its diagnosis. On the other hand, overexpression of multidrug transporters (P-gp, MRP2, MRP5, BCRP) may explain intrinsic epileptogenicity and resistance to antiepileptogenic drugs. Recurrences are rare even in subtotally resected cases; thus, aggressive therapy should be avoided.

Cytologic Features

The smear findings include a dual population of small, oligodendrocyte-like cells and scattered normal-looking neurons, which are loosely arranged in a mucoid background with slim capillaries. The oligo-like cells are monomorphic with round regular nuclei and dark chromatin. Because of this cellularity, this tumor can easily be overgraded as oligodendroglioma infiltrating the cortex. A clue suggesting DNT is the absence of any appreciable cytologic atypia (Fig. 11.1c).

Ganglion Cell Tumors (Ganglioglioma/Gangliocytoma)

Ganglioglioma is probably most common of the neuronal and glioneural tumors, whereas pure gangliocytomas are rare. Ganglion cell tumors have been described at all levels of the central neuroaxis, but most are supratentorial with a predilection for the temporal lobes (greaterthan70%). The usual clinical picture varies, depending on the location of the tumor, from local compression symptoms to a long history of seizures, which may precede diagnosis by several years. Therefore, ganglion cell tumors are the most frequent entities observed in patients undergoing surgery for control of epilepsy. Neuroimaging usually shows a well-demarcated, enhancing mass devoid of perilesional edema; extensive cystic change, leading to a cystic lesion with mural nodule, also is a common finding. Some cases extend to the nearby subarachnoid space and originate scalloping of the overlying calvaria (indicator of chronicity). These neoplasms are composed of variably sized neurons, some large and rotund, in a delicate fibrillary matrix that is prone to spongy rarefaction. Anomalous clustering, architectural disarray, and conspicuous dysplastic changes that can include striking pleomorphism, bi- or multinucleation, and gigantism also are characteristic features. These dysmorphic ganglion cells are the predominant component of gangliocytoma with a minimal glial component (Fig. 11.2a), whereas ganglioglioma, as their name implies, contains a variable neuronal component (sometimes inconspicuous) in combination with abundant glial cells, usually with pilocytic or fibrillary morphology (Fig. 11.2b). Focal collections of EGBs

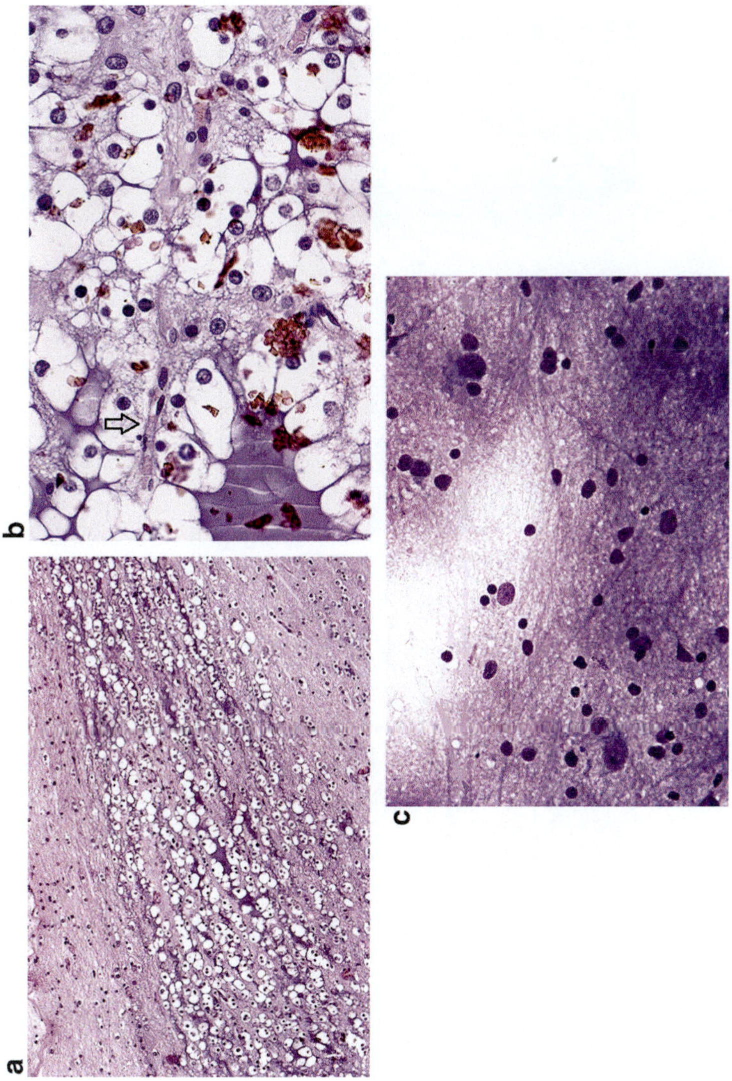

Fig. 11.1 *Dysembryoplastic neuroepithelial tumor (DNT)*. **(a)** The histoarchitecture of "specific glioneural elements" is characterized by the presence of "patterned" glioneuronal units (columns) with small, oligo-like cells lining vascular elements and neuronal processes. **(b)** High-power view displaying the characteristic components of DNTs: oligo-like cells, small neurons, mucinous pools, and slim capillaries (*arrow*). **(c)** This cytologic preparation displays remarkably uniform oligo-like cells and small neurons loosely arranged in a mucoid background (Smear, Romanowsky)

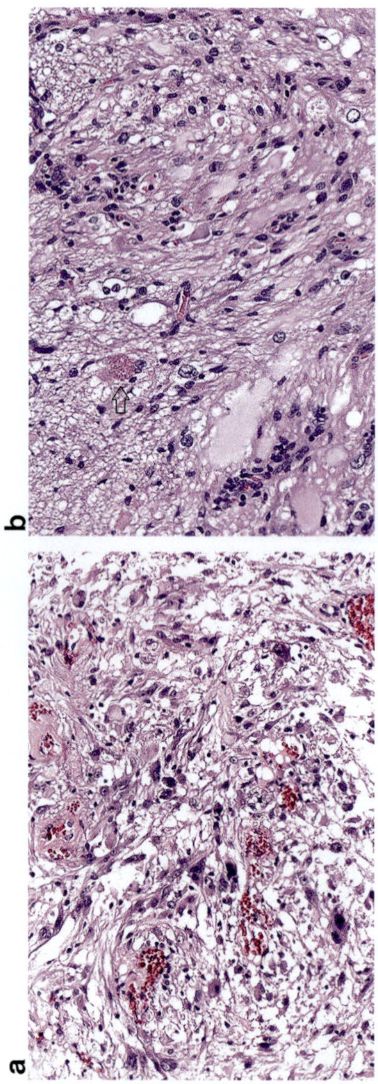

Fig. 11.2 *Ganglion cell tumors, histology*. (**a**) *Gangliocytoma*. This tumor is composed of irregular groups of large, dysplastic neurons in a delicate fibrillary matrix with spongy rarefaction. Also note hyalinized blood vessels (*above*). (**b**) *Ganglioglioma*. In this case large, dysmorphic and unoriented ganglion cells are seen admixed with mildly pleomorphic astrocytic glial element. Also note an eosinophilic granular body (*arrow*) suggesting the lesion's chronicity

represent a diagnostically important feature in both tumors. Malignant transformation is reported to occur in about 8% to 10% gangliogliomas (*anaplastic ganglioglioma,* WHO grade III) and almost invariably involves the glial component, which displays features of anaplastic astrocytoma. Almost 80% of gangliogliomas reveal immunoreactivity for CD34 (a stem cell epitope not expressed in normal brain). On the other hand, a *BRAF* V600E mutation occurs in about 20–30% of gangliogliomas, whereas IDH mutations are not (useful differential feature with diffuse gliomas). The vast majority of ganglion cell tumors behave in a benign fashion (WHO grade I neoplasms); therefore, therapy is limited to surgery. Because brainstem gangliogliomas are frequently inoperable, the targeted inhibitor vemurafenib can be used successfully in *BRAF* V600E mutated cases. Anaplastic, WHO grade III gangliogliomas have dismal clinical outcomes regardless therapy, with median overall survival of 25 months.

Cytologic Features

The defining feature of both gangliocytoma and ganglioglioma is dysmorphic neurons, which are better preserved in smears than in frozen sections. In *gangliocytoma,* these dysmorphic ganglion cells, which are usually larger and more rotund than normal neurons, are haphazardly arranged in a loose neuropil-rich background. Distorted features include bizarre shapes with several oddly oriented processes and anomalous tight clustering (Fig. 11.3a). The presence of bi- or multinucleated dysplastic cells with prominent nucleoli is a key diagnostic feature (Fig. 11.3b). In *ganglioglioma,* the dysmorphic ganglion cells are intermixed with glial cells in a fibrillary background. The glial cells can display features of fibrillar or pilocytic astrocytoma or even appear oligodendroglial. A diagnostically important feature of both gangliocytoma and ganglioglioma is the presence of EGBs that bespeaks about the indolent behavior of these tumors (Fig. 11.4a, b).

Desmoplastic Infantile Astrocytoma and Ganglioglioma

Desmoplastic infantile astrocytoma and desmoplastic infantile ganglioglioma (DIA/DIG) are rare, supratentorial tumors of infancy (nearly all cases are present in patients under the age of 2 years). They are remarkably large, solid and cystic hemispheric masses that may replace much of the brain on one side. Clinically, DIA/DIG produce manifestations associated with increased intracranial pressure that includes vomiting, bulging fontanels, lethargy, and macrocephaly. Seizures and forced downward deviation of the eyes (the "sunset" sign) may also be observed. Imaging studies are quite characteristic, exhibiting a large heterogeneous and partially cystic mass compressing a cerebral hemisphere and abutting the dura. Grossly, they are unilocular or multilocular lesions with a firm to rubbery superficial cortical/

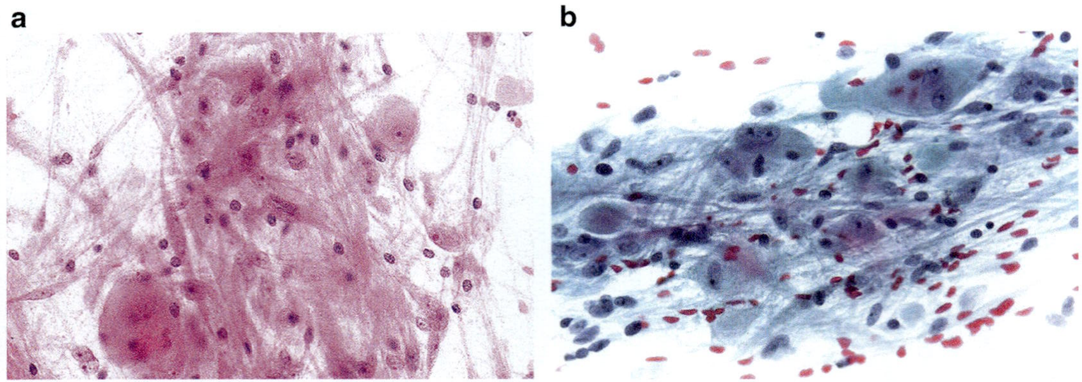

Fig. 11.3 *Gangliocytoma, cytologic features*. (**a**) This preparation shows different size neurons in a fine, fibrillary background of neuropil. Note the rotund appearance of some cells (smear, H&E). (**b**) The presence of large, dysmorphic neurons with frequent binucleation is a key diagnostic feature (Smear, Papanicolaou)

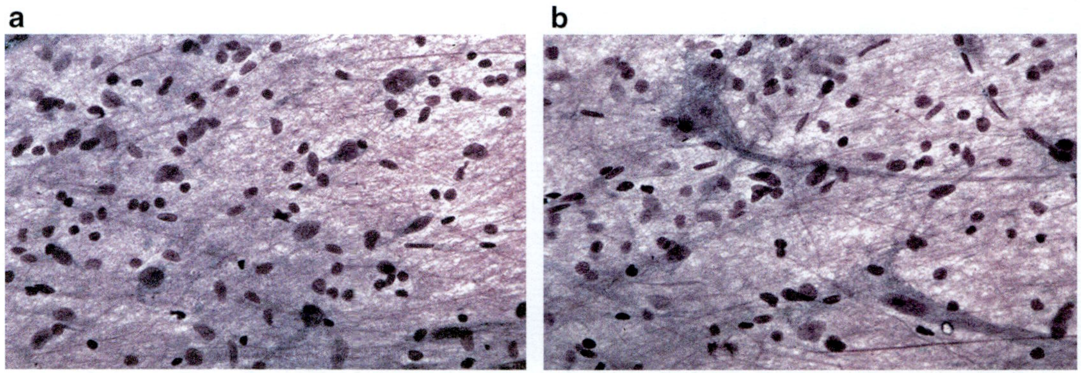

Fig. 11.4 *Ganglioglioma, cytologic features*. (**a**) A biphasic pattern with large neurons and mildly pleomorphic glial cells in a fibrillary background characterizes this variant. (**b**) In this preparation dysplastic ganglion cells with large, vesicular nuclei, and macronucleoli are well seen (**a**, **b**; Smears, Papanicolaou)

meningeal solid component. Microscopically, DIA/DIG are tumors composed of spindle-shaped cells and attendant pericellular stroma, with a population of neoplastic astrocytes (DIA) or astrocytes together with a variable neuronal component (DIG). In addition, aggregates of poorly differentiated neuroepithelial cells can be present in both. A similar molecular profile suggests that DIA and DIG represent a histologic spectrum of the same tumor rather than two separate entities (gain of 7q31 involving *MET* is found in more than 40% of DIAs/DIGs).These neoplasms have a generally good prognosis after surgical resection with the possibility of long-term survival (WHO grade I tumors).

Cytologic Features

Because of associated fibroplasia, this tumor is often difficult to smear and resist disaggregation remaining as fibrotic tissue fragments. It is necessary to perform additional smears of different zones of the specimen in order to see a complex cellularity, which includes spindle-shaped cells and pleomorphic astrocytes in DIA, associated with neuronal elements in DIG. Astrocytes may appear gemistocyte-like or spindle-shaped, whereas the neuronal elements vary greatly, ranging from atypical ganglion-like cells to smaller polygonal cells. The occasional presence of cytoplasmic polarization, binucleation, and prominent nucleoli may aid in identification of the neuronal component. Sometimes this pleomorphic cellularity is accompanied by atypical cells that can be either embryonal-like or display an astroglial morphology (Fig. 11.5a, b).

Central Neurocytoma

Central neurocytomas present primarily in the second to third decades of life with and equal predilection for males and females. They are typically located supratentorially in the lateral ventricles or third ventricle, with the vast majority attached to the septum pellucidum close to foramen of Monro. Due to its location, most patients present with symptoms of increased intracranial pressure, including headaches and visual disturbances from papilledema. In neuroimaging they tend to be circumscribed, often calcified, heterogeneously enhancing masses, which typically protrude into the ventricular system near the foramen of Monro. Occasionally, cases with an extraventricular location (*extraventricular neurocytomas*) are observed affecting the brain parenchyma of the cerebral hemispheres, well demarcated from the surrounding tissue. Both tumors are composed of small and remarkably uniform neurocytes in a fine, neuropil-like fibrillar matrix (Fig. 11.6a). *Cerebellar liponeurocytoma* is a rare variant with focal aggregates of lipoma-like cells, which consist of lipid-laden neuroepithelial cells that resemble mature adipocytes (Fig. 11.6b). The extent of resection is the most important prognostic factor, with possible role for radiotherapy in recurrent, subtotally excised tumors (about 50% of cerebellar liponeurocytomas recur).

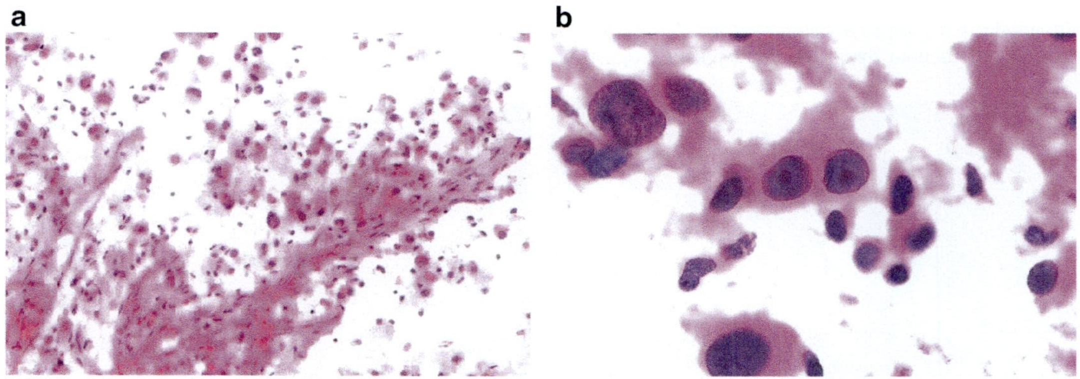

Fig. 11.5 *Desmoplastic infantile ganglioglioma*. (**a**) Pleomorphic cell population, including atypical cells that can be either astroglial or ganglioid in morphology and bundles of spindle cells. (**b**) Neuronal elements range from atypical ganglion-like cells to smaller polygonal cells. Some display cytoplasmic polarization, binucleation, and prominent nucleoli that aid in identification as neuronal (**a**, **b**; Smears, H&E)

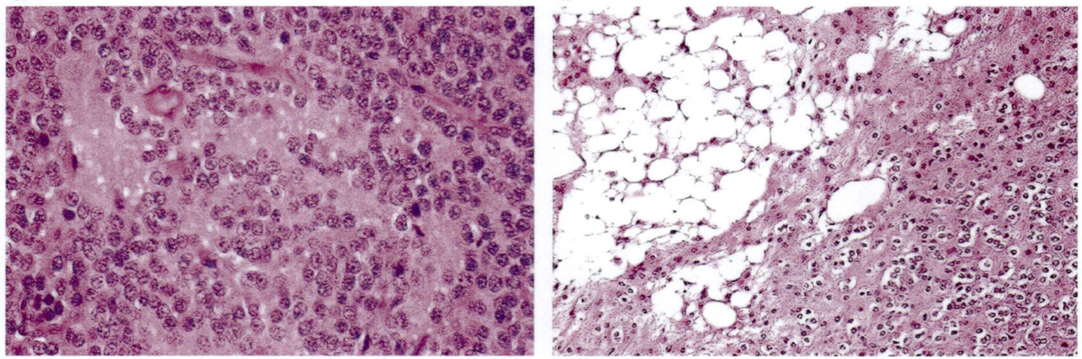

Fig. 11.6 *Neurocytic tumors, histologic features*. (**a**) *Central neurocytoma*. Typical histology includes sheets of small, monomorphous neurocytes and nucleus-free areas of delicate fibrillary matrix. (**b**) *Cerebellar liponeurocytoma*. In this case there is focal accumulation of lipidized (lipoma-like) tumor cells on a background of typical neurocytes, which often show perinuclear halos

Cytologic Features

Smears are highly cellular displaying a discohesive pattern of small, round cells with remarkable uniformity in size and shape. Nuclei have a neuroendocrine appearance with delicate speckled chromatin and variably present nucleoli. The cytoplasm is scant and wispy, but occasional perinuclear "empty-appearance" halos may be present. The background is finely granular with a delicate capillary network. A frequent finding is the presence of conglomerates of light neuropil matrix (Fig. 11.7a, b). Because of their cellular appearance, these tumors are easily confused with oligodendroglioma, but oligodendroglioma lacks conglomerates of neuropil matrix and perinuclear halos in smears.

Rosette-Forming Glioneuronal Tumor

Rosette-forming glioneural tumors (RGNTs) usually arise in the posterior fossa occupying the fourth ventricular compartment and/or cerebral aqueduct, from where they can extend to involve adjacent brain stem and cerebellar vermis. Rare examples may manifest in the pineal gland/tectal region, hypothalamus/optic chiasm, and spinal cord. Most of the reported cases have occurred within the second to fourth decades of life with no significant sex predilection. Patients usually present with headache or ataxia, and neuroimaging studies often reveal a solid and partially cystic circumscribed midline mass with mild enhancement. Microscopically, tumors are biphasic with clearly defined neurocytic and glial components. Uniform neurocytes forming diminutive rosettes and narrow perivascular pseudorosettes that often seem to float within microcavities represent a distinct neuronal component (Fig. 11.8a, b), whereas the glial one is often largely piloid closely resembling pilocytic astrocytoma, including Rosenthal fibers and eosinophilic granular bodies (Fig. 11.9a, b). RGNTs lack of *BRAF* alterations, but *PIK3CA* and *FGFR1* mutations have been reported. Because of the difficulty of surgical resection, the morbidity carried by this lesion is most often related to surgical intervention, with disabling postoperative deficits in about half of cases.

Cytologic Features

Smears show distinctive dual cell morphology. One of the components is composed of small neurocytes with uniform round nuclei and occasional small nucleoli, which may form neuropile core rosettes (Fig. 11.8c); the other is often pilocytic, with large "piloid" cells in a faint myxoid background (Fig. 11.9c). Due to its biphasic nature, RGNT must be differentiated from pilocytic astrocytoma, oligodendroglioma, and DNT.

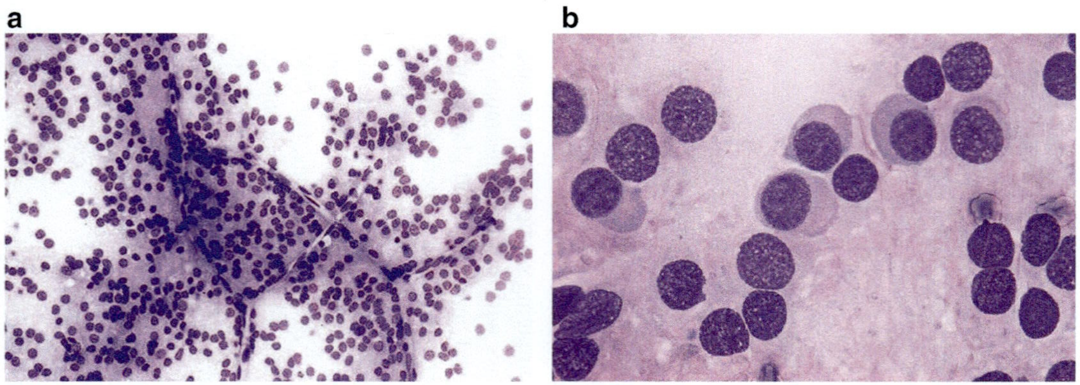

Fig. 11.7 *Neurocytoma, cytologic features.* (**a**) This preparation shows a population of round monomorphic cells, nuclei-free areas of neuropil, and branching thin-walled capillaries. (**b**) High-magnification view demonstrating a remarkable uniformity in nuclear size and shape. Note stippled chromatin and some perinuclear halos (**a**, **b**; Smears, Romanowsky)

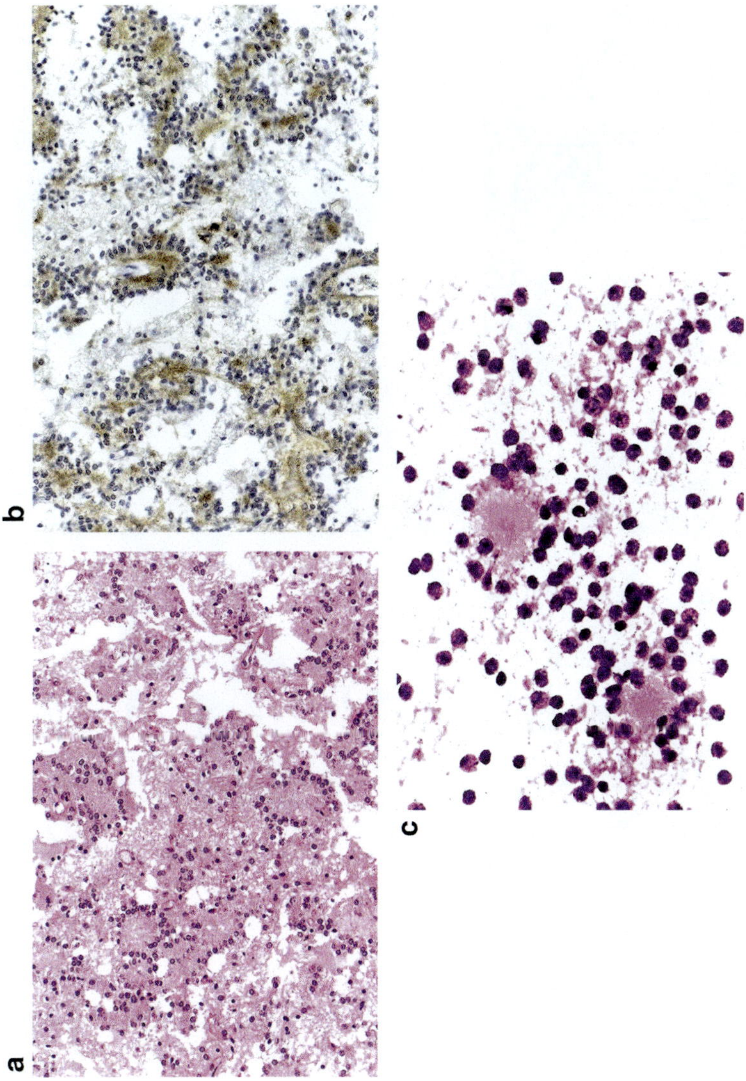

Fig. 11.8 *Rosette-forming glioneuronal tumor, neurocytic element.* **(a)** Histology. Neurocytic rosettes of small diameter that often appear free floating are defining components of this entity. **(b)** The neuropil component of rosettes and perivascular pseudorosettes exhibit immunolabeling for synaptophysin stain. **(c)** Population of small neurocytes with uniform round nuclei and small nucleoli. Although slightly distorted by the smearing process, rosettes with eosinophilic neuropile cores are still evident (Smear, H&E)

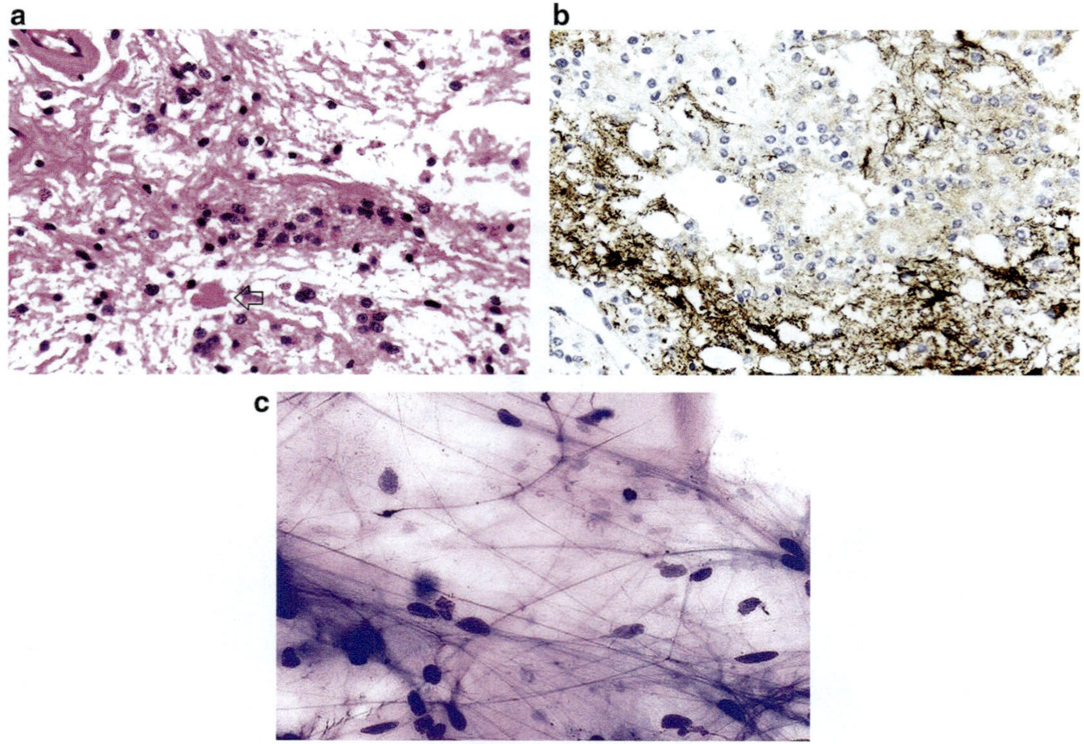

Fig. 11.9 *Rosette-forming glioneuronal tumor, glial element*. (**a**) Histology. The glial element often has the appearance of pilocytic astrocytoma, including the presence of eosinophilic granular bodies (*arrow*). (**b**) Glial fibrillary acidic protein stain expression is present in the glial component, but absent in neurocytic areas. (**c**) Like pilocytic astrocytoma, preparations from this element display very long "piloid" cells and a faint myxoid background (Smear, Romanowsky)

Spinal Paraganglioma

Extra-adrenal paragangliomas arise from neuroendocrine cells associated with autonomic ganglia (paraganglia) of the sympathetic and parasympathetic chains throughout the body. In the craniospinal axis, they typically arise in either the jugulotympanic area or in the filum terminale/cauda equina region of the spinal cord (spinal paraganglioma), at the levels of vertebrae L1 to L3. This tumor usually affects adults, with a peak incidence in the fourth through sixth decades of life, but has been reported in all age groups. Clinical symptoms include a long history of low back pain, sciatica, legs weakness, sphincter dysfunction, and, rarely, hypertension. Radiologically, most cases appear as a discrete, avidly enhancing "sausage-shaped" mass in the filum terminale/cauda equina region (intradural), or attached to a nerve root (extradural); there may be erosion of the surrounding vertebral laminae. Grossly, spinal paragangliomas are well-circumscribed, delicately encapsulated masses allowing total resection (the treatment of choice). Microscopically, the tumor is composed by solid nests or lobules (*Zellballen*) of round to polygonal chief cells within a fibrovascular stroma (Fig. 11.10a). Extensive gangliocytic differentiation is present in nearly one-third of cases, which are termed *gangliocytic paragangliomas*.

Cytologic Features

Smears of paraganglioma are largely discohesive and spread easily, displaying discrete and mildly pleomorphic cells – plasmacytoid, triangular, and polygonal – in a clear, no fibrillary background. Nuclei are round to oval and slightly eccentric with stippled chromatin. As with other endocrine tumors, nuclear atypia (anisokaryosis and larger hyperchromatic nuclei) is common, but this nuclear pleomorphism is not an indicator of biological behavior (Fig. 11.10b). In *gangliocytic paraganglioma*, a high proportion of tumor cells have ganglion morphology (Fig. 11.10c). With a so well-defined clinical picture and location, the main diagnostic dilemmas arise with myxopapillary ependymoma and schwannoma, but because of the epithelial appearance and the occasional cell atypia, it may also be confused with metastatic carcinoma, particularly neuroendocrine carcinoma (both tumors have stippled chromatin).

Differential Diagnosis Considerations of Neuronal and Mixed Neuronal-Glial Tumors

In spite of their nonaggressive clinical behavior, this is the group of tumors that is most easily overgraded during intraoperative consultation, frequently being mistaken for infiltrating gliomas. A careful correlation with clinical and imaging data is essential to avoid a diagnosis of malignancy. A clinical history of long progression and imaging features of well-demarcated tumors are not compatible with aggressive gliomas (Fig. 11.11a, b). With respect to cytomorphology, the frequent presence of

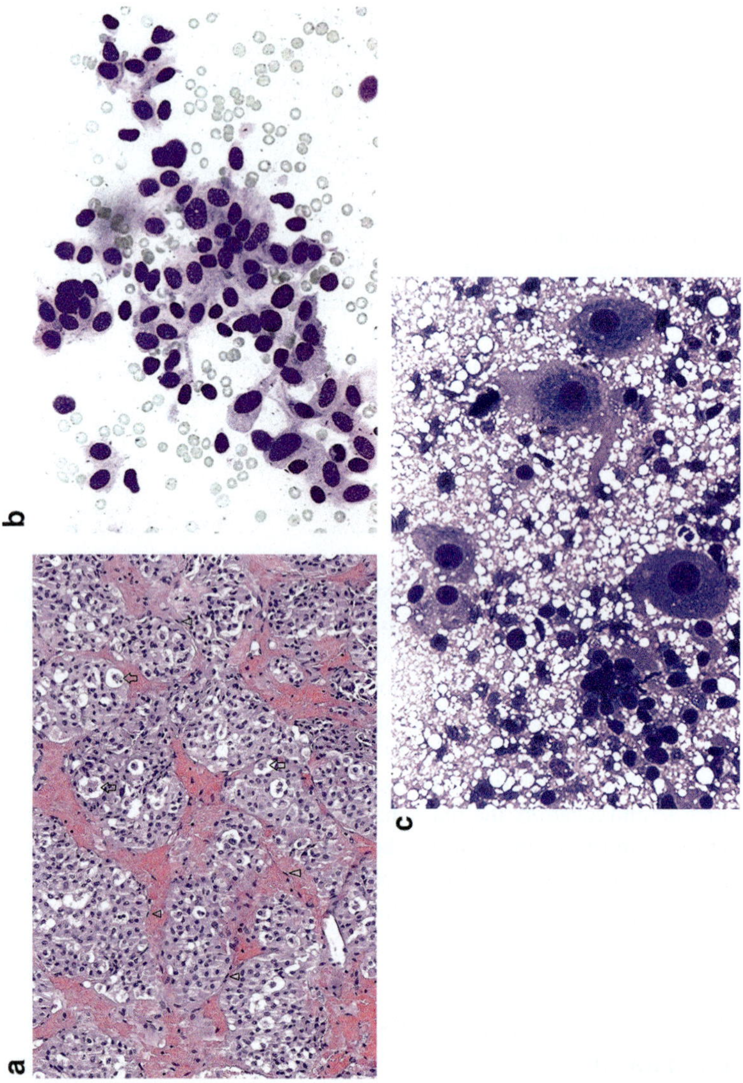

Fig. 11.10 *Spinal paraganglioma*. (**a**) Tissue section displaying a hypervascular tumor with a *Zellballen* pattern consisting of small nests of epithelioid cells. Also note ganglion cell differentiation (*arrows*) and sustentacular cells with a thin bipolar morphology (*arrowheads*). (**b**) Discohesive cluster of medium-size cells exhibiting a rim of cytoplasm and oval nuclei with stippled chromatin. Although some small cytoplasmic bridges span between cells, these tumors lack fine glial processes. Also note endocrine nuclear pleomorphism. (**c**) *Gangliocytic paraganglioma*. Numerous ganglion cells with large, vesicular nuclei and macronucleoli characterize this variant (**b**, **c**; Smears, Romanowsky)

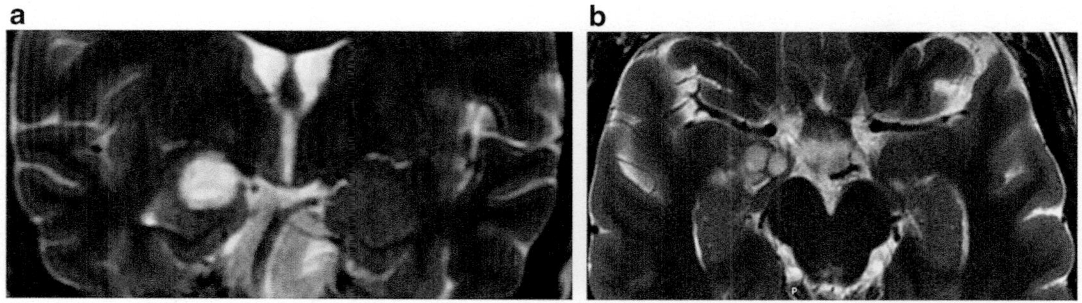

Fig. 11.11 *Imaging features of neuroglial tumors*. (**a**) *Ganglioglioma*. A coronal T2 MR image shows a hyperintense mesiotemporal lesion well-demarcated from surrounding tissue. (**b**) *Dysembryoplastic neuroepithelial tumor*. An axial T2 MR image shows a characteristic multinodular lesion expanding the right mesiotemporal cortex. In both cases there is minimal mass effect and surrounding edema, a useful differential diagnostic feature that helps distinguish them from more aggressive tumors, such as high-grade gliomas

Table 11.1 Differential diagnosis of neuronal and mixed neuronal-glial tumors

Easily overgraded tumors
DNT vs infiltrating glioma
Ganglioglioma vs infiltrating glioma
DIG/DIA vs infiltrating glioma
Neurocytoma vs infiltrating glioma
RGNT vs infiltrating glioma
Paraganglioma vs metastatic carcinoma
Relevant differential features
Clinical data and imaging
Neuronal/neurocytic differentiation
DNT, ganglioglioma, DIG/DIA, RGNT
Presence of eosinophilic granular bodies
Ganglioglioma, RGNT
Presence of Rosenthal fibers

DIG/DIA desmoplastic infantile ganglioglioma/astrocytoma, *DNT* dysembryoplastic neuroepithelial tumor, *RGNT* rosette-forming glioneuronal tumor

EGBs and/or FRs is suggestive of a well-circumscribed and slow-growing low-grade neoplasm (Table 11.1).

Suggested Reading

Bleggi-Torres LF, Netto MR, Gasparetto EL, Gonçalves E, Silva A, Moro M. Dysembryoplastic neuroepithelial tumor: cytological diagnosis by intraoperative smear preparation. Diagn Cytopathol. 2002;26:92–4.

Blümcke I, Wiestler OD. Gangliogliomas: an intriguing tumor entity associated with focal epilepsies. J Neuropathol Exp Neurol. 2002;61:575–84.

Chiang JCH, Ellison DW. Molecular pathology of paediatric central nervous system tumours. J Pathol. 2017;241:159–72.

Donson AM, Kleinschmidt-DeMasters BK, Aisner DL, Bemis LT, et al. Pediatric brainstem gangliogliomas show BRAF(V600E) mutation in a high percentage of cases. Brain Pathol. 2014;24:173–83.

Daumas-Duport C, Scheithauer BW, Chodkiewicz JP, Laws ER, Vedrenne C. Dysembryoplasic neuroepithelial tumor: a surgically curable tumor of young patients with intractable partial seizure. Report of thirty-nine cases. Neurosurgery. 1988;23:545–56.

Chappé C, Padovani L, Scavarda D, Forest F, et al. Dysembryoplastic neuroepithelial tumors share with pleomorphic xanthoastrocytomas and gangliogliomas BRAF (V600E) mutation and expression. Brain Pathol. 2013;23:574–83.

Ellezam B, Theeler BJ, Luthra R, Adesina AM, Aldape KD, Gilbert MR. Recurrent PIK3CA mutations in rosette-forming glioneuronal tumor. Acta Neuropathol. 2012;123:285–7.

Fadare O, Mariappan MR, Hileeto D, Zieske AW, Kim JH, Ocal IT. Desmoplastic infantile ganglioglioma: cytologic findings and differential diagnosis on aspiration material. Cytojournal. 2005;2:1–4.

Gessi M, Moneim YA, Hammes J, Goschzik T, et al. FGFR1 mutations in rosette-forming glioneuronal tumors of the fourth ventricle. J Neuropathol Exp Neurol. 2014;73:580–4.

Gessi M, Zur Mühlen A, Hammes J, Waha A, Denkhaus D, Pietsch T. Genome-wide DNA copy number analysis of desmoplastic infantile astrocytomas and desmoplastic infantile gangliogliomas. J Neuropathol Exp Neurol. 2013;72:807–15.

González-Cámpora R, Otal-Salaverri C, Panea-Flores P, Lerma-Puertas E, Galera-Davidson H. Fine needle aspiration cytology of paraganglionic tumors. Acta Cytol. 1988;32:386–90.

Ghosal N, Furtado SV, Hegde AS. Rosette forming glioneuronal tumor pineal gland and tectum: an intraoperative diagnosis on smear preparation. Diagn Cytopathol. 2010;38:590–3.

Hasegawa Y, Hayabuchi Y, Namba I, Watanabe T, et al. Cytologic features of desmoplastic ganglioglioma. A report of two cases. Acta Cytol. 2001;45:1037–42.

Hernández-Martínez SJ, De Leíja-Portilla JO, Medellín-Sánchez R. Cytologic features during intraoperative assessment of central neurocytoma: a report of three cases and review of the literature. Acta Cytol. 2013;57:400–5.

Horbinski C, Kofler J, Yeaney G, Camelo-Piragua S, et al. Isocitrate dehydrogenase 1 analysis differentiates gangliogliomas from infiltrative gliomas. Brain Pathol. 2011;21:564–74.

Hsu C, Kwan G, Lau Q, Bhuta S. Rosette-forming glioneuronal tumour: imaging features, histopathological correlation and a comprehensive review of literature. Br J Neurosurg. 2012;26:668–73.

Jaiswall S, Vij M, Jaiswal AK, Behari S. Squash cytomorphology of central neurocytoma. A study of five cases. Diagn Cytopathol. 2012;40:678–83.

Kinno M, Ishizawa K, Shimada S, Masaoka H, et al. Cytology is a useful tool for the diagnosis of rosette-forming glioneuronal tumour of the fourth ventricle: a report of two cases. Cytopathology. 2010;21:194–7.

Klysik M, Gavito J, Boman D, Miranda RN, Hanbali F, De Las Casas LE. Intraoperative imprint cytology of central neurocytoma: The great oligodendroglioma mimicker. Diagn Cytopathol. 2010;38:202–7.

Kobayashi TK, Bamba M, Ueda M, Nishino T, et al. Cytologic diagnosis of central neurocytoma in intraoperative squash preparations: a report of 2 cases. Acta Cytol. 2010;54:209–13.

Koelsche C, Wöhrer A, Jeibmann A, Schittenhelm J, et al. Mutant BRAF V600E protein in ganglioglioma is predominantly expressed by neuronal tumor cells. Acta Neuropathol. 2013;125:891–900.

Komori T, Arai N. Dysembryoplastic neuroepithelial tumor, a pure glial tumor? Immunohistochemical and morphometric studies. Neuropathology. 2013;33:459–68.

Komori T, Scheithauer BW, Hirose T. A rosette-forming glioneuronal tumor of the fourth ventricle: infratentorial form of dysembryoplastic neuroepithelial tumor? Am J Surg Pathol. 2002;26:582–91.

Loesel LS. Fine needle aspiration cytology of a cerebral ganglioglioma. Report of a case. Acta Cytol. 1988;32:391–4.

Moran CA, Rush W, Mena H. Primary spinal paragangliomas: a clinicopathological and immunohistochemical study of 30 cases. Histopathology. 1997;31:167–73.

Ng H. Cytologic features of central neurocytomas of the brain. A report of three cases. Acta Cytol. 1999;43:252–6.

Park J, Suh Y, Han J. Dysembryoplastic neuroepithelial tumor. Features distinguishing it from oligodendroglioma on cytologic squash preparations. Acta Cytol. 2003;47:624–9.

Rivera B, Gayden T, Carrot-Zhang J, Nadal J, et al. Germline and somatic FGFR1 abnormalities in dysembryoplastic neuroepithelial tumors. Acta Neuropathol. 2016;131:847–3.

Schild SE, Scheithauer BW, Haddock MG, Schiff D, et al. Central neurocytomas. Cancer. 1997;79:790–5.

Sugita Y, Tokunaga O, Morimatsu M, Abe H. Cytodiagnosis of central neurocytoma in intraoperative preparations. Acta Cytol. 2004;48:194–8.
Varma K, Jain S, Mandal S. Cytomorphologic spectrum in paraganglioma. Acta Cytol. 2008;52:549–56.
Wolf HK, Wietsler OD. Surgical pathology of chronic epileptic seizure disorders. Brain Pathol. 1995;3:371–80.
Zanello M, Pages M, Tauzi̇̀ede-Espariat A, Saffroy R, et al. Clinical imaging, histopathological and molecular characterization of anaplastic ganglioglioma. J Neuropathol Exp Neurol. 2016;75:971–80.

Chapter 12
Embryonal (Primitive) Tumors

Although there is significant histological variability, embryonal tumors are grouped together because they are, at least partially, composed of poorly differentiated neuroepithelial cells resembling the cells that make up the most primitive or embryonal stages of the CNS – the germinal matrix stem cell population. These tumors characteristically occur in children and adolescents (0–14 years) and together comprise 15–20% of all CNS tumors in this age group. All embryonal neoplasms are characterized by an aggressive behavior with a high frequency of local recurrence, spread through the CSF and, even, can spread as extraneural metastasis (WHO grade IV tumors). Molecular studies have substantiated the differences between tumors arising in different areas of the brain and give credence to the following 2016 WHO classification approach: *medulloblastoma*, an embryonal tumor arising in the cerebellum or, rarely, dorsal brainstem, with four major molecular subgroups based on differences in the gene expression profiles; *embryonal tumor with multilayered rosettes, C19MC-altered*, an embryonal tumor arising in both the supratentorial and infratentorial regions and characterized by C19MC locus amplification or fusion; *atypical teratoid/rhabdoid tumor (AT/RT)*, an embryonal neoplasm that may be located throughout the neuroaxis and characterized by loss of *INI1* or, rarely, *BRG1* expression; and *other CNS embryonal tumors*, a group of rare embryonal neoplasms that lack the specific histopathological features or molecular alterations that define other CNS tumors, which are typically located in the cerebral hemispheres with rare examples occurring in the brain stem and spinal cord. Except for AT/RT, the rest of embryonal tumors are all considered poorly differentiated tumors of neuronal lineage.

C. R. Lacruz et al., *Central Nervous System Intraoperative Cytopathology*, Essentials in Cytopathology 13, https://doi.org/10.1007/978-3-319-98491-9_12

Medulloblastoma

Medulloblastoma is the most common embryonal tumor (over 60–70% of all cases), with a peak age at diagnosis of 7–9 years and a male-to-female ratio around 1.5:1. It is more often vermian in children, whereas in young adults it is more often hemispheric. The etiology for this tumor is unclear, except for a small fraction of children who harbor a germline mutation of a tumor-suppressor gene, i.e., Gorlin syndrome or, even more rarely, type 2 Turcot syndrome or Li-Fraumeni syndrome.

Patients often present with irritability, lethargy, and loss of appetite, followed by symptoms of increase intracranial pressure (headache, morning emesis) and cerebellar signs – truncal ataxia and disturbed gait (midline lesions) or appendicular ataxia and dysmetria (hemispheric lesions). The radiologic appearance is that of large, T2-hyperintense masses with heterogeneous enhancement and peritumoral edema. Striking nodularity ("bunch of grapes") is characteristic in the extensively nodular type. Distant seeding of the subarachnoid space may be identified on neuroimaging and is associated with decreased rates of survival (one-third of cases will already have seeded the cerebrospinal fluid at diagnosis, especially as spinal drop metastases).

Macroscopically, medulloblastomas are soft, pink-gray masses with small foci of necrosis and sometimes hemorrhagic areas, whereas desmoplastic tumors tend to be firm. They frequently invade the subarachnoid space, forming whitish granular aggregates often referred to as "sugar coating" or "icing" (see Chap. 3, Fig. 3.1c).

Microscopically, they are composed of densely packed small cells with hyperchromatic nuclei and minimal cytoplasm, even though there is considerable intertumoral variation. About 70% of cases consist of small, uniform cells that vary little in size and shape (*classic medulloblastoma*; Fig. 12.1a). In 20–25% of cases, conspicuous neurocytic differentiation occurs, which may take place in the form of isolated nodes (pale islands) surrounded by densely packed proliferative cells with a dense intercellular reticulin network (*desmoplastic/nodular medulloblastoma*; Fig. 12.1b) or else in an extended fashion producing large, lobular, and elongated free-reticulin zones (*medulloblastoma with extensive nodularity*). The remaining others – approximately 10% – are composed, either focally or globally, of extremely malignant larger or more anaplastic cells (*large-cell/anaplastic medulloblastomas*; Fig. 12.1c). A subset of classic medulloblastomas (roughly 10%) displays nodules similar to those in desmoplastic/nodular type, but no perinodular reticulin (*biphasic classic medulloblastoma*).

Based on differences in the gene expression profiles, the current consensus considers four principal molecular categories of medulloblastoma (Table 12.1).

The SHH-activated, *TP53*-mutant and the group 3 variants are the most lethal, requiring more aggressive therapeutic strategies. On the other hand, large-cell/anaplastic histology may be a prognostic factor independent of molecular grouping. Thus, histopathological and molecular classifications complement each other in order to provide optimal prognostic and predictive information.

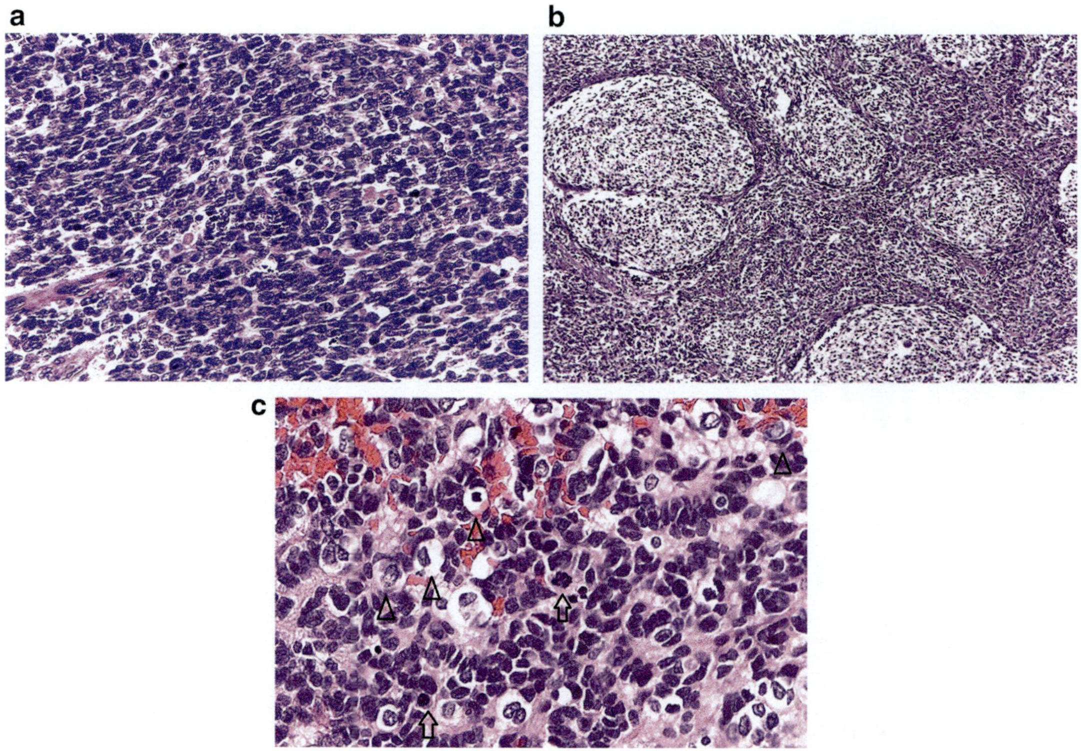

Fig. 12.1 *Medulloblastoma, histology*. (**a**) *Classic*. Typical appearance composed of a monotonous sea of undifferentiated tumors cells. (**b**) *Desmoplastic/nodular*. Pale nodular areas of neurocytoma-like cells that appear demarcated by densely packed hyperchromatic cells characterize this variant. (**c**) *Large cell/anaplastic*. Increased nuclear size, pleomorphism, mitosis (*arrows*), and cell wrapping (*arrowheads*) are features of anaplasia in medulloblastoma

Table 12.1 Characteristics of medulloblastoma molecular groups and surrogate IHC

Medulloblastoma, WNT-activated (around 11%)
IHC: nuclear β-catenin (+), YAP1 (+), GAB1 (−), INI1 retained
Predominant age(s): mostly older children, some adults
Virtually all cases classic histology
Excellent prognosis
Medulloblastoma, *SHH*-activated (around 28%)
IHC: cytoplasmic β-catenin (+), YAP1 (+), GAB1 (+), INI1 retained
For this group, the presence of a *TP53* mutation should be reported
TP53-wild type (around 22%); IHC: p53 (−)
Predominant age(s): bimodal, infants, and adults
Desmoplastic, MBEN, classic, and LCA histology
Infants good prognosis, others intermediate
TP53-mutant (around 6%); IHC: p53 (+)
Predominant age: children
Classic and LCA histology
Poor prognosis
Medulloblastoma, group 3 (around 28%)
IHC: β-catenin (−), YAP1 (−), GAB1 (−), INI1 retained
Predominant age(s): infants and children, almost never in adults
LCA and classic histology; *MYC* overexpression/amplification
Poorest prognosis of all groups
Medulloblastoma, group 4 (around 34%)
IHC: β-catenin (−), YAP1 (−), GAB1 (−), INI1 retained
All age groups (peak incidence 5–15 years)
Majority classic histology, LCA rare
Intermediate prognosis (standard-risk)

IHC (immunohistochemistry) cannot distinguish between group 3 and group 4 tumors (both designated as non-SHH/WNT subgroup by ICH analysis), *LCA* large cell/anaplastic, *MBEN* medulloblastoma with extensive nodularity

Currently, by using a combination of therapies including surgical resection, risk-adjusted irradiation and adjuvant chemotherapy, about 70% of pediatric medulloblastomas can be cured.

General Diagnostic Approach

Because an incomplete gross surgical resection is a significant negative prognostic factor (patients with greaterthan1.5 cm^2 cross-sectional area residual tumor have a worse prognosis), an accurate intraoperative diagnosis of medulloblastoma is crucial for management. On the other hand, intraoperative cytological evaluation allows one to distinguish large-cell/anaplastic variants from classic/nodular variants, and this can be of prognostic value during surgery.

Cytologic Features

Classic medulloblastoma exfoliates cells very easily. Smear preparations are highly cellular and evenly distributed with discohesive sheets of small, rounded or wedge-shaped cells with minimal cytoplasm. Nuclei have a slightly coarse "salt-and-pepper" chromatin and lack nucleoli, whereas nuclear membranes show folds and indentations, but they are not highly convoluted (Fig. 12.2a). In contrast to completely discohesive tumors like lymphomas, medulloblastoma nuclei often stick together forming short chains or circles or conform around each other, giving the characteristic nuclear molding (Fig. 12.2b). The *desmoplastic/nodular variant* elaborates an extensive neuropil matrix and remains less cellular than their more primitive counterparts. In the smear, its neuropil matrix leads to the finely granular background that hosts the tumor cells. Neurocytic differentiation is common (Fig. 12.3a, b). *Large-cell/anaplastic variants* give cellular smears with large nuclei, coarser chromatin, and/or prominent nucleoli. Nuclear molding, brisk mitosis, numerous apoptotic bodies, and the presence of nuclei that appear to wrap around or encompass other nuclei (cell wrapping) are also useful features for these variants (Fig. 12.4a, b).

CNS Embryonal Tumors Replacing PNET

Tumors formerly designated CNS PNETs are now separated into two groups: *embryonal tumor with multilayered rosettes (ETMR), C19MC-altered*, and *other CNS embryonal tumors*.

The genetic basis for ETMR, C19MC-altered, as a novel category of embryonal neoplasms is an amplification or fusion of a small segment of DNA on 19q13.42 that contains the largest cluster of miRNAs in humans. This segment is referred to as C19MC, which abbreviates "chromosome 19 microRNA cluster." The term ETMR encompasses three histologic patterns: (1) *embryonal tumor with abundant neuropil and true rosettes (ETANTR)*, a biphasic neoplasm featuring clusters of small, undifferentiated cells and fibrillary/neuropil-like areas with well-formed epithelial rosettes (Fig. 12.5a); (2) *medulloepithelioma*, a tumor composed of glands or

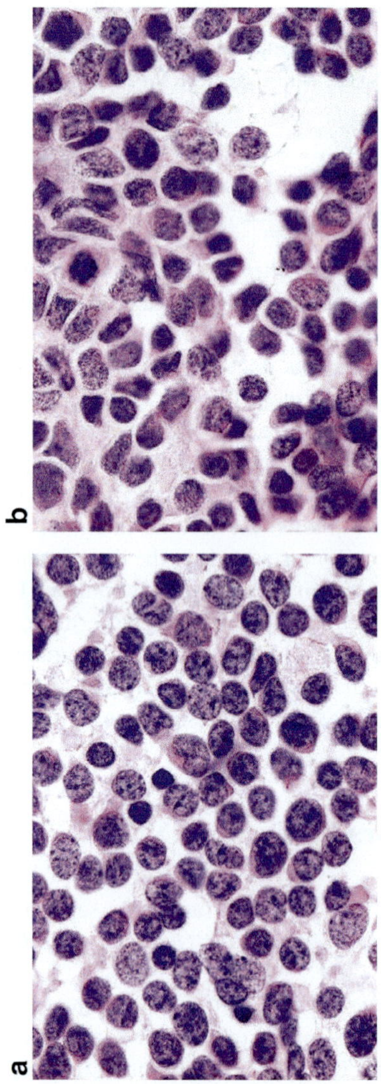

Fig. 12.2 *Classic medulloblastoma, cytologic features.* (**a**) Characteristic discohesive pattern of small, round cells with hyperchromatic nuclei and minimal cytoplasm. (**b**) Nuclei often conform around each other, giving the characteristic nuclear molding. Also a small numbers of nuclei stick together, forming short chains or circles (**a**, **b**; Smears, H&E)

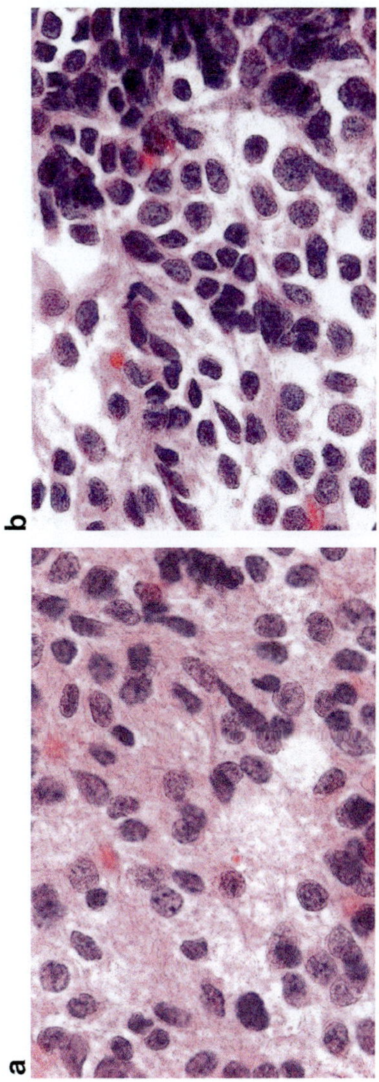

Fig. 12.3 *Desmoplastic/nodular medulloblastoma, cytologic features*. (**a**) Rather than having no background, this variant displays abundant pink neuropil. (**b**) Tumor cells with neurocytic differentiation contrast with the densely packed hyperchromatic cells in the upper right corner, which show nuclear moldings and angulations (**a**, **b**; Smears, H&E)

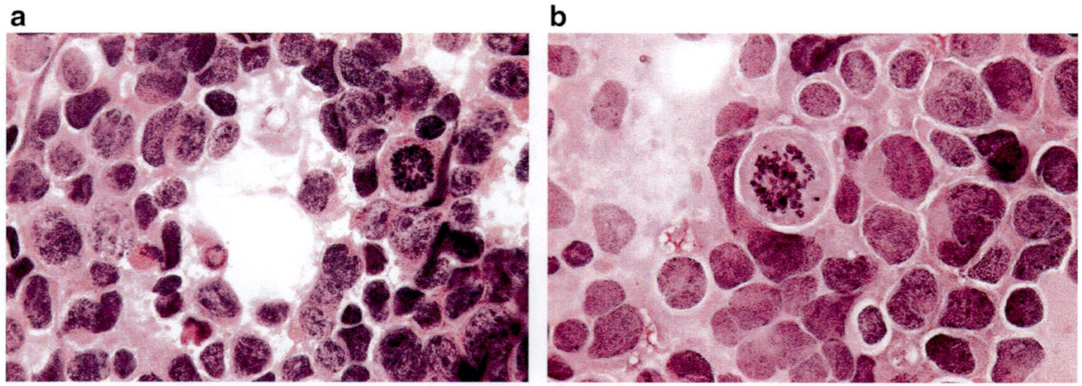

Fig. 12.4 *Large-cell/anaplastic medulloblastoma, cytologic features.* (**a**) This preparation displays large pleomorphic cells, mitotic figures, and frequent apoptotic bodies. (**b**) Additionally, "cannibalistic" cell wrapping, wherein some tumor cells phagocytose the neighbor just in mitosis, is well seen here (**a**, **b**; Smears, H&E)

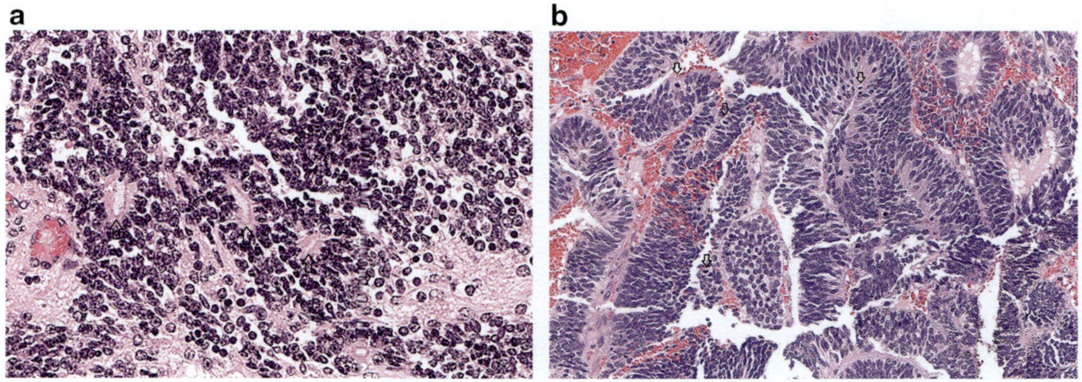

Fig. 12.5 *Embryonal tumors with multilayered rosettes (ETMR), histology.* (**a**) Characteristic features of *embryonal tumor with abundant neuropil and true rosettes (ETANTR)* combine fibrillar neuropil and true, lumen-containing rosettes (*arrows*). (**b**) The rare *medulloepithelioma* neoplasm recapitulates the embryonic neural tube with epithelioid ribbons and glands. Mitoses are characteristically located superficially, near the lumen (*arrows*)

tubules of primitive appearing epithelium that resembles the epithelium of the developing brain (Fig. 12.5b); and (3) *ependymoblastoma*, a neoplasm with innumerable true ependymal rosettes and no perivascular pseudorosettes. This group of embryonal tumors exclusively affects infants and young children under the age of 3 years, can develop in both the supratentorial and infratentorial compartments, and has a distinctly dismal prognosis (overall survival about 10 months). Immunohistochemically, C19MC-altered ETMR varieties share strong and diffuse LIN 28A cytoplasmic positivity; however, due to LIN 28A lack of specificity (also found in AT/RT, GCTs, teratomas, and some gliomas), interphase fluorescence in situ hybridization (iFISH) for C19MC is now routinely used for the diagnosis of this group of aggressive embryonal neoplasms. Of note, up to one quarter of medulloepitheliomas analyzed genetically has not shown C19MC alterations (*medulloepithelioma, C19MC-unaltered*).

The term "other CNS embryonal tumors" comprises a group of rare, poorly differentiated embryonal neoplasms that lack the specific histopathological features or molecular alterations that define other CNS tumors. Histologically, three varieties are recognized: (1) *CNS neuroblastoma*, zones of neurocytic differentiation are formed among sheets of densely packed embryonal cells (Fig. 12.6a); (2) *CNS ganglioneuroblastoma*, zones of neurocytic and ganglion cell differentiation are formed among sheets of densely packed embryonal cells (Fig. 12.6b); and (3) *CNS embryonal tumor, NOS*, only sheets of densely packed embryonal cells. These neoplasms occur primarily in children and young people (rare in adults), are typically located in the cerebral hemispheres with occasional examples reported in the brain stem and spinal cord, and have a worse prognosis as a group than medulloblastoma (5-year survival 29–57%). Recent genomic studies suggest that many of the CNS neuroblastomas and ganglioneuroblastomas correspond to a newly designated molecular subtype, known as *"CNS neuroblastoma with FOXR2 activation"*; such cases are associated with complex chromosomal rearrangements converging on forkhead box R2 (FOXR2) and show strong OLIG2 expression.

Cytologic Features

The cytomorphologic features are similar to those of medulloblastoma, with tumors smearing out into a diffuse monolayer of small-to-midsize primitive-looking cells. Nuclei are round to oval or carrot-shaped with granular chromatin, whereas the cytoplasm is minimal (Fig. 12.7a, b). Additionally, some cases may show better differentiated neuroepithelial/neuronal features, i.e., neuroepithelial "true" rosettes, Homer-Wright rosettes, or neurocytic to ganglionic cytomorphology, which are very useful findings to confirm the neuroepithelial nature of an otherwise undifferentiated process. For example, the presence of neuroepithelial "true" rosettes is the

a b

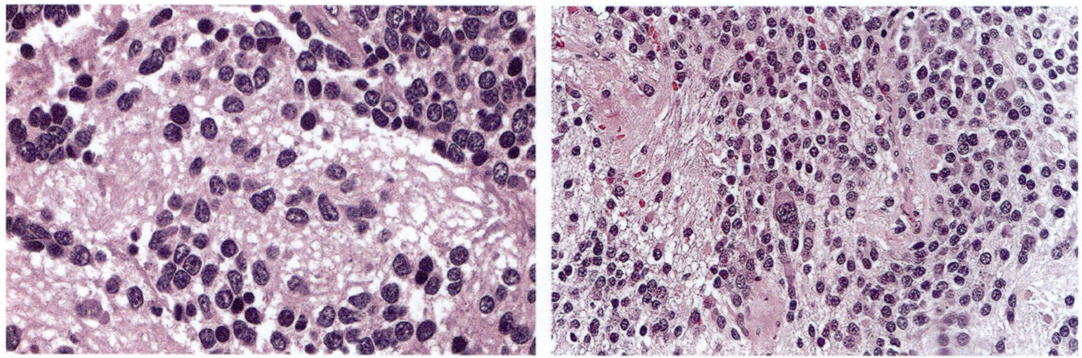

Fig. 12.6 *Other CNS embryonal tumors, histology*. (**a**) *CNS neuroblastoma*. Neuroblastic tumor cells surrounding nuclei-free areas of neuropil characterize this embryonal tumor. (**b**) *CNS ganglioneuroblastoma*. This tumor has similar histologic features to CNS neuroblastoma, except that groups of dystrophic-appearing ganglion cells are also present

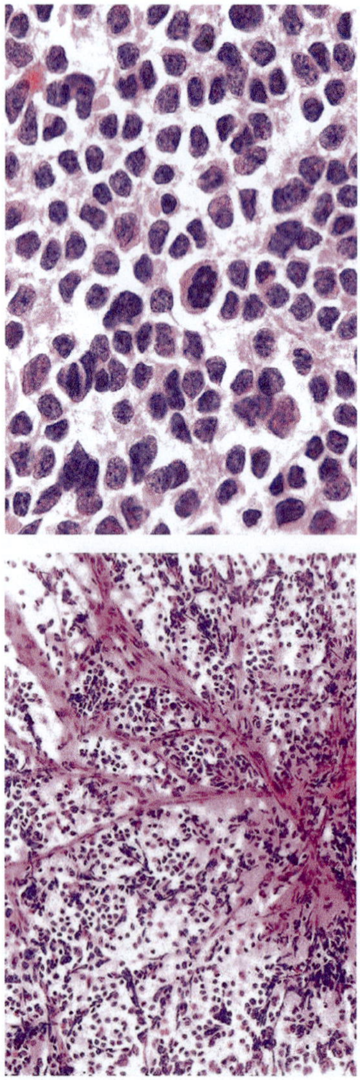

Fig. 12.7 *CNS embryonal tumors replacing PNET, cytologic features.* (**a**) This preparation from a supratentorial example shows a discohesive pattern of small, undifferentiated cells and prominent fibrovascular stroma. (**b**) A high-magnification view displays a monotonous population of primitive-looking cells with round or carrot-shaped nuclei and stippled chromatin. Also note a mitotic figure in the central region (**a**, **b**; Smears, H&E)

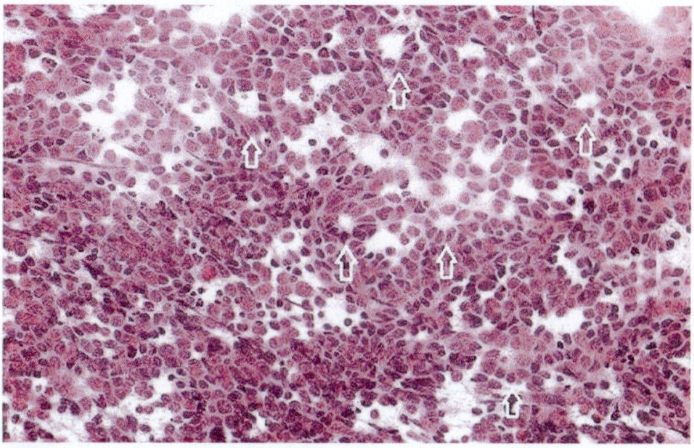

Fig. 12.8 Preparation from an *ependymoblastoma* showing numerous lumen-containing rosettes (*arrows*) in a small-cell (primitive) background of embryonal neoplasm. Unlike anaplastic ependymoma, fibrillary processes are lacking (Smear, H&E)

characteristic feature of *ETMR varieties* (Fig.12.8); *CNS neuroblastoma* often displays Homer-Wright rosettes with central tangles of neuropil and neuroblastic cells with unipolar cytoplasmic processes (Fig. 12.9a, b), whereas in *CNS ganglioneuroblastoma*, both neurocytic and ganglion cell differentiation can be identified (Fig.12.10).

Differential Diagnosis Considerations of Medulloblastoma/ CNS Embryonal Tumors Replacing PNET

Age is clearly a critical factor to consider when encountering embryonal-appearing tumors. Therefore, the most important differential diagnosis includes small-cell gliomas (mainly anaplastic ependymoma) in children and adolescents and metastatic small-cell lung carcinoma in adults. Embryonal tumors do not show an obvious fibrillary background and often smear out into a diffuse monolayer, unlike ependymomas, which often show tissue fibrillary fragments and perivascular pseudorosettes. On the other hand, in adults, an extra-cerebellar location, the presence of multiple lesions, the existence of a lung lesion, and the absence of neuronal differentiation point toward a metastatic small-cell lung tumor. In addition, small-cell carcinomas tend to smear in aggregates with frequent crush artifact. Lymphoma may also be a consideration, although abundant lymphoglandular bodies are absent. Differentiation from a PNET-like AT/RT is a particularly difficult issue covered in the description of this tumor. In the chapter of normal brain cytology, we already mentioned that the inexperienced must be aware of interpreting smears with normal cerebellar cortex as medulloblastoma, but granular cells can be distinguished by

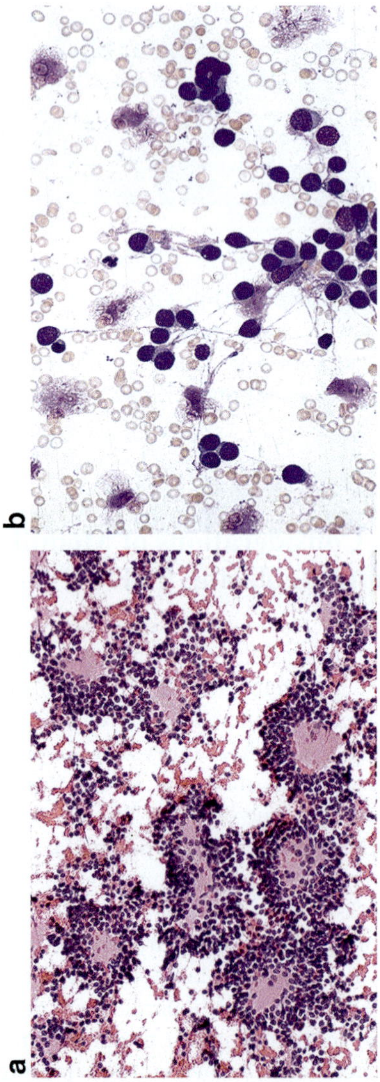

Fig. 12.9 *CNS neuroblastoma.* (**a**) One of the most characteristic cytomorphologic features is the presence of neuroblastic rosettes with fibrillary cores of neuropil (smear, H&E). (**b**) Typical primitive neuronal (neuroblastic) cells with unipolar cytoplasmic extensions (smear, Romanowsky)

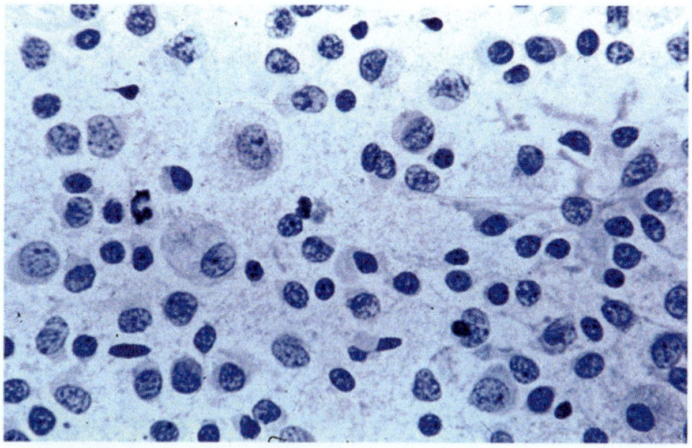

Fig. 12.10 *CNS ganglioneuroblastoma.* In this case a differentiated cellular population with clearly neurocytic and neuronal features is well seen (Smear, toluidine blue)

their small size (similar to a small lymphocyte) and uniformity (Fig. 12.11a, b). Table 12.2 summarizes the characteristics of medulloblastoma/CNS embryonal tumors replacing PNET.

Atypical Teratoid/Rhabdoid Tumor

Atypical teratoid/rhabdoid tumor (AT/RT) is a highly malignant polyphenotypic neoplasm (EMA, GFAP, SMA, and CK +) that is pathogenetically and morphologically similar to the malignant rhabdoid tumors of the kidney and soft tissue and represents about 15% of CNS embryonal tumors. AT/RT primarily affects children, with most patients younger than 3 years, and can occur anywhere along the neuroaxis including the cerebral hemispheres, the ventricular system, the suprasellar and pineal regions, the brain stem, the cerebellum, the cerebellopontine angle (typical location), and the spinal cord (rare). AT/RT is now defined by alterations (mutation or loss) of either *INI1/SMARCB1* or, very rarely, *BRG1/SMARCA4* tumor-suppressor genes on chromosome 22q11.2. Familial cases may occur in a condition known as *rhabdoid tumor predisposition syndrome* in which germline inactivation of 1 allele of a gene occurs.

Symptoms depend on location, with seeding along CSF pathways (i.e., drop metastases) found in as many as one quarter of all patients at presentation. The imaging and gross findings are similar to those for other embryonal tumors: large, variably enhancing masses with frequent hemorrhage and necrosis.

Microscopically, these are heterogeneous lesions that contain a combination of rhabdoid cells and epithelioid cells with pale or clear cytoplasm. Additionally, tumors may contain variable components with embryonal (primitive), sarcomatoid, and/or epithelial features, but unlike others embryonal tumors in this chapter, the AT/RT usually lacks neuronal differentiation (Fig. 12.12a, b). In some examples, the small-cell (primitive) component is predominant with scant representation of diagnostic rhabdoid cells (PNET-like AT/RT). In this respect, loss of nuclear immu-

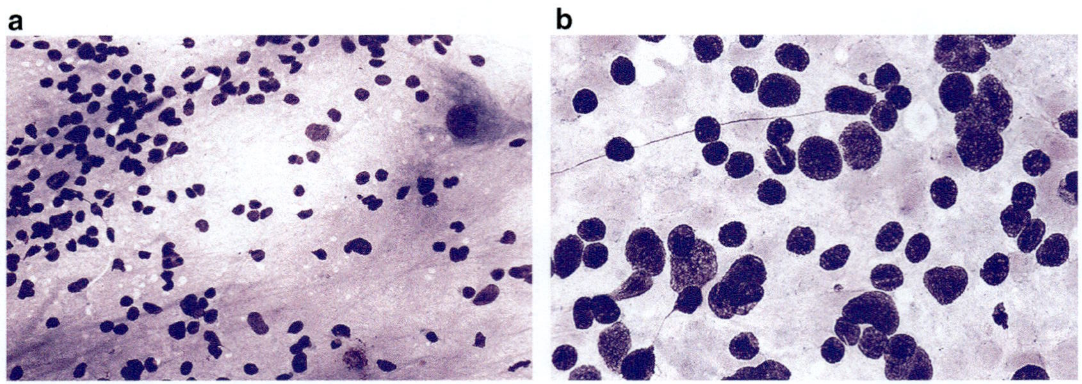

Fig. 12.11 *Medulloblastoma infiltrating cerebellar cortex.* (**a**) Mixed cellular pattern with small and very small hyperchromatic cells. Also note a large Purkinje's neuron in the upper right corner. (**b**) A high-magnification view reveals significant differences between tumor cells and neurons from the granular cell layer, which are smaller and more uniform (**a**, **b**; Smears, Romanowsky)

Table 12.2 Characteristics of medulloblastoma/CNS embryonal tumors replacing PNET

Cytologic features		
	Highly cellular smears with discohesive pattern	
	Small, primitive-looking cells with minimal cytoplasm	
	Clear or finely granular background, sometimes necrotic	
	Features of neuroepithelial/neuronal differentiation	
		Neuroepithelial "true" rosettes
		Homer Wright rosettes
		Neurocytic to ganglionic cytomorphology
	Conspicuous neuronal differentiation in	
	Desmoplastic/nodular medulloblastoma and MBEN	
	CNS neuroblastoma and ganglioneuroblastoma	
	Features of anaplasia	
	Large and pleomorphic cells	
	Coarser chromatin or prominent nucleoli	
	Brisk mitosis and apoptosis	
	Cell-to-cell wrapping	
Differential diagnosis and pitfalls		
	Small-cell gliomas	
	Metastatic small-cell lung carcinoma	
	Lymphoma	
	PNET-like atypical teratoid/rhabdoid tumor	
	Normal cerebellar cortex	

MBEN medulloblastoma with extensive nodularity, *PNET* primitive neuroectodermal tumor

noreactivity for INI1 (antibody BAF47) is now routinely used to confirm or rule out AT/RT in embryonal neoplasms (Fig. 12.12c). In the rare event that one has a tumor that is strongly suspicious for AT/RT but has retained SMARCB1/INI1 expression, consideration should be given to testing for loss of SMARCA4/BRG1 expression (can also be detected by IHC).

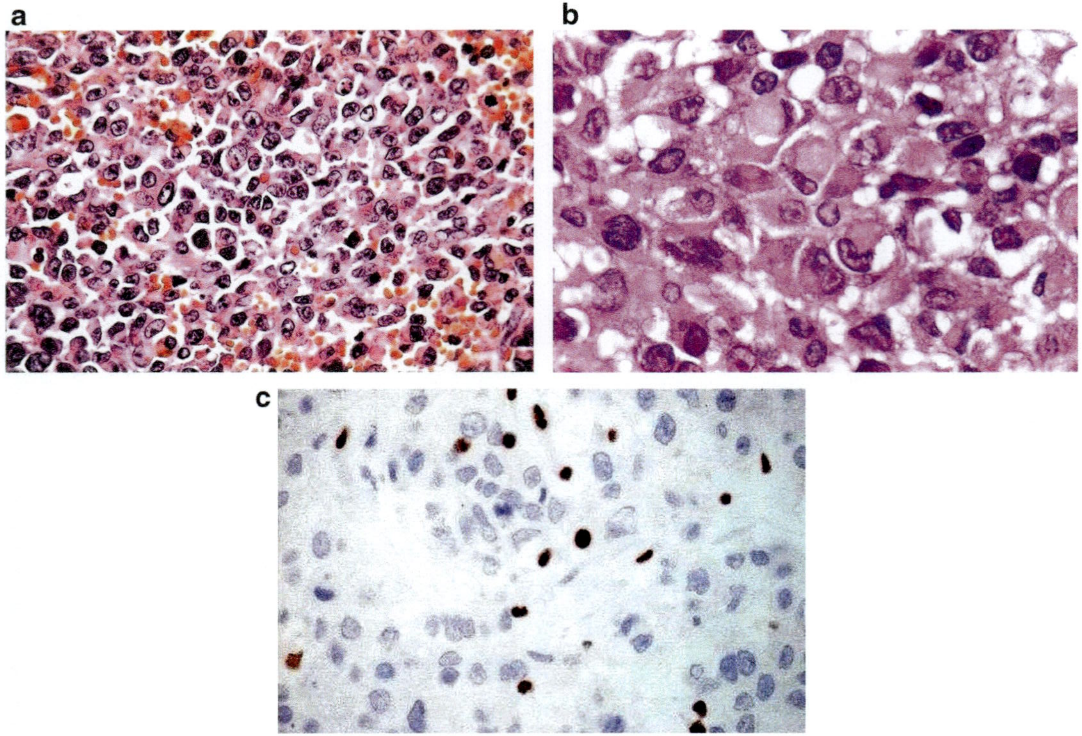

Fig. 12.12 *Atypical teratoid/rhabdoid tumor (AT/RT), histology.* (**a**) Fields of monotonous cells with large, round nuclei and prominent nucleoli (seen here) are a common feature. (**b**) Large jumbled cells, some with rhabdoid features, as these also are characteristic. (**c**) The immunohistochemical absence of INI1 protein expression in a suspected AT/RT is diagnostic, along with characteristic immunopositivity for tumor blood vessels as an internal positive control

They are differences in survival by age at diagnosis, treatment pattern, and location of tumor in the brain, but overall this tumor carries a distinctly poor prognosis with a mean survival after surgery generally less than 1 year. However, gross total resection/debulking and intensive multimodal therapy may improve it.

Cytologic Features

Intraoperative squash preparations have a mixture of pseudopapillary and diffuse smearing patterns with isolated elements, loose clusters, and perivascular aggregates around branching vessels (unlike other embryonal tumors, the AT/RT cells often show a high affinity for blood vessels). Tumor cells show a range of features from embryonal (primitive) to epithelioid. Diagnostic cells are of medium/large size with rhabdoid, polygonal, or elongated features and distinct borders. Nuclei are located eccentrically, with pale chromatin and prominent nucleoli. The cytoplasm is eosinophilic to pale with occasional paranuclear inclusion bodies that represent intermediate filaments whorls. Also bi−/multinucleated cells, mitosis, apoptotic bodies, and granular (necrotic) background may be seen (Fig. 12.13a–c). In some examples, the small-cell component is predominant (e.g., simple nuclei with minimal cytoplasm), being indistinguishable from other embryonal tumors.

Differential Diagnosis Considerations

Based on age and location, the differential diagnosis must be made with the other embryonal tumors, but the cytological picture described above, if present, is so defining that allows an accurate diagnosis of AT/RT. However, in cases with predominance of small-cell component, an intraoperative diagnosis of rhabdoid tumor may be unreliable. In such circumstances a preliminary report of "high-grade, neuroepithelial small-cell neoplasm" is preferable. We also must include in the differential diagnosis other tumors with rhabdoid phenotype, such as rhabdoid meningioma and metastatic tumor with rhabdoid features (carcinoma, melanoma, or sarcoma) whose appearance may be almost identical. In such cases, clinico-radiologic correlation is necessary; in the absence of these data, a descriptive report of "high-grade, malignant tumor with rhabdoid features" is adequate. Germinoma may also be a consideration, although the combination of a dual cell population (large germ cells and small lymphocytes) in a striped "tigroid" background allows an accurate diagnosis of germinoma. We already mentioned that an intraoperative differentiation from solid, anaplastic choroid plexus carcinoma may be unreliable (Table. 12.3).

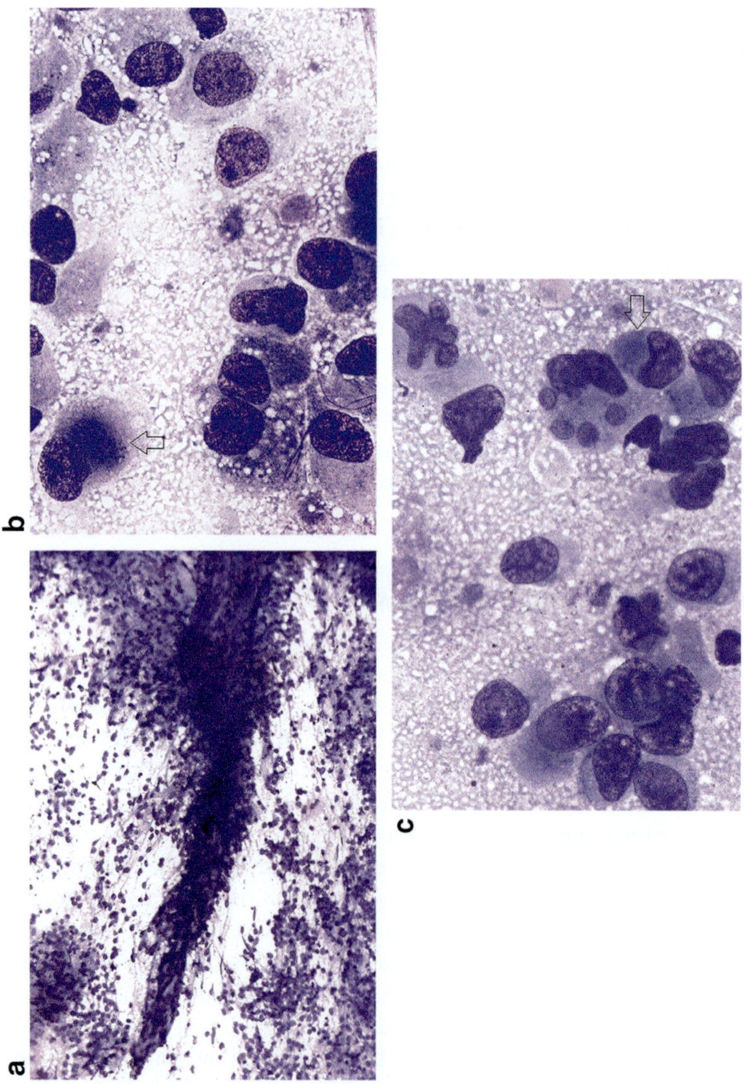

Fig. 12.13 *Atypical teratoid/rhabdoid tumor (AT/RT), cytologic features.* (**a**) Unlike other embryonal tumors, the AT/RT cells often show a high affinity for blood vessels. In this preparation, they form ragged collars around rigid vessels. (**b**) A high-power view display characteristics rhabdoid cells with open chromatin and prominent nucleoli. The eccentricity of cytoplasm in some of these cells is a clue. Also note a dense paranuclear inclusion body that pushes the nucleus to the side (*arrow*). (**c**) Along with typical rhabdoid cells (*arrow*), this preparation shows larger multinucleated cells (**a–c**; Smears, Romanowsky)

Table 12.3 Characteristics of atypical teratoid/rhabdoid tumor

Cytologic features	
	Highly cellular smears
	Isolated cells, loose clusters, and perivascular aggregates
	Tumor cells show a range of features
	Rhabdoid (eccentric nuclei and condensed cytoplasm)
	Epithelial (large, pale cytoplasm)
	Primitive (simple nuclei with minimal cytoplasm)
	Large multinucleated
	Apoptotic and mitotic figures
Differential diagnosis and pitfalls	
	Medulloblastoma[a]
	CNS embryonal tumors replacing PNET
	Rhabdoid meningioma
	Metastatic tumor with rhabdoid features
	Germinoma
	Choroid plexus carcinoma

[a]consider possibility of AT/RT, no medulloblastoma, if patient is below the age of 3 years

Suggested Reading

Burger PC, Yu IT, Tihan T, Friedman HS, et al. Atypical teratoid/rhabdoid tumor of the central nervous system: a highly malignant tumor of infancy and childhood frequently mistaken for medulloblastoma: a Pediatric Oncology Group study. Am J Surg Pathol. 1998;22:1083–92.

Chiang JCH, Ellison DW. Molecular pathology of paediatric central nervous system tumours. J Pathol. 2017;241:159–72.

DeSouza RM, Jones BRT, Stephen P, Lowis SP, Kurian KM. Pediatric medulloblastoma – Update on molecular classification driving targeted therapies. Front Oncol. 2014;4:176.

Eberhart CG. Molecular diagnostics in embryonal brain tumors. Brain Pathol. 2011;91:96–112.

Edmonson CA, Weaver KJ, Kresak J, Pincus DW. Embryonal tumor with multilayered rosettes of the fourth ventricle: case report. J Neurosurg Pediatr. 2015;7:1–5.

Ellison DW, Dalton J, Kocak M, Nicholson SL, et al. Medulloblastoma: clinicopathological correlates of SHH, WNT, and non-SHH/WNT molecular subgroups. Acta Neuropathol. 2011;121:381–96.

Frühwald MC, Biegel JA, Bourdeaut F, Roberts CWM, Chi SN. Atypical teratoid/rhabdoid tumors—current concepts, advances in biology, and potential future therapies. Neuro Oncol. 2016;18:764–78.

Gandolfi A. The cytology of cerebral neuroblastoma. Acta Cytol. 1980;24:344–6.

Güner G, Önder S, Söylemezoğl F. Cytomorphological features of atypical teratoid/rhabdoid tumor: an account of 12 years' experience. Diagn Cytopathol. 2014;42:856–62.

Ho C-Y, VandenBussche CJ, Huppman AR, Chaudhry R, Ali SZ. Cytomorphologic and clinico-radiologic analysis of primary nonhematologic central nervous system tumors with positive cerebrospinal fluid. Cancer Cytopathol. 2015;123:123–35.

Judkins AR, Burger PC, Hamilton RL, Kleinschmidt-DeMasters B, et al. INI 1 protein expression distinguishes atypical teratoid/rhabdoid tumor from choroid plexus carcinoma. J Neuropathol Exp Neurol. 2005;64:391–7.

Korshunov A, Ryzhova M, Jones DT, Northcott PA, et al. LIN28A immunoreactivity is a potent diagnostic marker of embryonal tumor with multilayered rosettes (ETMR). Acta Neuropathol. 2012;124:875–81.

Korshunov A, Sturm D, Ryzhova M, Hovestadtet V, et al. Embryonal tumor with abundant neuropil and true rosettes (ETANTR), ependymoblastoma, and medulloepithelioma share molecular similarity and comprise a single clinicopathological entity. Acta Neuropathol. 2014;128:279–89.

Kumar PV, Hosseinzadeh M, Bedayat GR. Cytologic findings of medulloblastoma in crush smears. Acta Cytol. 2001;45:542–6.

Lu L, Wilkinson E, Yachnis A. CSF cytology of atypical teratoid/rhabdoid tumor of the brain in a two-year-old girl. A case report. Diagn Cytopathol. 2000;23:329–32.

Massimino M, Biassoni V, Gandola L, Garrè ML, et al. Childhood medulloblastoma. Cri Rev Oncol Hematol. 2016;105:35–51.

Northcott PA, Shih DJ, Remke M, Cho YJ, Kool M, et al. Rapid, reliable, and reproducible molecular sub-grouping of clinical medulloblastoma samples. Acta Neuropatol. 2012;123:615–26.

Ostrom QT, Chen Y, de Blank P M, Ondracek A, et al. The descriptive epidemiology of atypical teratoid/rhabdoid tumors in the United States, 2001–2010. Neuro Oncol. 2014;16:1392–9.

Parwani A, Stelow E, Pambuccian SE, Burger PC, Ali SZ. Atypical teratoid/rhabdoid tumor of the brain: cytopathologic characteristics and differential diagnosis. Cancer Cytopathol. 2005;105:65–70.

Raisanen J, Hatanpaa KJ, Mickey BE, White CL III. Atypical teratoid/rhabdoid tumor: cytology and differential diagnosis in adults. Diagn Cytopathol. 2004;31:60–3.

Riazmontazer N, Beddayat GR. A case of calcified cerebral neuroblastoma diagnosed cytologically in intraoperative imprint smears. Acta Cytol. 1991;35:253–4.

Riazmontazer N, Daneshbod Y. Cytology of desmoplastic medulloblastoma in imprint smears: a report of 2 cases. Acta Cytol. 2006;50:97–100.

Spence T, Sin-Chan P, Picard D, Barszczyk M, et al. CNS-PNETs with C19MC amplification and/or LIN28 expression comprise a distinct histogenetic diagnostic and therapeutic entity. Acta Neuropathol. 2014;128:291–303.

Sredni ST, Tomita T. Rhabdoid tumor predisposition syndrome. Pediatr Dev Pathol. 2015;18:49–58.

Sturm D, Orr BA, Toprak UH, Hovestadt V, et al. New brain tumor entities emerge from molecular classification of CNS-PNETs. Cell. 2016;164:1060–72.

Takei H, Dauser RC, Adesina AM. Cytomorphologic characteristic, differential diagnosis and utility during intraoperative consultation for medulloblastoma. Acta Cytol. 2007;51:183–92.

Taylor MD, Northcott PA, Korshunov A, Remke M, et al. Molecular subgroups of medulloblastoma: the current consensus. Acta Neuropathol. 2012;123:465–72.

Tena-Suck ML, Gomez-Amador JL, Ortiz-Plata A, Salina-Lara C, Rembao-Bojorquez D, Vega-Orozco R. Rhabdoid choroid plexus carcinoma. A rare histological type. Arq Neuropsiquiatr. 2007;65:705–9.

Chapter 13
Meningiomas

Meningiomas are common tumors (greaterthan30% of all primary CNS tumors), generally benign, arising from the arachnoid cap cells. These most commonly occur in middle-aged and elderly adults (peak at 65–75 years) and are rare in children, where they tend to pursue a more aggressive course. Meningiomas show a marked predominance in women (60–70%); this percentage increases to 90% for spinal locations. They may develop anywhere along the neuroaxis, particularly in the convex and parasagittal regions of the cerebral hemispheres, skull base (olfactory grooves, optic nerve sheaths, sphenoid wings, para–/suprasellar regions), posterior fossa (tentorium, clivus, petrous bone), and spinal canal (mostly in the thoracic region); some examples are intraventricular (mainly in lateral ventricles). Monosomy 22 or chromosome 22q deletions are the most frequent abnormalities in meningioma (reported in 60–80% of the cases), whereas inactivating mutations in the *NF2* gene (chromosome 22) are detected in most meningiomas associated with *neurofibromatosis type 2* and more than a half of sporadic cases. Meningiomas may also develop in the setting of *schwannomatosis* with germline mutations in *SMARCB1*. Other germline mutations associated with meningiomas have included *SUFU* and *BAP1*. Additionally, *SMARCE1* germ line mutations have been identified in both familial and sporadic clear cell meningiomas, whereas combined *KLF4* and *TRAF7* somatic mutations characterize the secretory meningioma variant.

Clinically, meningiomas cause symptoms resulting from the compression of adjacent structures, but they can be asymptomatic and an incidental finding. Unspecific headache has been reported as the most common single symptom. The frequent expression of progesterone and, less commonly, estrogen receptors in meningiomas explains why some clinically silent tumors grow rapidly and give rise to progressive symptoms during pregnancy, particularly blindness due to compression of chiasm/optic nerves. In neuroimaging, meningiomas are usually globular, iso- or hypodense avidly enhancing masses due to external carotid blood supply. Although no specific, the "dural tail" sign (extension of contrast-enhancing tissue along the dura) provides with a reasonably reliable means of identifying a menin-

C. R. Lacruz et al., *Central Nervous System Intraoperative Cytopathology*, Essentials in Cytopathology 13, https://doi.org/10.1007/978-3-319-98491-9_13

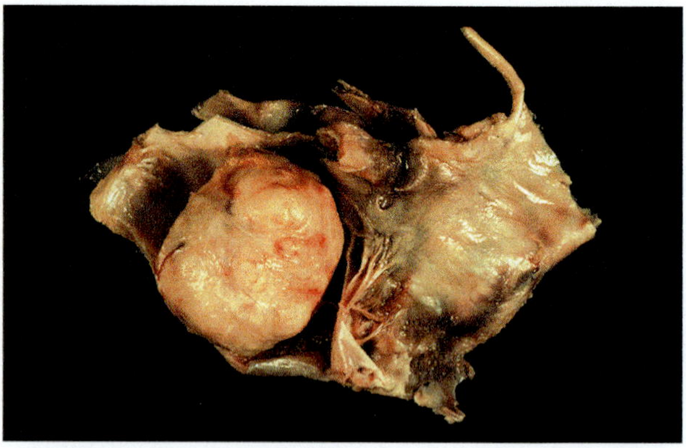

Fig. 13.1 *Meningioma resection specimen*. This large tumor is attached to the resected sleeve of the dura and shows a smooth external surface

Table 13.1 WHO 2016 classification scheme for meningiomas

WHO grade I	**WHO grade II**
Meningothelial	Atypical (any variant plus criteria)
Fibrous	Chordoid
Transitional	Clear cell
Psammomatous	
Angiomatous (vascular)	
Microcystic	**WHO grade III**
Secretory	Anaplastic (any variant plus criteria)
Lymphoplasmacyte-rich	Papillary
Metaplastic	Rhabdoid

gioma. Other features that signal meningioma are hyperostosis of adjacent skull bone and calcification (on CT). Angiomatous, microcystic, secretory, atypical, and anaplastic meningiomas typically cause considerable vasogenic edema.

Grossly, most meningiomas are rubbery or firm, rounded to lobulated masses, which are broadly attached to the inner surface of the dura (Fig. 13.1). Some, usually found over the sphenoid wing, grow as flat carpet-like masses termed "en plaque" meningioma. Meningeal tumors usually compress rather than infiltrate the underlying brain parenchyma, even though they may invade the dura (frequently) and even the cranial bones and scalp (occasionally) in benign cases.

Microscopically, meningioma can have an impressive array of patterns (Table 13.1), but meningothelial, transitional, and fibrous meningiomas are the most common variants.

Tumor cells are polygonal (epithelial-like) or elongated (mesenchymal-like) with ill-defined cytoplasmic borders. Nuclei are slightly oval, with delicate chromatin and solitary discrete nucleoli. Nuclear pseudoinclusions, consisting of invaginated pockets of cytoplasm in the nuclei and clear "washed out" chromatin also are characteristic. In *meningothelial meningioma*, these cells group together in lobules with a tendency to form typical whorls at the center (Fig. 13.2a). In *fibrous meningioma*, there is a marked predominance of elongated cells associated in fascicles,

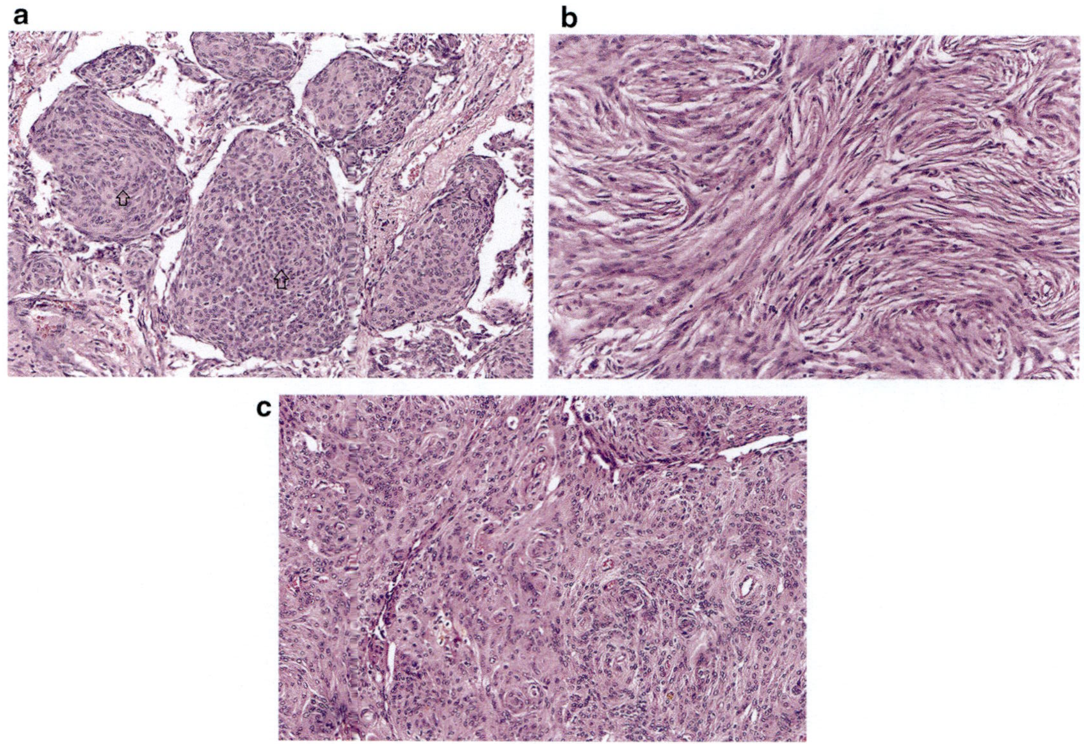

Fig. 13.2 *Common histologic patterns*. (**a**) Meningothelial meningioma. Characteristic lobular growth pattern with syncytium-like appearance due to poorly defined cell borders. Note a tendency to form typical whorls at the center (*arrows*). (**b**) Fibrous meningioma. Cellular spindling and a fascicular or storiform architecture are the hallmark of this variant. (**c**) Transitional meningioma with prominent whorl formation

Table 13.2 WHO 2016 grading criteria for meningioma and associated recurrence rates

Benign meningioma (WHO grade I); recurrence rates of 7–20%
Any predominant histology other than clear cell, chordoid, papillary, or rhabdoid
Lacks criteria of grade II or III tumors
Atypical meningioma (WHO grade II); recurrence rates of 29–50%
Any of the following three major criteria:
Mitotic index ≥4 mitoses per 10 high-power fields
Brain invasion
At least three of the following five features:
Sheeting architecture or patternless pattern
Small-cell population
Hypercellularity
Prominent nucleoli
Foci of spontaneous (not induced) necrosis
Anaplastic meningioma (WHO grade III); recurrence rates of 50–90%
Either of the following two criteria:
Overt anaplasia (frank sarcomatous, carcinomatous, or melanomatous histology)
Mitotic index ≥20 mitoses per 10 high-power fields

Note: Invasion of dura, bone, or soft tissues and pleomorphic or atypical nuclei do not affect grade

whereas cell whorls are infrequent (Fig. 13.2b). In *transitional meningioma*, lobules and fascicles are combined in variable proportions, with a noticeable number of cell whorls (Fig. 13.2c). Occasionally, psammoma bodies formed by hyalinization and subsequent mineralization of whorls are also observed. In some cases, these concentric laminar calcifications are so frequent that they justify the term *psammomatous meningioma*. The histopathologic grading, however, is of greater prognostic interest. Most meningiomas are benign (WHO grade I), with a low risk of recurrence and of aggressive growth; a group of meningiomas, comprising between 5% and 6%, have a greater likelihood of recurrence and/or aggressive behavior (WHO grade II); and overt anaplastic/malignant meningiomas (WHO grade III) account for between 1% and 3%. Table 13.2 lists the grading criteria and the average recurrence rates of these three groups.

Regarding *immunomarkers*, diffuse membranous cytoplasmic immunoreactivity for somatostatin receptor 2a (SSTR2a) and dual immunoreactivity for D2–40 (podoplanin) and E-cadherin may be superior to classic EMA/vimentin IHC. Progesterone receptors are also recommended.

Most variants have an excellent prognosis and are curable by gross total resection, but malignant histology is associated with shorter survival times: 2–5 years depending largely on the extent of resection. In spite of the histologic grade, tumor location is the most important feature regarding therapy since it practically defines the terms of surgical intervention. Stereotactic radiosurgery (gamma knife) may be used in cases where complete resection cannot be achieved, such as skull base tumors or recurrent lesions.

Cytologic Features of Common Meningioma Variants

Intraoperative cytology is more accurate than frozen sections in meningioma. The freezing artifact produces a clear distortion of the meningothelial cells, giving rise to disturbing images that resemble both metastatic carcinoma and other aggressive neoplasias.

Despite their variable histologic appearance, the cytomorphologic features of meningiomas are remarkably consistent. Specimens spread with a moderate grade of difficulty to form speckled, uneven preparations with large irregular clusters, small cell groups, and single cells in a clear background. With the exception of overly fibrous meningioma, tumor cells have slightly oval nuclei with delicate chromatin, solitary discrete nucleoli, and frequent intranuclear pseudoinclusions/clearings. A special characteristic is the copious "tissue paper" cytoplasm with broad, borderless processes, which often interconnect tumor cells or groups (Fig. 13.3a), but can also display a more streaked, fibrillary appearance (Fig. 13.3b). In most types, there are at least a few cell whorls, which are the most characteristic diagnostic feature of meningioma (Fig. 13.3c). Psammoma bodies, although less common, also have a highly characteristic appearance and tend to be particularly abundant in *psammomatous meningioma* (Figs. 13.4a, b). However, even in the absence of cell whorls and psammoma bodies, the combination of high cellularity and uniform, benign cytologic features is characteristic of meningioma. Within the most frequent variants, *fibrous meningioma* is the only one that departs to a great extent from this common picture. Smears show a more uniform aspect of fusiform cells with elongated nuclei and long, tapering cytoplasmic processes. This appearance, together with the frequent absence of cell whorls, may cause it to be confused with other fusiform neoplasms, such as schwannoma or solitary fibrous tumor. However, in spite of elongation, the nuclei of fibrous meningioma preserve the typical appearance of meningothelial cells, even with nuclear pseudoinclusions (Fig. 13.5a, b).

Cytologic Features of Uncommon Meningioma Variants

To the cytologic appearances described above, in a number of uncommon variants of meningioma, characteristic features are added that must be taken into account for the differential diagnosis.

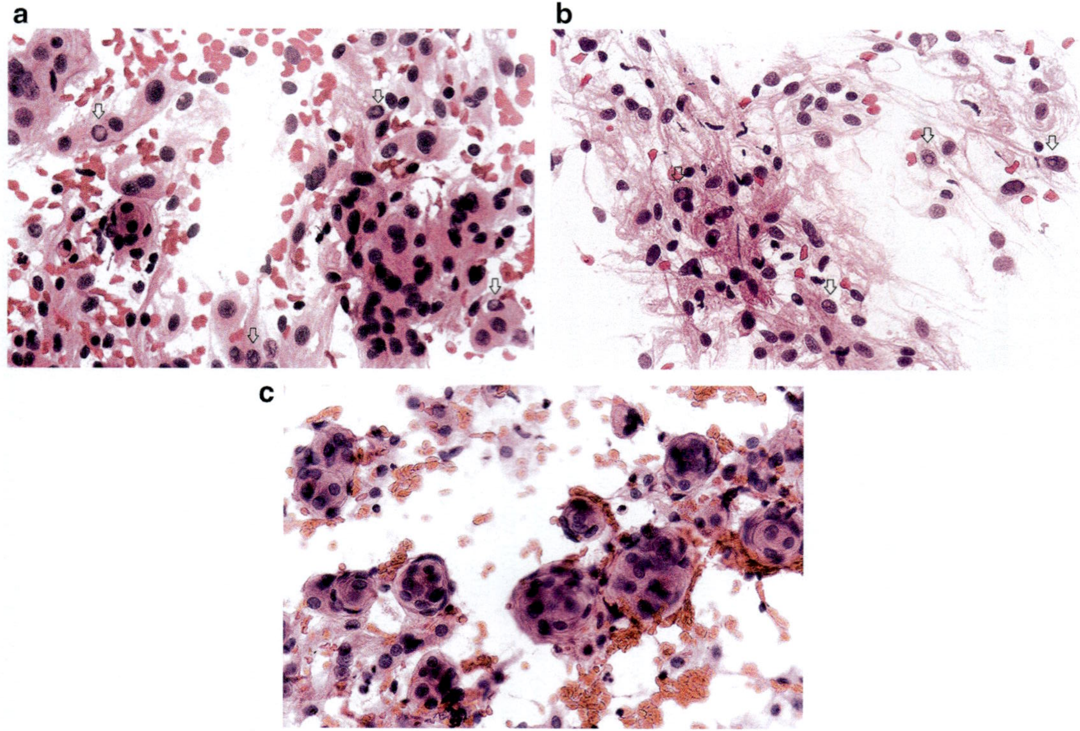

Fig. 13.3 *Meningioma, cytologic features*. (**a**) Characteristic smear pattern with irregular clusters, small groups, and single cells in a clear background. Tumor cells have copious cytoplasm with broad, borderless processes. Nuclei are slightly oval with frequent intranuclear pseudoinclusions or clearings (*arrows*). (**b**) In this case, the cells have streaked fibrillary cytoplasm reminiscent of astrocytoma, but the nuclei retain meningioma features including intranuclear pseudoinclusions (*arrows*). (**c**) Cellular whorls such as these are highly distinctive features of meningioma and, when present, confirm the diagnosis beyond doubt (**a–c**; Smears, H&E)

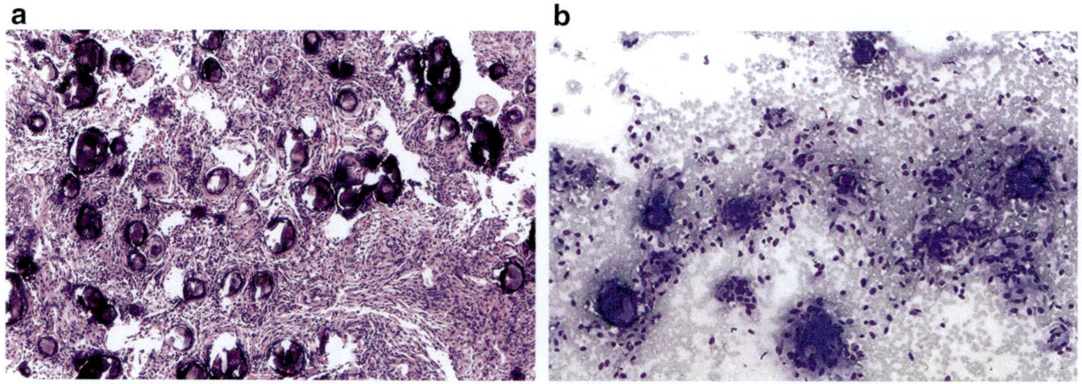

Fig. 13.4 *Psammomatous meningioma*. (**a**) Histology. This spinal meningioma displays numerous hyalinized and calcified cell whorls. (**b**) Cellular preparation showing many calcified psammoma bodies (Smear, Romanowsky)

a
b
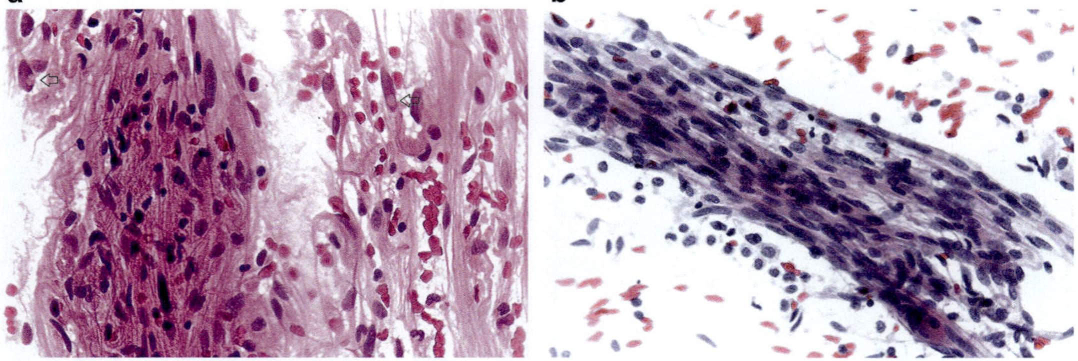

Fig. 13.5 *Fibrous meningioma*. (**a**) This preparation shows fusiform cells with tapering cytoplasmic processes. Despite elongation, nuclei show characteristic meningothelial features including nuclear pseudoinclusions (*arrows*; Smear, H&E). (**b**) In contrast to schwannoma, the fusiform cells of fibrous meningioma tend to appear dispersed with visible cytoplasmic boundaries (Smear, Papanicolaou)

Secretory Meningioma This tumor that commonly arises at the cranial base contains the distinctive feature of discrete eosinophilic cytoplasmic spheres that represent CEA deposits (patients may have elevated serum CEA levels). The presence of such cytoplasmic inclusions makes it possible to confuse secretory meningioma with metastatic adenocarcinoma, but, with the exception of this feature, the rest of the characteristics are the same as those of conventional meningioma (Fig. 13.6a, b).

Microcystic Meningioma This variety exhibits a distinctive histologic "sponge-like" appearance created by both intra- and intercellular microcystic spaces. Smears reveal small cystic spaces within the clusters and sheets of an otherwise typical meningioma. The cytoplasm of tumor cells may also appear finely vacuolated confirming that many of microcystic spaces are intracellular (Fig. 13.7a–c).

Angiomatous Meningioma This tumor is characterized by the presence of an exuberant stromal vasculature, among which groups of meningioma tumor cells are arranged. The vascular-rich pattern may lead us to confuse it with hemangioblastoma or vascular malformations if we do not pay attention to the presence of the diagnostic meningothelial cell groups (Fig. 13.8a, b).

Lymphoplasmacyte-Rich Meningioma The chronic infiltrates of this variety is so prominent that it may overshadow the meningothelial pattern of the tumor. Clinically, it may be associated with hyperglobulinemia or iron-refractory anemia. From the cytologic point of view, its confusion with an inflammatory/reactive process is quite easy. Only careful examination of the smears, when intraoperative findings do not match the clinico-radiologic picture, enables us to find cells with unequivocal meningothelial morphology in the infiltrate (Fig. 13.9a, b). However, it is likely that some examples diagnosed as "lymphoplasmacyte-rich meningioma" represent inflammatory disorders with associated meningothelial hyperplasia instead.

Metaplastic Meningiomas These are variants in which the presence of xanthomatous, cartilaginous, bony, myxoid, or lipomatous tissue, individually or in combination, stands out in an otherwise classic meningioma. Its cytologic appearance does not differ from that of the more common varieties except for the presence of these added-on elements (Fig. 13.10a, b).

Cytologic Features of Grade II Meningiomas

Atypical Meningiomas Considerable pleomorphism can be seen in any of the meningioma variants without necessarily connoting a more aggressive behavior (Figs. 13.11a, b). Nevertheless, in comparison to a grade I lesion, atypical meningiomas are more cellular with loss of whorls and lobules. Small-cell population with a high nuclear-to-cytoplasmic ratio, prominent nucleoli, and presence of

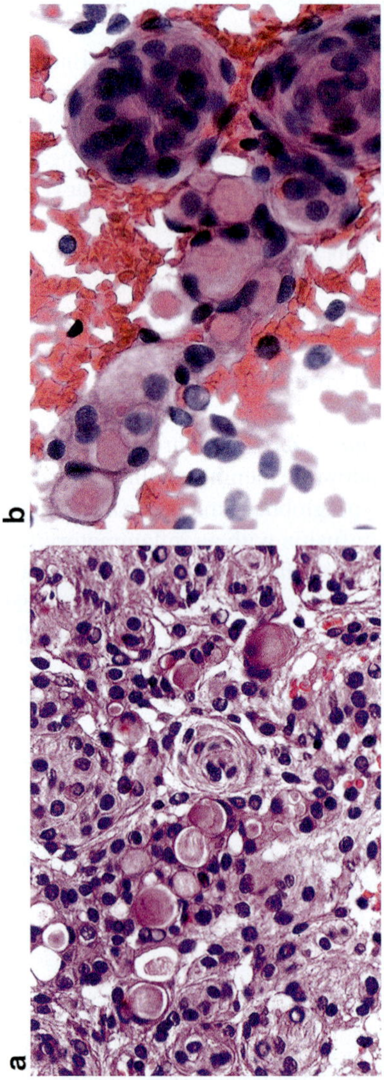

Fig. 13.6 *Secretory meningioma.* (**a**) Histology. Numerous intracellular lumens containing eosinophilic globules are typically present in this variant. (**b**) Preparation from this tumor displaying target-like intracytoplasmic bodies and cell whorls (Smear, H&E)

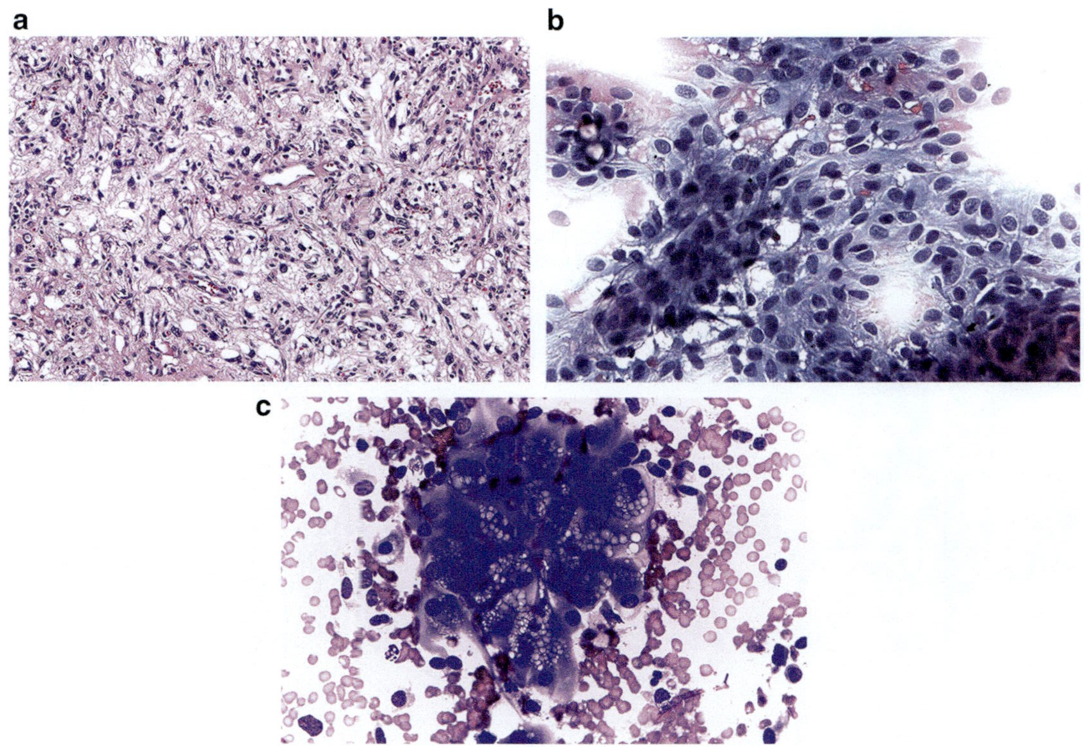

Fig. 13.7 *Microcystic meningioma*. (**a**) Histology. This variant exhibits numerous tiny holes (sponge-like appearance), scattered bizarre nuclei, and prominent vasculature. (**b**) Cytologic preparation revealing cystic spaces of variable sizes within the cell clusters and sheets of an otherwise typical meningioma (Smear, Papanicolaou). (**c**) The tumor cells exhibit numerous tiny cytoplasmic vacuoles. This finding confirms that many microcystic spaces are intracellular (Smear, Romanowsky)

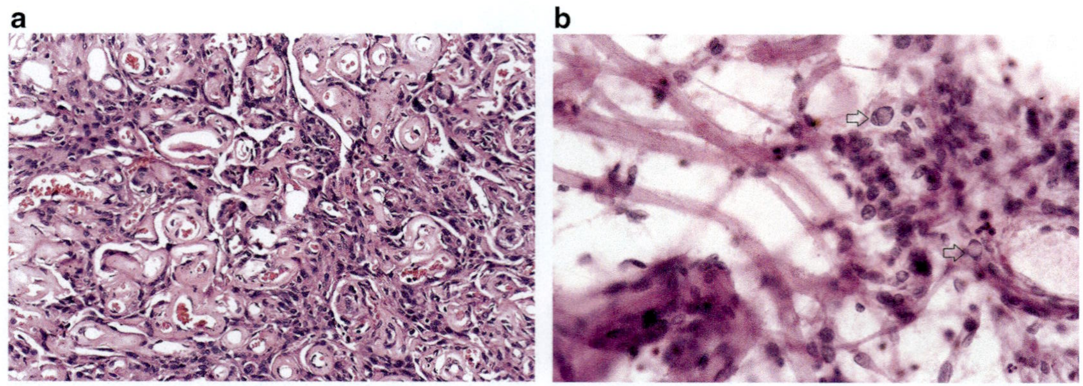

Fig. 13.8 *Angiomatous meningioma*. (**a**) Histology. Blood vessels constitute most of the mass. The intervening tumor cells are difficult to recognize as meningothelial. (**b**) This preparation shows a dense network of mature vessels and small clumps of meningothelial cells with characteristic nuclear pseudoinclusions (*arrows*; Smear, H&E)

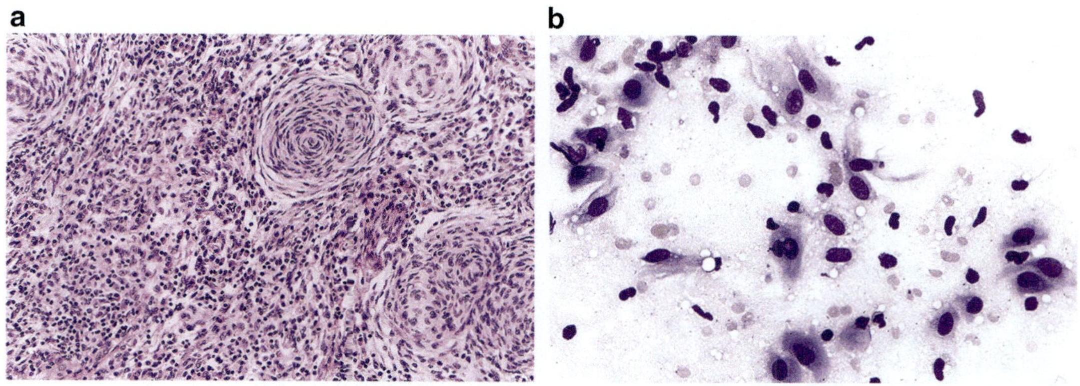

Fig. 13.9 *Lymphoplasmacyte-rich meningioma*. (**a**) Tissue section showing an extensive chronic inflammatory infiltrate overshadowing the meningothelial component. (**b**) Very few areas in this case showed meningothelial cells intermixed with the inflammatory infiltrate (Smear, Romanowsky)

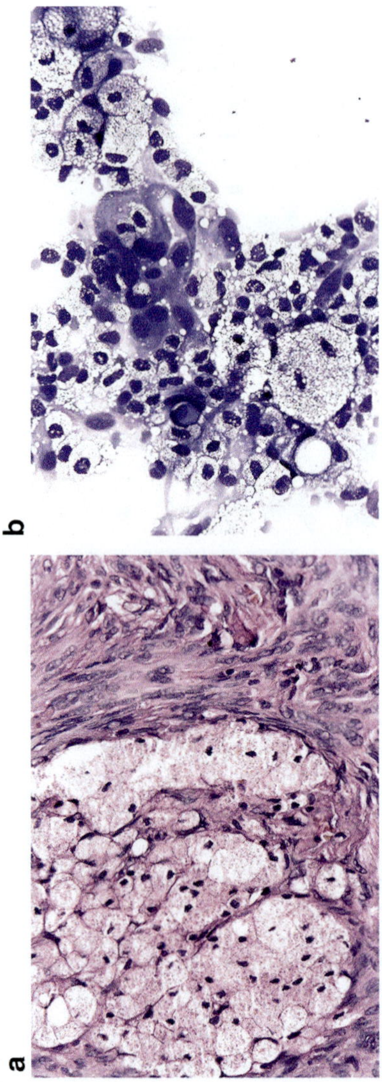

Fig. 13.10 *Metaplastic meningioma.* **(a)** Histology. Presence of xanthomatous cell aggregates in this case of metaplastic meningioma. **(b)** Large, foamy xanthomatous cells admixed with smaller meningothelial cells (Smear, Romanowsky)

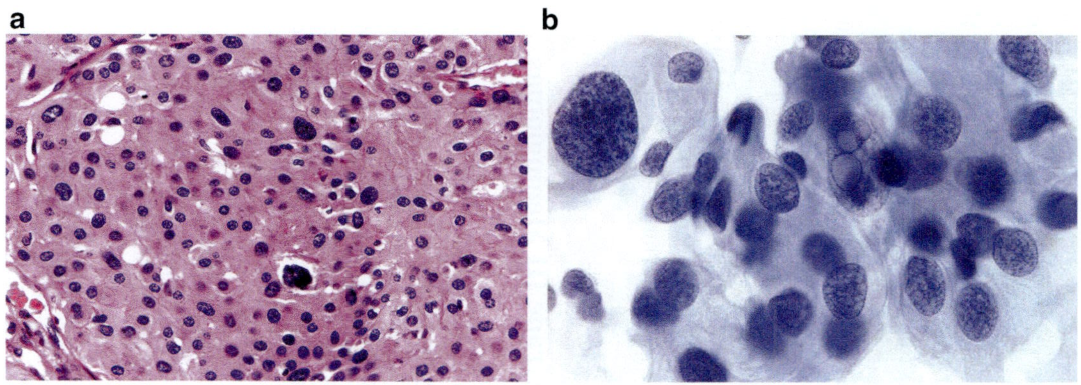

Fig. 13.11 *Pleomorphic meningioma*. (**a**) Histology. Some, otherwise, completely benign meningiomas may show conspicuous nuclear pleomorphism, which should not be misinterpreted as signifying a potentially aggressive behavior. (**b**) Similarly, the presence of bizarre pleomorphic cells in cytological preparations is not an indicator of high-grade tumor (Smear, Papanicolaou)

necrotic debris are also features to be taken into account independently of the morphologic variety (Fig. 13.12a, b).

Chordoid Meningioma This variant show lobules or trabeculae of cells in an abundant mucoid matrix background (chordoma-like appearance). Smears show cell groups and single cells with the characteristic nuclear features of meningioma (including pseudoinclusions) embedded in a myxoid background. Due to the presence of this matrix and occasional cell vacuolization, smears may closely resemble the cytomorphology of chordoma. To resolve this dilemma it is necessary to look for the presence of meningioma nuclear features and cell whorls (Fig. 13.13a, b).

Clear Cell Meningioma This tumor most commonly arises in the spinal canal, cerebellopontine angle, or foramen magnum region and tends to occur in younger patients than most other meningioma variants. Tumor cells display abundant clear cytoplasm due to increased glycogen accumulation. Mild nuclear pleomorphism and nuclear overlap also are frequent features. This appearance may cause it to be confused with oligodendroglioma or clear cell ependymoma in histologic sections. In smears, confusion is more difficult because the broad and clear appearance of some cells is preserved, which does not happen in oligodendroglioma, whereas the characteristic fibrillary matrix of ependymoma is lacking (Fig. 13.14a–c).

Cytologic Features of Grade III Meningiomas

Anaplastic (Malignant) Meningioma In the case of overt anaplastic meningiomas the diagnosis of malignancy is simple; what is complicated is to determine the nature of the tumor. Anaplastic cell features and brisk mitosis can closely resemble carcinoma, sarcoma, or amelanotic melanoma. Thus, a descriptive appellation such as "spindle cell," "pleomorphic," or "undifferentiated" malignant tumor, followed by the possible diagnostic considerations, may be all that the pathologist can give (Fig. 13.15a, b).

Papillary Meningioma The cytomorphologic features of this variant may be no distinct than those of classic meningioma. However, the presence of perivascular papillary clusters with discohesive tumor cells is characteristic (Fig. 13.16a, b).

Rhabdoid Meningioma More distinctive is the cytomorphology of this variant, consisting of abundant single or loosely clustered plump cells with rhabdoid features. The presence of associated cellular component of meningothelial appearance is of great value for diagnosing the nature of the lesion. Tumors with combined papillary, clear cell, and rhabdoid features may also be seen (Fig. 13.17a, b).

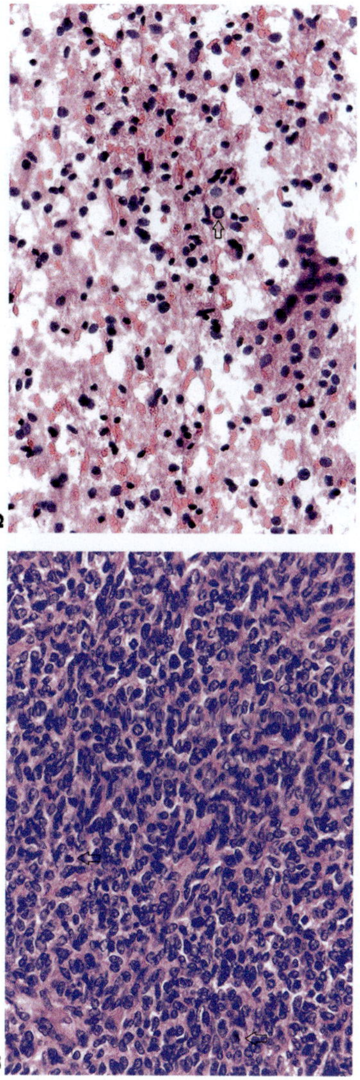

Fig. 13.12 *Atypical meningioma*. (**a**) Hypercellularity, patternless pattern, and small cell population are characteristic features of this histologic variant. Also note mitotic figures (*arrows*). (**b**) Preparation from this tumor showing a discohesive pattern of small, lymphocyte-like cells and many naked nuclei. Note a nuclear pseudoinclusion (*arrow*; Smear, H&E)

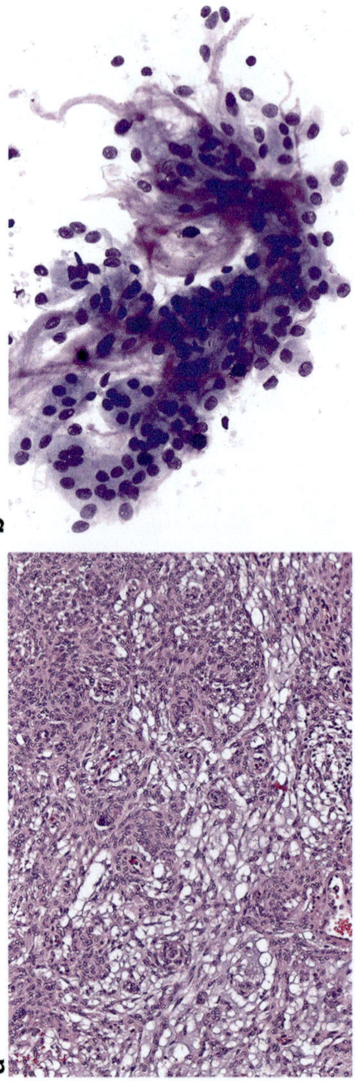

Fig. 13.13 *Chordoid meningioma*. (**a**) Histology. Nests and cords of epithelioid cells in a basophilic, myxoid-rich matrix characterize this variant. (**b**) Undoubted meningothelial cell group embedded in a metachromatic myxoid matrix. Note the characteristic nuclear features including frequent pseudoinclusions (Smear, Romanowsky)

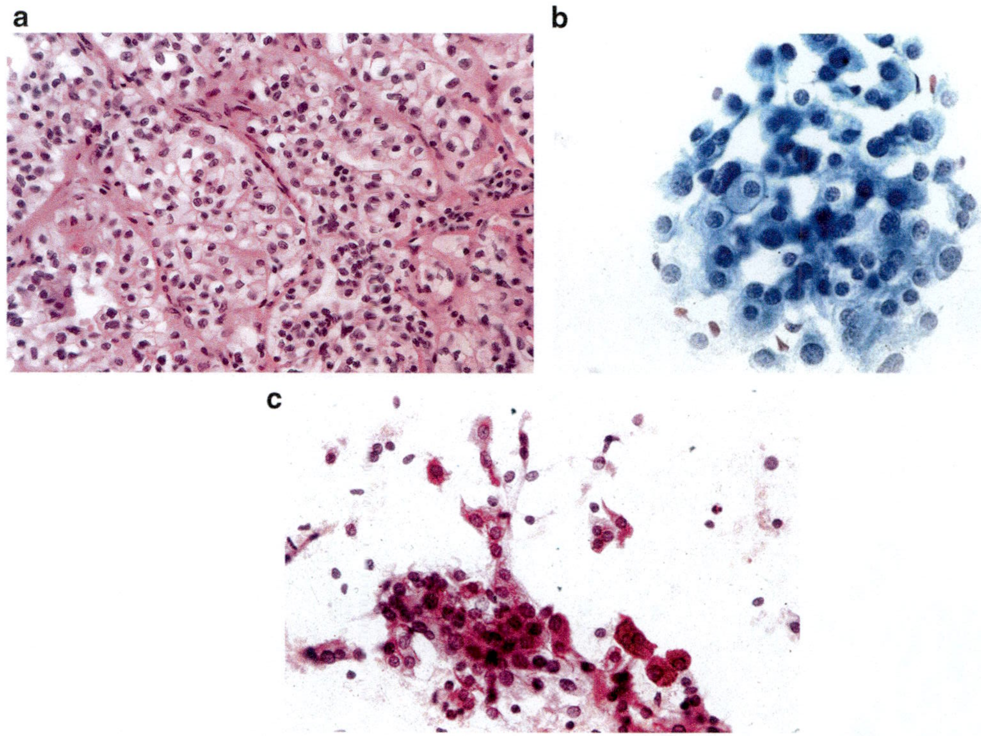

Fig. 13.14 *Clear cell meningioma*. (**a**) Characteristic histology pattern includes sheets of cells with cleared cytoplasm due to increased glycogen accumulation and strands of collagen scattered throughout. (**b**) Preparation from this tumor displaying round clear cells with nuclear features of meningioma (Smear, Papanicolaou). (**c**) A cytochemical stain nicely reveals cytoplasmic accumulation of glycogen (Smear, PAS stain)

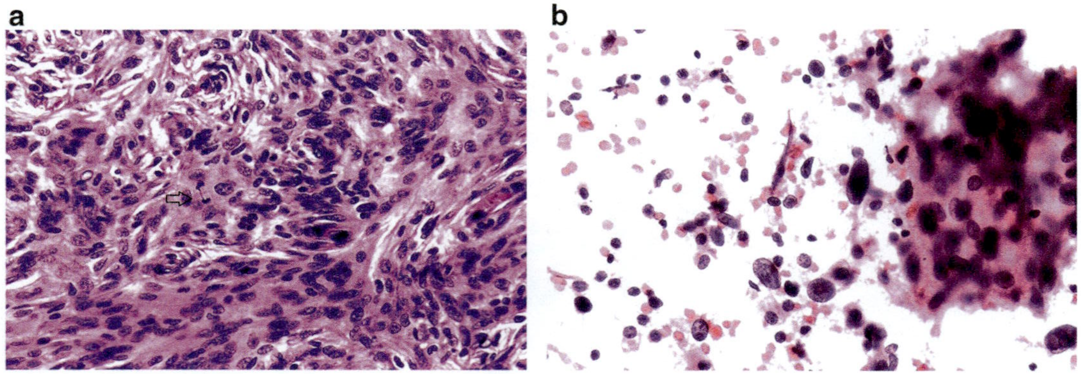

Fig. 13.15 *Anaplastic meningioma*. (**a**) Histology. Sarcomatous-like anaplastic meningioma with spindled morphology, poorly differentiated cytology, and mitosis (*arrow*). (**b**) Preparation from this tumor showing crowded tissue fragments and individual cells with anaplastic features (Smear, H&E)

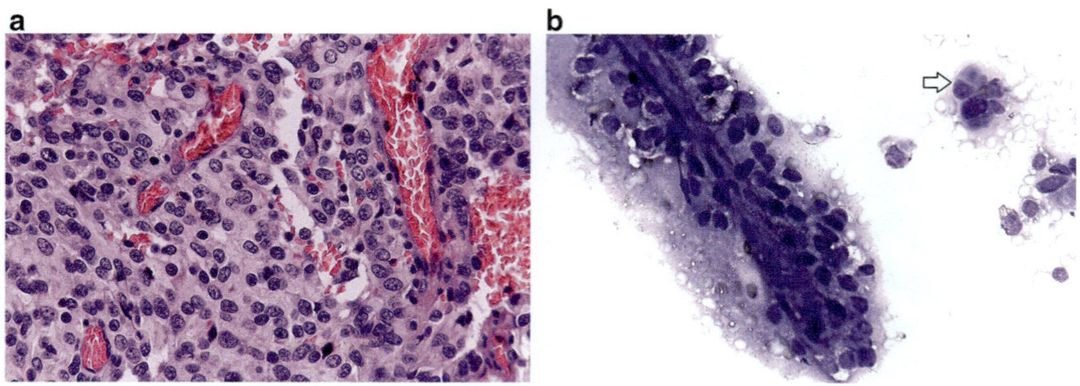

Fig. 13.16 *Papillary meningioma*. (**a**) The histologic pattern consists of a perivascular pseudopapillary arrangement of cells on a vascular-fibrous stroma. (**b**) Preparation from this tumor showing a papillary cluster and single cells. Note that some cells have rhabdoid features (*arrow*) or clear cytoplasm (Smear, Romanowsky)

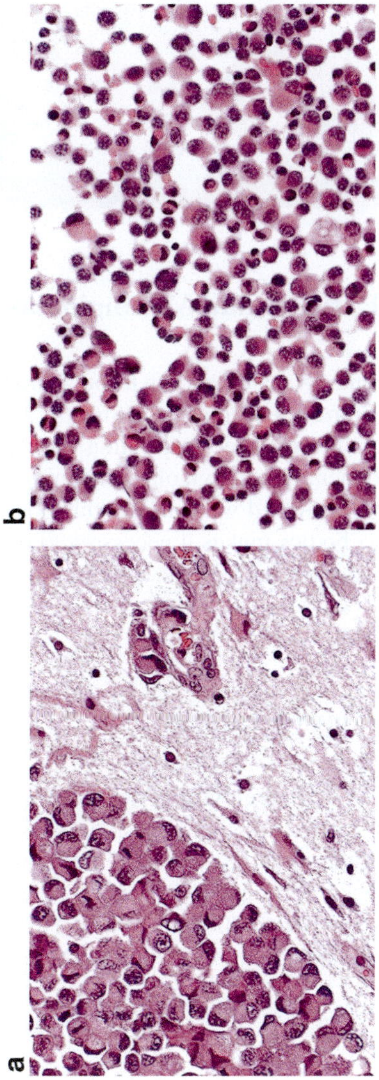

Fig. 13.17 *Rhabdoid meningioma.* (**a**) Tissue section showing an area of cortical infiltration indicating aggressive tumor behavior. This variant loses the syncytial appearance of most meningiomas. (**b**) Highly cellular preparation with a discohesive pattern of rhabdoid cells (Smear, H&E)

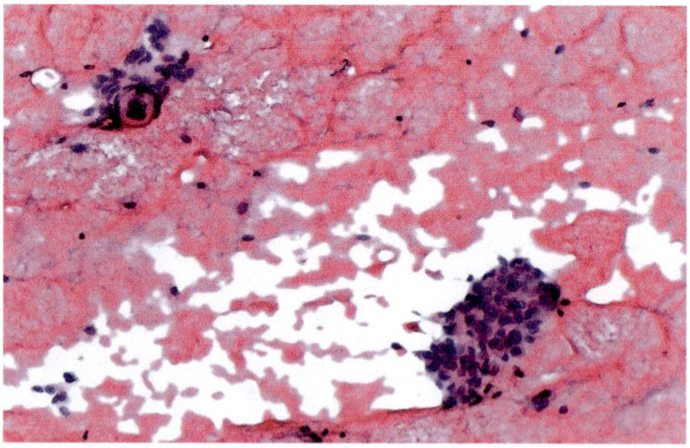

Fig. 13.18 *Extracranial meningioma*, direct fine-needle aspiration cytology. This preparation from a latero-cervical mass shows a bloody background with aggregates of meningothelial cells. Note a psammoma body in the left upper cell aggregate (Smear, Papanicolaou)

Cytologic Features of Extracranial Meningiomas

Whether ectopic or, more frequently, by extending through cranial sutures or foramina of the skull base, meningiomas may present clinically as extracranial tumors, which is why they are accessible to direct aspiration biopsy. These extracranial lesions, preferentially located facially or cervicolaterally, may be diagnosed without the use of ancillary techniques provided we consider this possibility. The presence of cell whorls and psammoma bodies makes it necessary to rule out squamous carcinoma (whorls) and thyroid papillary carcinoma (psammoma bodies) at these locations (Fig. 13.18).

Differential Diagnosis Considerations

The astonishing array of patterns of meningioma requires the differential diagnosis to include many types of neoplastic and nonneoplastic processes (Table 13.3).

As a general rule, meningioma should be included in the differential diagnosis of any intracranial/intraspinal mass, particularly in the presence of dura-based, extra-axial masses in patients between 40 and 70 years of age. This diagnosis will not be difficult if the characteristic cytologic features mentioned here are taken into account (Table 13.4).

Table 13.3 Common differential diagnosis for meningioma variants

Variant	Differential diagnosis
Meningothelial/transitional	Metastatic carcinoma
	Melanoma
Psammomatous	Calcifying pseudoneoplasm of the neuraxis
Fibroblastic	Schwannoma
	Solitary fibrous tumor
Secretory	Metastatic adenocarcinoma
Microcystic	Diffuse/pilocytic astrocytoma
Angiomatous	Hemangioma
	Vascular malformation
Lymphoplasmacyte-rich	Inflammatory pseudotumor
	Rosai-Dorfman disease
	MALT-lymphoma of the dura
Metaplastic	Soft tissue tumors
	Histiocytic disorders
Chordoid	Chordoma
	Chordoid glioma of the third ventricle
Clear cell	Oligodendroglioma
	Clear cell ependymoma
	Hemangioblastoma
	Metastatic renal cell carcinoma
Anaplastic	Metastatic carcinoma/melanoma
	Other meningeal sarcomas
Papillary	Papillary ependymoma
	Astroblastoma
	Hemangiopericytoma
	Metastatic malignancy
Rhabdoid	Atypical teratoid/rhabdoid tumor
	Choroid plexus carcinoma
	Metastatic tumors with rhabdoid features

MALT-lymphoma marginal zone lymphoma of mucosa-associated lymphoid tissues (MALT)

Table 13.4 Characteristics of meningioma

Cytologic features
High cellularity and clear background
Uniform, benign cellular aspect with
Oval nuclei with delicate chromatin
Nuclear pseudoinclusions and clearings
Copious cytoplasm with broad or streaked processes
Cell whorls and psammoma bodies
Characteristic morphologic variants (fibrous, secretory, chordoid….)
Differential diagnosis and pitfalls
Consider meningioma in any intracranial/intraspinal mass, particularly if
Long-standing clinical history
Middle-aged and elderly patients
Intradural, extra-axial location
Women

Suggested Reading

Ali S, Nassar A, Siddiqui MT. Crush preparations of meningiomas. Can grading be accomplished? Diagn Cytopathol. 2008;36:827–31.

Bansal M, Pathak VP, Kishore S, Bansal KK. Rhabdoid meningioma: rapid intraoperative diagnosis on squash smears. Diagn Cytopathol. 2010;38:594–6.

Batoroev YK, Nguyen G. Rhabdoid meningioma diagnosed by imprint cytology. Acta Cytol. 2005;49:464–5.

Fukuoka K, Hirokawa M, Kanahara T, Ishii N, Ishii R, Shirabe T. Cytology of microcystic meningioma in crush preparation. Diagn Cytopathol. 2000;23:275–8.

Hinton DR, Kovacs K, Chandrasoma PT. Cytologic features of secretory meningioma. Acta Cytol. 1999;43:121–5.

Imlay SP, Snider TE, Raab SS. Clear-cell meningioma: diagnosis by fine-needle aspiration biopsy. Diagn Cytopathol. 1998;18:131–6.

Inagawa H, Ishizawa K, Shimada S, Shimada T, et al. Cytologic features of chordoid meningioma. A case report. Acta Cytol. 2004;48:397–401.

Jeong J, Kim NR, Lee SG. Crush cytology of a primary intraspinal rhabdoid papillary meningioma: a case report. Acta Cytol. 2013;57:528–33.

Kirby PA. Rhabdoid meningioma: Intraoperative diagnosis using smear preparation. Diagn Cytopathol. 2003;29:292–6.

Kobayashi S. Meningioma, neurilemmoma and astrocytoma specimens obtained with the squash method for cytodiagnosis. A cytologic and immunochemical study. Acta Cytol. 1993;37:913–22.

Lui PC, Chau TK, Wong SS, Lau PP, Tse GM, Thomas TM, Ng HK. Cytology of chordoid meningioma: a series of five cases with emphasis on differential diagnoses. J Clin Pathol. 2007;60:1024–8.

Menke JR, Raleigh DR, Gown AM, Thomas S, Perry A, Tihan T. Somatostatin receptor 2a is a more sensitive diagnostic marker of meningioma than epithelial membrane antigen. Acta Neuropathol. 2015;130:441–3.

Nagaishi M, Nobusawa S, Tanaka Y, Ikota H, Yokoo H, Nakazato Y. Slug, twist, and E-cadherin as immunohistochemical biomarkers in meningeal tumors. PLoS One. 2012;7(9):e46053.

Nguyen GK, Johnson ES, Mielke BW. Cytology of meningiomas and neurilemomas in crush preparations. A useful adjunct to frozen sections. Acta Cytol. 1988;32:362–5.

Ocque R, Khalbuss WE, Monaco SE, Michelow PM, Pantanowitz L. Cytopathology of extracranial ectopic and metastatic meningiomas. Acta Cytol. 2014;58:1–8.

Reuss DE, Piro RM, Jones DT, Simon M, et al. Secretory meningiomas are defined by combined KLF4 K409Q and TRAF7 mutations. Acta Neuropathol (Berl). 2013;125:351–8.

Riazmontazer N, Bedayat G. Cytodiagnosis of meningioma with atypical cytologic features. Acta Cytol. 1991;35:501–4.

Salinero E, Beltran L, Costa JR. Intraoperative cytologic diagnosis of chordoid meningioma. A case report. Acta Cytol. 2004;48:259–63.

Sangoi AR, Dulai MS, Beck AH, Brat DJ, Vogel H. Distinguishing chordoid meningiomas from their histologic mimics: an immunohistochemical evaluation. Am J Surg Pathol. 2009;33:669–81.

Siddiqui MT, Mahon BM, Cochran E, Gattuso P. Cytologic features of meningiomas on crush preparations: a review. Diagn Cytopathol. 2008;36:202–6.

Smith MJ, Wallace AJ, Chris Bennett C, Hasselblatt M, et al. Germline SMARCE1 mutations predispose to both spinal and cranial clear cell meningiomas. J Pathol. 2014;234:436–40.

Solares J, Lacruz CR. FNAC diagnosis of an extracranial meningioma presenting as a cervical mass. Acta Cytol. 1987;31:502–4.

Vogelsang PJ, Nguyen G, Mielke BW. Cytology of atypical and malignant meningiomas in intraoperative crush preparations. Acta Cytol. 1993;37:884–8.

Chapter 14
Non-meningothelial Mesenchymal Tumors

CNS mesenchymal, non-meningothelial tumors arise from craniospinal meninges, supporting tissues, vasculature, or surrounding osseous structures, representing the homologous of neoplasms encountered far more frequently in the somatic soft tissues or bones. They're extremely rare, with the exception of hemangioblastoma and solitary fibrous tumor/hemangiopericytoma; the remaining mesenchymal tumors represent less than 1% of all CNS tumors in the Central Brain Tumor Registry of the United States (CBTRUS). These neoplasms can occur in patients of any age and may arise anywhere along the neuroaxis and its coverings, with tumors arising in the meninges more common than the ones originating within the CNS parenchyma or in the choroid plexus. Histologically, they present a broad gradient of malignancy ranging from benign neoplasms (WHO grade I) to highly malignant sarcomas (WHO grade IV), with many tumor types featuring both benign and malignant variants (Table 14.1). Benign tumors may be completely resected with a favorable prognosis, while sarcomas have a high risk of recurrence and metastasis despite extensive surgical debulking and the use of adjuvant radiation therapy, chemotherapy, or both.

Hemangioblastoma

Hemangioblastoma is a benign, highly vascular, well-demarcated, slowly growing, solid or cystic neoplasm that represents 1–3% of total brain tumors and approximately 7% of posterior fossa tumors. The lesion may arise at any age, although it has a peak incidence during the third and fourth decades, and no gender preference is apparent. This tumor is strongly associated with mutations of the von Hippel-Lindau gene (*VHL*) at 3p25-p26, either as part of von Hippel-Lindau disease (20–25% of hemangioblastomas) or due to a sporadic mutation or other inactivating abnormalities. Inactivation of the *VHL* tumor-suppressor gene causes increased production of vascular endothelial growth factor, leading to richly vascular tumors such

C. R. Lacruz et al., *Central Nervous System Intraoperative Cytopathology*, Essentials in Cytopathology 13, https://doi.org/10.1007/978-3-319-98491-9_14

Table 14.1 CNS mesenchymal, non-meningothelial tumors

Benign	Malignant
Solitary fibrous tumor	Hemangiopericytoma
Lipoma	Liposarcoma
Fibromatosis	Fibrosarcoma
Benign fibrous histiocytoma	Undifferentiated pleomorphic sarcoma
Leiomyoma	Leiomyosarcoma
Rhabdomyoma	Rhabdomyosarcoma
Chondroma	Chondrosarcoma
BNCT (*ecchordosis physaliphora*)	Chordoma
Osteoma	Osteosarcoma
Hemangioma	Angiosarcoma
	Epithelioid hemangioendothelioma
	Kaposi sarcoma
Hemangioblastoma	(No malignant counterpart)
Inflammatory myofibroblastic tumor	(Malignant behaviour very rare)
(No benign counterpart)	Ewing sarcoma

BNCT benign notochordal cell tumor

as hemangioblastoma, pheochromocytoma, and clear cell type of renal cell carcinoma. Patients with von *Hippel-Lindau disease* have a propensity for the development of multiple tumors.

Clinically, hemangioblastoma frequently causes symptoms of intracranial hypertension and hydrocephalus due to the obstruction of the CSF flow. Approximately 10% of tumors produce an erythropoietin-like protein, and the resulting polycythemia serves as a tumor indicator. The typical radiologic image is that of a cystic lesion with a contrast-enhancing mural nodule, preferentially located in the cerebellum, brainstem, or spinal cord (usually dorsal); "flow voids" (vascular patency) may be encountered.

Grossly, they are often well-circumscribed mural nodules, at times diminutive, within a large, fluid-filled cyst that abuts the pial surface.

Histologically, the tumor has two components: (1) an anastomosing network of thin-walled vascular channels / capillaries and (2) intervening stromal cells, which have an ample cytoplasm that varies from vacuolated with clear lipid droplets to faintly eosinophilic and finely granular. The stromal cells' nuclei may show conspicuous pleomorphism and hyperchromatism. It is not unusual to find gliotic parenchyma with a considerable number of Rosenthal fibers at the periphery of the tumor. A clear demarcation from adjacent native tissues also is typical (Fig. 14.1a).

Brachyury is weakly expressed in the cytoplasm of stromal cells (not nuclear as in chordoma) and is highly specific for hemangioblastoma, distinguishing it from metastatic clear cell renal carcinoma. Also inhibin alpha positivity in the cytoplasm of stromal cells distinguishes hemangioblastoma from clear cell renal carcinoma.

a b c
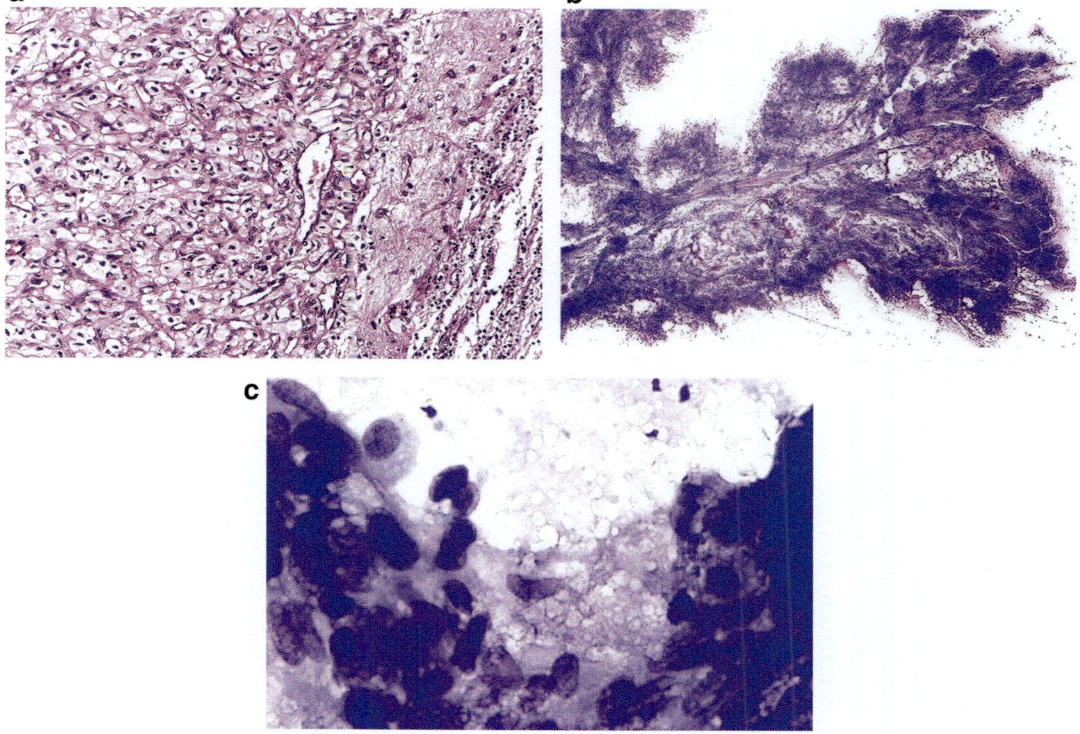

Fig. 14.1 *Hemangioblastoma.* (**a**) Histology. Hemangioblastoma consists of an intricate network of vascular channels and capillaries with a component of stromal lipid-rich cells. Note a sharp interface between the tumor and the adjacent gliotic cerebellum. (**b**) Cohesive vascular core tissue fragment with associated coarse stromal cells. (**c**) A high-magnification view reveals the characteristic lipid-rich cytoplasm and pleomorphic nuclei of the stromal cells. Also note a granular-vacuolated background with lipid droplets (**b, c**; Smears, Romanowsky)

Hemangioblastomas are slowly growing tumors corresponding to WHO grade I, being curable with gross total resection. Antiangiogenic therapy (bevacizumab) can be used successfully in recurrent or nonresectable tumors.

Cytologic Features

Hemangioblastoma can closely resemble diffuse astrocytoma in frozen sections, but not in smears. Preparations are made with difficulty because of the tenacity with which the vascular network, rich in reticulin, resists smearing. Thus, smears show compact tissue fragments and few single cells. These tissue fragments are composed by an intricate network of thin-walled vascular channels and capillaries, surrounded by interstitial (stromal) cells with indistinct or foamy cytoplasm. Nuclei of endothelial cells are oval to elongated and remarkably uniform, whereas the stromal cells' nuclei may show atypical changes including prominent pleomorphism, chromatin smudging, and irregular outlines. The characteristic cytoplasmic vacuoles of the stromal cells, representing dissolved lipids, are best identified at the group edges where there is less cellular density. Cytoplasm often shears apart during the preparation, leaving membranous debris and lipid droplets (granular-vacuolated background). Frequently, just as in other vascular tumors, the presence of siderophages and mast cells is observed, which, although not specific, may be a diagnostic clue (Fig. 14.1b, c).

Differential Diagnosis Considerations

Because it shares similar location and radiologic features, pilocytic astrocytoma ought to be taken into a consideration. This problem may be accentuated if the biopsy sample originates from the hemangioblastoma cyst wall, which consists of reactive gliosis with Rosenthal fibers (pilocytic gliosis). Further smears from the mural nodule will be necessary to enable one to observe the characteristic vascular framework and lipidized stromal cells from hemangioblastoma. On the other hand, the presence of clear, vacuolated cells may lead to confusion with metastatic renal clear cell carcinoma or clear cell meningioma, even though these dilemmas come up more frequently in frozen sections. Smears of the three tumors show quite different aspects. (Table 14.2)

Solitary Fibrous Tumor/Hemangiopericytoma

Because of clinical, histological, and molecular overlap, solitary fibrous tumor (SFT) and hemangiopericytoma (HPC) are currently considered a histologic spectrum of the same tumor rather than two separate entities. Both neoplasms share the

Table 14.2 Characteristics of hemangioblastoma

Cytologic features
Specimens difficult to smear
Tissue fragments and few single cells
Intricate network of thin-walled vascular channels and capillaries
Coarse interstitial cells (often lipid-laden)
Granular-vacuolated background
Differential diagnosis and pitfalls
Diffuse astrocytoma
Pilocytic astrocytoma (surrounding piloid gliosis)
Metastatic renal clear cell carcinoma
Clear cell meningioma

same genomic inversion at the 12q13 locus that fuses *NAB2* and *STAT6* genes, resulting in nuclear translocation of the STAT6 protein that can be readily identified by nuclear immunoreactivity (a useful diagnostic biomarker that separates this tumor from its mimics). SFT/HPC is rare, accounting for lessthan1% of all primary CNS tumors. This neoplasm almost always occurs in adults and, like meningioma, is usually attached to the inner surface of cranial and spinal dura, but occasional examples may arise in lateral ventricles, cerebellum, and spinal cord.

Radiologic and clinical features are indistinguishable from those of meningioma, but HPC has a high incidence of local recurrence and late distant metastases outside the CNS, particularly in the lungs, liver, and bone.

Grossly, SFT is well circumscribed, rubbery to firm mass with white-tan coloration. HPC is a solid, plaque-like to lobulated mass with gray-pink coloration and a fleshy cut surface; it may invade and destroy the adjacent bone.

Microscopically, *SFT* (now SFT/HPC; WHO grade I) is composed of uniform oval to spindle cells invested in a variably but often dense collagenous background (Fig. 14.2a). *HPC* (now SFT/HPC, WHO grade II) is a more cellular lesion (blue-staining tissue section at low microscopic magnification) composed of closely packed, round-to-oval small cells arranged in "jumbled-up" architecture. In both tumors the elaborate vascular network may be composed of thin-walled branching "staghorn" vessels (Fig. 14.2b). *Anaplastic hemangiopericytoma* (now SFT/HPC, WHO grade III) shows high cellularity, increased mitotic activity (five or more per ten HPFs), and necrosis.

Cytologic Features

Due to desmoplasia, *SFT* often resists smearing, and preparations show compact cell groups that alternate with few spindle-shaped single cells. Tumor cells are uniformly bland, with oval to fusiform nucleus and scant elongated cytoplasm. The clear or

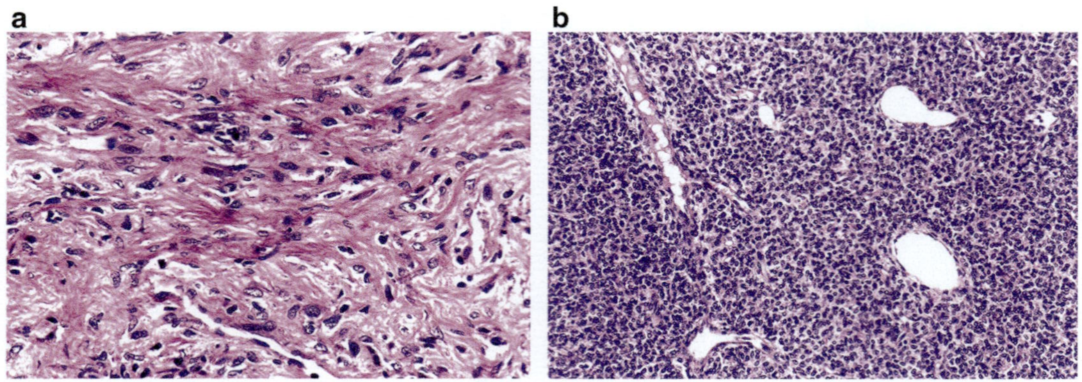

Fig. 14.2 *Solitary fibrous tumor* (*SFT*)/*hemangiopericytoma* (*HPC*). (**a**) Typical *SFT* histology with a patternless architecture of elongate cells in an intercellular background of eosinophilic collagen. Note characteristic thin-walled, slit-like vascular channels. (**b**) Characteristic *HPC* histology showing closely opposed cells with round to oval nuclei arranged in a haphazard pattern. Note limited intervening stroma and thin-walled, gaping vascular spaces

bloody background may contain ropy collagen fibers (Fig. 14.3a). Smear preparations from *HPC* are more cellular, showing a mixed pattern with smeared fragments and numerous single cells. Perivascular arrangements are common, as are arborizing vascular channels associated with tumor cell aggregations. Tumor cells are typically uniform with inconspicuous cytoplasm and small, dark oval nuclei. Many cells may appear as naked nuclei (Fig. 14.3b, c).

Differential Diagnosis Considerations

SFT should be differentiated from meningioma, with which it may share clinical, radiologic, and morphologic data. Particularly, the typical smear pattern of SFT often resembles a fibrous meningioma and is probably quite frequently misdiagnosed as such. However, SFT lacks the characteristic nuclear features of meningioma, including pseudoinclusions and clearings. The differential diagnosis of *HPC* includes meningioma and hemangioblastoma, but HPC lacks well-formed whorls, psammoma bodies, and nuclear pseudoinclusions as seen in meningiomas or the lipid-laden, coarse interstitial cells of hemangioblastoma (Table 14.3).

Lipoma

Lipoma is usually a malformative (lipomatous hamartoma) or occasionally neoplastic mass composed of mature adipose tissue. As dysembryoplastic errors, lipomas typically occur at midline and are often associated with developmental anomalies, particularly partial or complete agenesis of the corpus callosum and spinal dysraphism with tethered cord. Cranial examples involve the interhemispheric region (callosal examples may be massive), tectal plate, cerebellopontine angle, internal auditory canal (lipoma of eighth cranial nerve), sylvian cisterns (may encase middle cerebral artery branches), and suprasellar/hypothalamic region, whereas spinal cord examples usually involve the conus medullaris-filum terminale (known as lipomeningocele), the thoracic level (known as leptomyelolipoma), or the epidural space (spinal epidural lipoma). Clinically, lipomas may cause headache, seizures, and focal symptoms or may be asymptomatic. The MRI characteristics of lipoma are virtually diagnostic, as precontrast T1 images show fat having high (white) signal intensity. Grossly, lipomas are yellow, soft, lobulated masses often attached to meninges. Adherence to adjacent brain/spinal cord, local nerves, and vasculature is not uncommon, and attempts at en bloc resection may result in severe neurologic injury, so lipomas are generally not removed. Microscopically, *lipoma* is composed by mature adipose tissue; also Schwann cells, bone, cartilage, and hamartomatous blood vessels have been described. *Lipomeningocele* is a complex lipomatous lesion consisting of lobulated adipose tissue, often associated with fibrous tissue, vascular proliferation, smooth muscle elements, and neuroglial tissue (fibrolipomatous

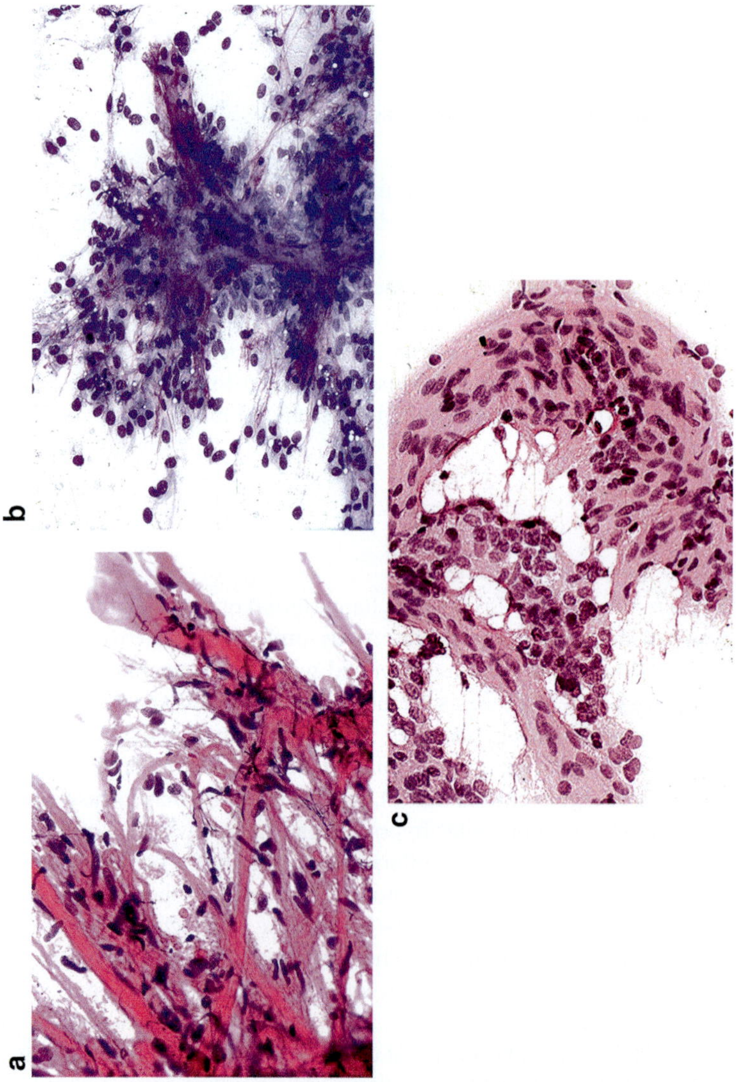

Fig. 14.3 *Solitary fibrous tumor* (*SFT*)/*hemangiopericytoma* (*HPC*), *cytologic features*. (**a**) *SFT* preparation showing oval to spindle-shaped cells and numerous bundles of brightly eosinophilic collagen (Smear, H&E). (**b**) *HPC* preparation showing a vascular channel with "staghorn" branching surrounded by tumor cell aggregates (Smear, Romanowsky). (**c**) A high-magnification view reveals the appearance of *HPC* tumor cells with rounded nuclei, dense chromatin, and inconspicuous cytoplasm. Note the clear difference with endothelial cells nuclei, which are elongated, bland, and remarkably uniform (Smear, H&E)

Table 14.3 Characteristics of solitary fibrous tumor/hemangiopericytoma

Cytologic features
Solitary fibrous tumor pattern
A meshwork of irregular fascicles and individual cells
Bland spindle cells with fusiform nuclei
Ropy collagen fibers
Hemangiopericytoma pattern
Cellular smears with perivascular clusters and single cells
Thin-walled "arborizing" vascular channels
Monotonous small cells with dark, oval nuclei
Many naked nuclei
Differential diagnosis and pitfalls
Solitary fibrous tumor pattern
Meningioma (particularly fibrous type)
Hemangiopericytoma pattern
Hemangioblastoma
Meningioma (particularly angiomatous type)

hamartoma). *Leptomyelolipomas* present as a subpial mass of mature adipose tissue, plastered over a variable length of the spinal cord. *Spinal epidural lipomas* may be markedly vascular, showing intimate admixture of vascular channels and mature adipose tissue (angiolipoma). It has been suggested that intracranial lipomas containing various other tissue types represent a transition between lipoma and teratoma.

Cytologic Features and Differential Diagnosis

Occasionally, smears can be prepared from lipoma specimens that show tissue fragments of large, balloon-like cells with clear cytoplasm and eccentric nuclei (Fig. 14.4a). Scattered foamy macrophages with ingested lipid (lipophages) are common in tumors with regressive changes, and it is important not to confuse these lipophages with lipoblasts from a liposarcoma (Fig. 14.4b).

As any lipomatous tissue is abnormal within the cranial cavity, *differential diagnosis* arises mainly with undersampled teratoma or meningioma with adipocytic metaplasia.

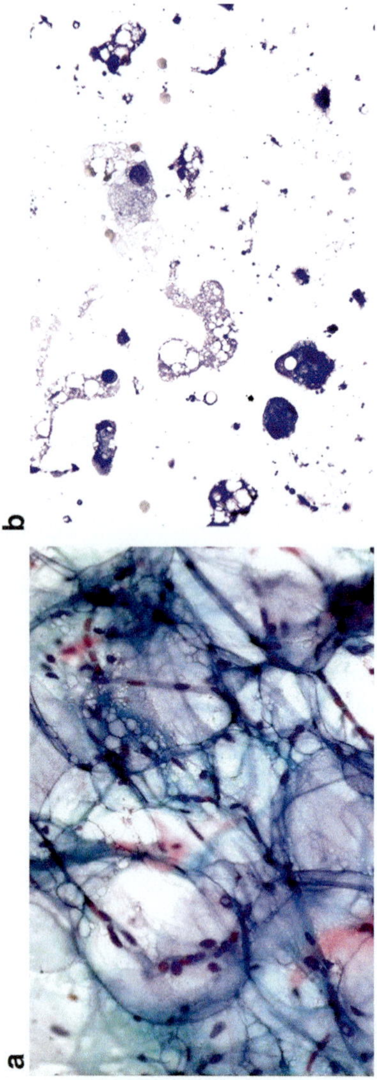

Fig. 14.4 *Lipoma*. (**a**) This tissue fragment is composed of large and uniform univacuolate adipocytes. Also note some capillaries (Smear, Papanicolaou). (**b**) Scattered foamy macrophages with ingested lipid are often seen in lipomas with regressive changes (Smear, Romanowsky)

Rhabdomyosarcoma

Rhabdomyosarcoma can arise throughout the neuroaxis, with a predilection for the skull base, nasal sinuses, and posterior fossa (cerebellum). However, medical literature describes more instances of metastatic rhabdomyosarcoma to the brain than of primary examples. It affects primarily infants and children, although tumors in adults may also occur. The clinical course is often rapidly progressive with proptosis, diplopia, unilateral deafness, or symptoms related to increased intracranial pressure. In neuroimaging, they are large, avidly enhancing masses, which may extend into orbital, paranasal, and intracranial compartments. Grossly, the tumor is poorly circumscribed, white, and soft. Whether meningeal or parenchymal, nearly all CNS rhabdomyosarcomas are of the embryonal type, consisting primarily of small, round to ovoid cells; distinctive strap cells with cross striation are only occasionally observed (Fig. 14.5a). Embryonal rhabdomyosarcoma with a dense pattern can mimic many other "small round blue cell" tumors. Despite aggressive radiation and chemotherapy, CNS rhabdomyosarcomas have been almost uniformly fatal within 2 years.

Cytologic Features and Differential Diagnosis

Smears are composed predominantly of isolated cells with occasional small cell clusters and, sometimes, a foamy "tigroid" background (release of intracytoplasmic glycogen). Tumor cells vary from round undifferentiated, to polygonal or spindle shaped. Larger cells may show rhabdomyoblastic differentiation with elongated, strap, or tadpole-shaped cytoplasm with cross striations (Fig. 14.5b, c).

Differential diagnosis should include CNS embryonal tumors (including medulloblastoma and AT/RT), Ewing sarcoma, and rhabdoid meningioma. The presence of rhabdomyoblastic differentiation (strap or tadpole cytomorphology) and the occasional presence of a frothy "tigroid" background are useful differential features.

Ewing Sarcoma

Ewing sarcoma (EWS) is a rare, small round cell tumor showing varying degrees of neuroectodermal differentiation. It may occur as either a primary dural neoplasm or by direct extension from contiguous bone/soft tissue, such as skull, vertebral bodies, or paraspinal soft tissues. Spinal examples are generally intradural and extramedullary often arising in association with nerve roots, whereas intracranial lesions are most often dura-based mimicking meningioma. The immunophenotype and biology are the same to that encountered in bone or soft tissue examples: CD99 strong

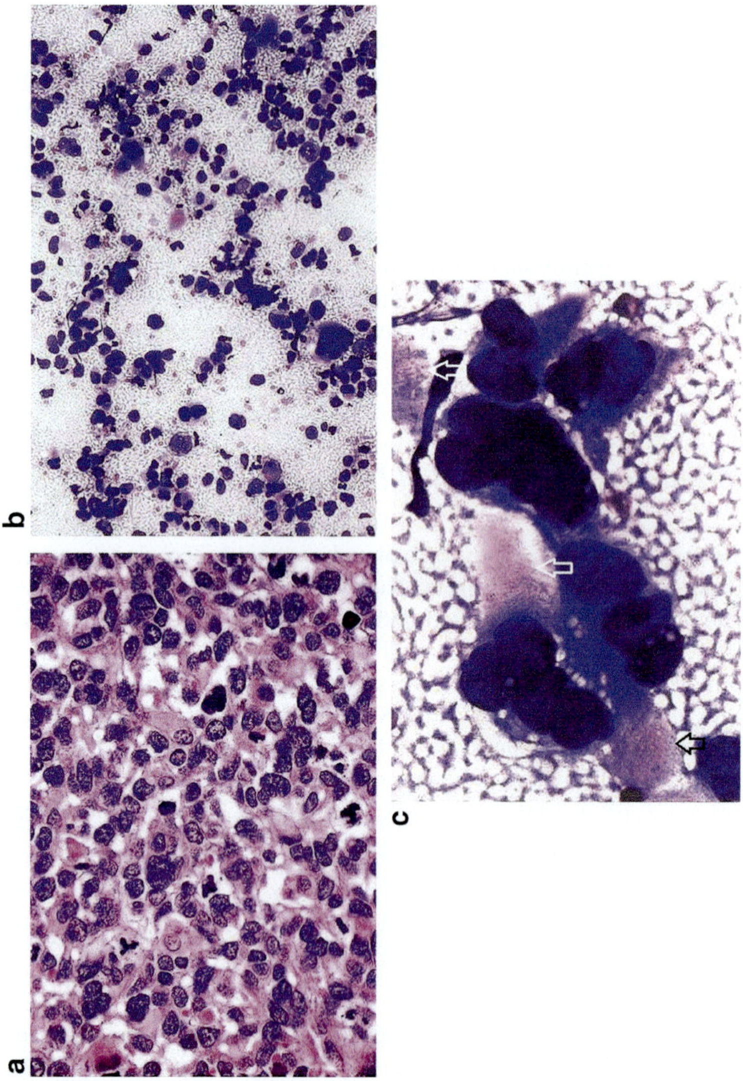

Fig. 14.5 *Embryonal rhabdomyosarcoma.* (**a**) Typical histology with round to ovoid to strap cells and numerous atypical mitoses. (**b**) This preparation displays dispersed tumor cells in a foamy background. (**c**) High-power view showing distinctive strap cells with cross striations (*arrows*). Also note the characteristic foamy "tigroid" background of glycogen-rich tumors (**b, c**; Smears, Romanowsky)

membranous immunoreactivity and somatic rearrangements between the *EWSR1* gene and members of the ETS gene family, more commonly the *EWSR1-FLI1* fusion transcript. A wide age range has been encountered with a peak incidence in the second decade. Clinically and radiologically, both spinal and intracranial examples may closely mimic meningioma. Microscopically, EWS consists of solid sheets of small, round primitive-appearing cells divided into irregular lobules by fibrous strands (Fig. 14.6a). Necrosis is common and may dominate the microscopic picture.

Cytologic Features and Differential Diagnosis

The morphologic features of the EWS can be recognized on cytologic examination, which represents an important diagnostic tool, both in bone/soft tissue examples and those involving the CNS. Smears are hypercellular, with clustered or dispersed small cells in a characteristic foamy "tigroid" background (release of intracytoplasmic glycogen). Two distinct cell types can be recognized: (1) the "light" (viable) cells have a rim of cytoplasm with clear spaces or vacuoles and rounded pale nuclei with finely chromatin texture and small nucleoli, whereas (2) the "dark" (dying) cells are smaller, with hyperchromatic smudged nuclei and scanty cytoplasm. Cytoplasm borders are typically ill-defined and wispy, whereas nuclear molding is usually prominent (Fig. 14.6b, c).

Differential diagnosis should include CNS embryonal tumors, lymphoma, rhabdomyosarcoma, and hemangiopericytoma; however, the diagnosis of EWS can be favored if the characteristic cytomorphologic features mentioned here are taken into account.

Fibrosarcoma

Primary CNS fibrosarcomas are extremely rare, being some related to prior radiation exposure (e.g., sellar fibrosarcoma in patients so treated for pituitary adenoma) with latent periods of 5–20 years. These tumors are commonly attached to the dura and leptomeninges, but some examples are situated within the cerebrum or cerebellum. Extensive involvement of the bone, dura, leptomeninges, and brain generally obscures the precise origin. Local recurrence is the rule even after gross total resection of circumscribed lesions, and patients with high-grade lesions usually succumb within several years of diagnosis developing leptomeningeal and distant extracranial metastases. Histologically, it is a malignant neoplasm composed of neoplastic spindle cells, variable collagen production, and at least focal v-shaped weaving "herringbone" pattern (Fig. 14.7a).

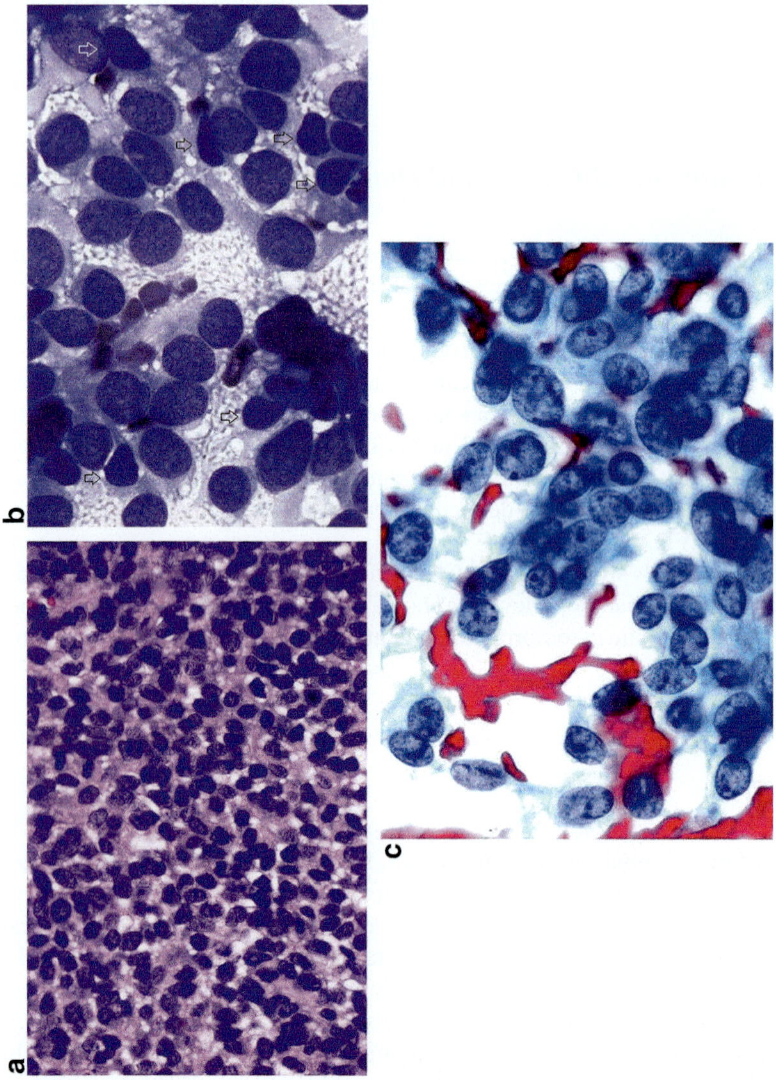

Fig. 14.6 *Ewing sarcoma*. (**a**) Histology. This tumor consists of solid sheets of small, undifferentiated cells. (**b**) Cytologic preparations are hypercellular, with clusters or dispersed small cells in a characteristic foamy "tigroid" background. Note two distinct cell types – "light" and "dark" (*arrows*) – and frequent nuclear molding (Smear, Romanowsky). (**c**) Viable "light" cells show small-to-medium-sized irregular nuclei with tiny nucleoli. Cytoplasmic borders are ill-defined and wispy (Smear, Papanicolaou)

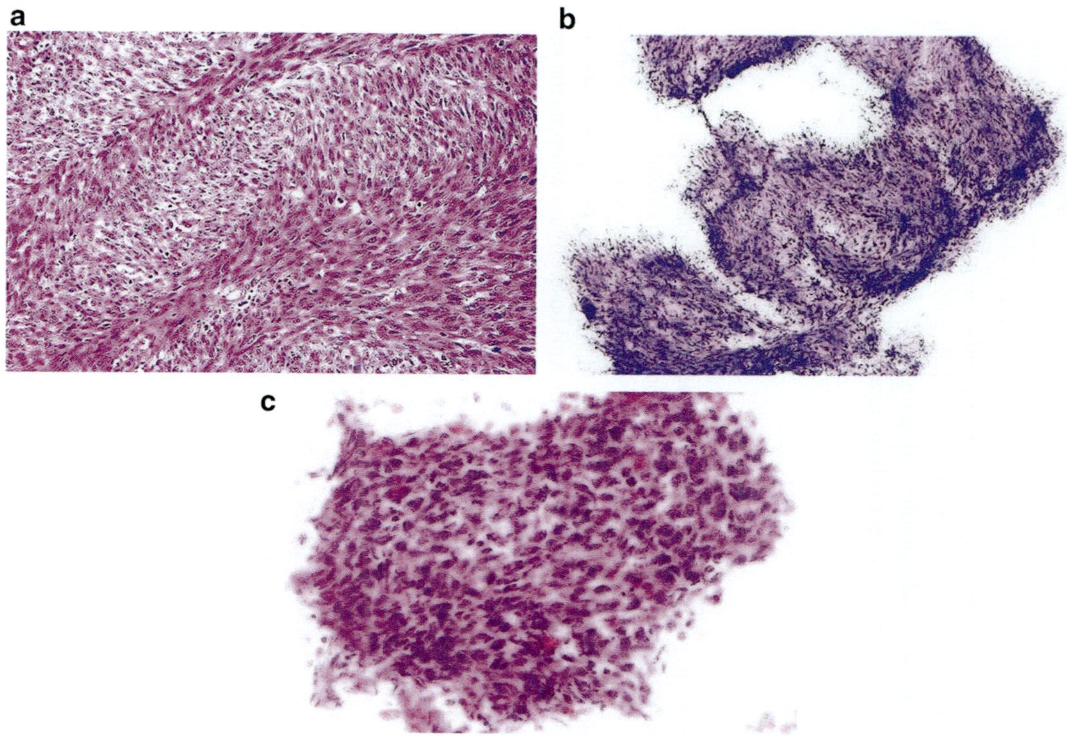

Fig. 14.7 *Fibrosarcoma*. (**a**) This radiation-induced neoplasm shows histologic features of fibrosarcoma, with intersecting fascicles of spindle cells, focal v-shaped "herringbone" pattern, and increased mitotic activity. (**b**) Cohesive tissue fragment composed of atypical spindle cells (Smear, Romanowsky). (**c**) High-power view showing closely packed hyperchromatic elongated cells (Smear, H&E)

Cytologic Features and Differential Diagnosis

The cytomorphologic features of fibrosarcoma are nonspecific; preparations display cohesive tissue fragments of hyperchromatic spindle cells in a clear or granular background (Fig. 14.7b, c).

Due to the fact that CNS fibrosarcomas often present as dura-based masses, the primary *differential diagnosis* is anaplastic meningioma, but gliosarcoma and malignant peripheral nerve cell tumor (MPNST) should also be considered. In such cases, we should look for conspicuous meningothelial, glial, or neural cell differentiation, and if these features cannot be identified, only an intraoperative descriptive appellation of "high-grade, spindle-cell malignant tumor" should be given. Even in permanent sections, fibrosarcoma is best regarded as a diagnosis of exclusion.

Chordoma

Chordoma is a rare, malignant midline bone tumor arising from notochord remnants. It usually affects adults, peaking around the fourth decade, but tumors in children may also occur. Chordoma has a very precise location in the axial skeleton, particularly in its cranial and sacral extremes: approximately half arise in the sacrum and one-third in the spheno-occipital region (skull base/clivus) whereas the remainder in articulating vertebrae. In these characteristic locations, scans show heterogeneous bulky masses that destroy the bone. Grossly, chordoma is a lobulated mass of translucent, gray tissue. Histologically, the tumor cells are arranged in sheets or cords or seen as single elements embedded in the background matrix. Their cytomorphology varies from cells with nonvaculoated eosinophilic cytoplasm, to ones containing one or several vacuoles, the so-called physaliphorous cells – from the Greek *physalis*, meaning *bubble* (Fig. 14.8a). Pediatric chordomas may be more cellular and poorly differentiated than adult cases and have a high rate of SMARCB1/INI1 loss by immunohistochemistry. Because chordoma has a high incidence of local recurrence and the possibility of late distant metastases (skin, bone), wide surgical excision at the time of initial surgery offers the best choice for cure. Large tumor size, performing an invasive diagnostic procedure in a nonspecialized tumor center, inadequate surgical margins, tumor necrosis, Ki-67 greaterthan5%, and local recurrence have been found to be adverse prognostic factors.

Cytologic Features and Differential Diagnosis

Smears preparations show abundant myxoid background matrix, characteristically encircling tumor cell groups and single tumor cells. The diagnostic cell is the physaliphorous one, which features abundant vacuolated (bubbly) cytoplasm with

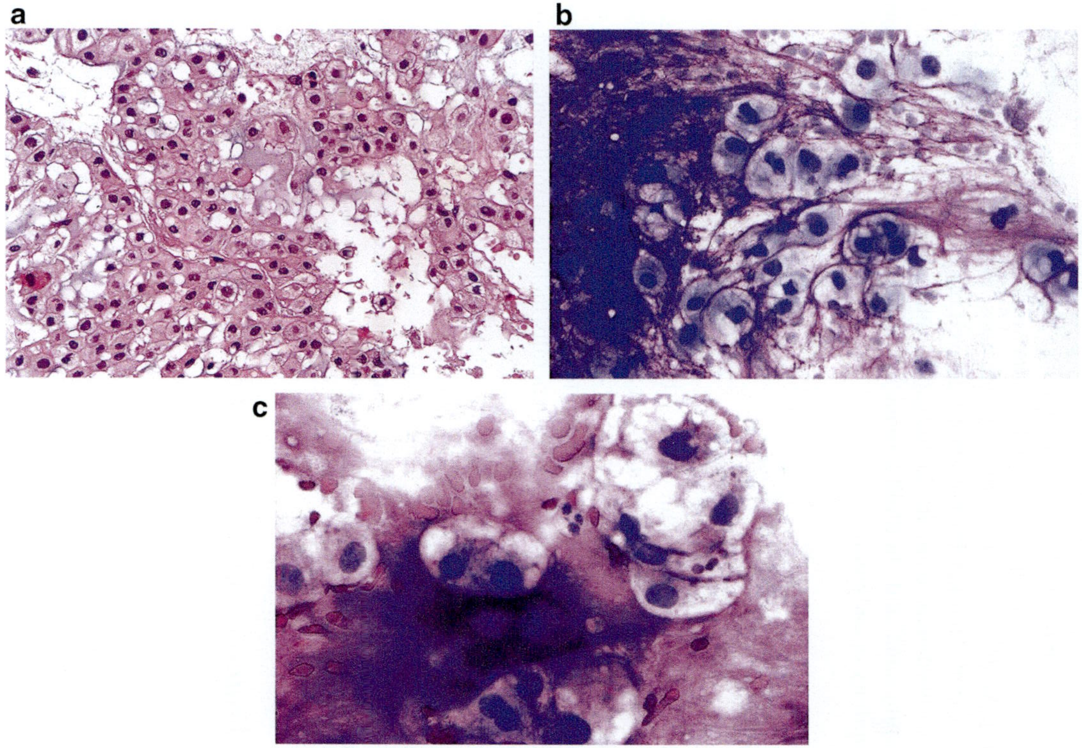

Fig. 14.8 *Chordoma.* (**a**) Histology. Characteristic cords and lobules of epithelioid vacuolated cells embedded in a dense myxoid stroma. (**b**) Small clusters of discrete tumor cells in a blue-violet myxoid matrix that encircles many single tumor cells. (**c**) Large cells corresponding to physaliforous cells with abundant multivacuolated cytoplasm. Nuclei are round with small nucleoli (**b, c**; Smears, Romanowsky)

well-defined cell borders. Nuclei are rather uniform with small nucleoli. Univacuolate "signet-ring" cells, smaller cuboidal cells, and spindly cells may be also present, which exemplifies the diverse histologic appearance of this tumor (Fig. 14.8b, c).

The differential diagnosis should include other tumors that may have vacuolated cells and myxoid-mucoid extracellular matrix, such as chondrosarcoma, chordoid meningioma, and metastatic mucinous adenocarcinoma, whereas in the sacrococcygeal region, we should also include the other characteristic myxoid regional tumor, the myxopapillary ependymoma (all already been covered in previous chapters). With respect to permanent sections, nuclear immunolabeling for brachyury (a specific marker for notochord-derived tissues and neoplasms) readily distinguishes chordomas from its histologic mimics including chondrosarcoma, chordoid meningioma, and chordoid glioma, as well as mucinous adenocarcinomas and myxopapillary ependymoma.

Osteosarcoma

Osteosarcoma can arise in the skull or facial bones and more rarely in the spine, the meninges, or the brain. It occurs primarily in adolescents and young adults (85% of cases arise before the age of 30 years). Most osteosarcomas arise de novo, but may also be seen as a consequence of radiation therapy or Paget's disease. Presenting symptoms of primary CNS osteosarcoma generally include a rapidly enlarged skull mass, headaches, or signs of increased intracranial pressure. Histologically, it is a malignant neoplasm composed of pleomorphic bizarre cells and multinucleated osteoclasts, but the key feature for the diagnosis is the presence of osteoid matrix. This homogeneous material is recognized by its eosinophilic quality, glassy appearance, and irregular contours (Fig. 14.9a). Craniospinal cases (e.g., skull, vertebrae) may be accessible to direct aspiration biopsy.

Cytologic Features and Differential Diagnosis

The cytomorphologic features of osteosarcoma are nonspecific, but combining these with the clinico-radiologic information, a high diagnostic accuracy can be reached. Smears are cellular with pleomorphic (rounded, ovoid, polygonal, spindle) bizarre cells. The nuclei are hyperchromatic, often multiple, and occasionally polylobulated. Multinucleated tumor giant cells and benign osteoclast-like cells may be seen sprinkled throughout the preparation. In some cases, distinctive osteoid matrix can be recognized as magenta (Romanowsky stain), pink (H&E stain), or green (Papanicolaou stain) hyaline homogeneous material (Fig. 14.9b, c).

Intracranial cases should be *differentiated* from high-grade pleomorphic neuroectodermal tumors, such as giant cell glioblastoma (presence of tumor cells with numerous cytoplasmic processes) and gliosarcoma with osteosarcomatous component (presence of conspicuous glial component).

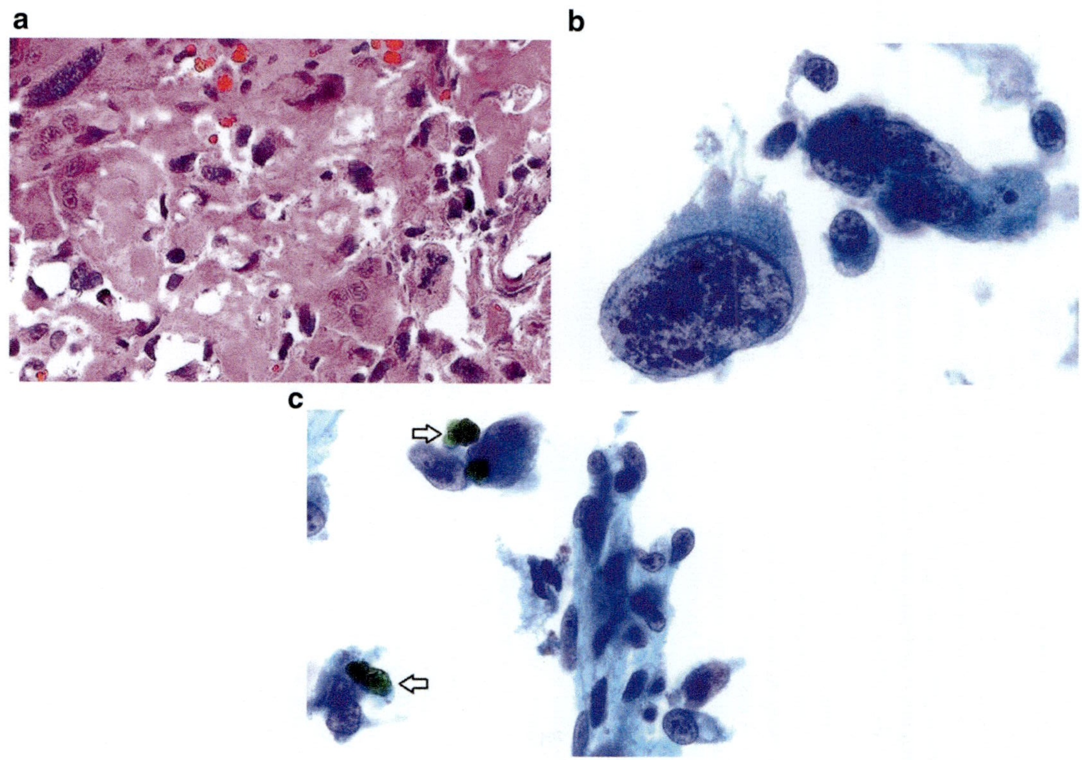

Fig. 14.9 *Osteosarcoma*, direct percutaneous needle aspiration from a skull lesion. (**a**) Malignant pleomorphic cells, multinucleated osteoclasts, and osteoid matrix in the right upper corner (Cell block). A population of pleomorphic tumor cells, some multinucleated (**b**), and green hyaline fragments of osteoid matrix (*arrows*; **c**) in the cytologic preparations (**b, c**; Thin Prep, Papanicolaou)

Suggested Reading

Ashraf MJ, Azarpira N, Shishegar M, Sepidbakht S. Fine needle aspiration cytology of intracranial peripheral-type primitive neuroectodermal tumor. Acta Cytol. 2010;54:740–2.

Barresi V, Ieni A, Branca G, Tuccari G. Brachyury: a diagnostic marker for the differential diagnosis of chordoma and hemangioblastoma versus neoplastic histological mimickers. Dis Markers. 2014;2014:514753.

Barthelmeß S, Geddert H, Boltze C, Moskalev EA, et al. Solitary fibrous tumors/hemangiopericytomas with different variants of the NAB2-STAT6 gene fusion are characterized by specific histomorphology and distinct clinicopathological features. Am J Pathol. 2014;184:1209–18.

Bergh P, Kindblom LG, Gunterberg B, Remotti F, Ryd W, Meis-Kindblom JM. Prognostic factors in chordoma of the sacrum and mobile spine: a study of 39 patients. Cancer. 2000;88:2122–34.

Bouvier D, Metellus P, de Paula AM, Vasiljevic A, et al. Solitary fibrous tumors and hemangiopericytomas of the meninges: overlapping pathological features and common prognostic factors suggest the same spectrum of tumors. Brain Pathol. 2012;22:511–21.

Commins DL, Hinton DR. Cytologic features of hemangioblastoma. Comparison with meningioma, anaplastic astrocytoma and renal cell carcinoma. Acta Cytol. 1998;42:1104–10.

Ghaffar H, Parwani A, Rosenthal DL. FNAC of hepatic metastasis from a meningeal hemangiopericytoma. A case report. Acta Cytol. 2003;47:281–6.

Gill SS, Bharadwaj R. Cytomorphologic findings of hemangiopericytoma of the meninges: a case report. Indian J Pathol Microbiol. 2007;50:422–5.

Hasselblatt M, Thomas C, Hovestadt V, Schrimpf D, et al. Poorly differentiated chordoma with SMARCB1/INI1 loss: a distinct molecular entity with dismal prognosis. Acta Neuropathol. 2016;132:149–51.

Hoang MP, Amirkhan RH. Inhibin alpha distinguishes hemangioblastoma from clear cell renal cell carcinoma. Am J Surg Pathol. 2003;27:1152–6.

Kay PA, Nascimento AG, Unni KK, Salomão DR. Chordoma. Cytomorphologic findings in 14 cases diagnosed by fine needle aspiration. Acta Cytol. 2003;47:202–8.

Kazmi SA, Perry A, Pressey JG, Wellons JC, et al. Primary Ewing sarcoma of the brain: a case report and literature review. Diagn Mol Pathol. 2007;16:108–11.

Lau SK, Cykowski MD, Desai S, Cao Y, et al. Primary rhabdomyosarcoma of the pineal gland. Am J Clin Pathol. 2015;143:728–33.

Mobley BC, Roulston D, Shah GV, Bijwaard KE, McKeever PE. Peripheral primitive neuroectodermal tumor/Ewing's sarcoma of the craniospinal vault: case reports and review. Hum Pathol. 2006;37:845–53.

Niwa T, de Vries LS, Manten GT, Lequin M, et al. Interhemispheric lipoma, callosal anomaly, and malformations of cortical development: a case series. Neuropediatrics. 2016;47:115–8.

Oliveira AM, Scheithauer BW, Salomao DR, Parisi JE, et al. Primary sarcomas of the brain and spinal cord: a study of 18 cases. Am J Surg Pathol. 2002;26:1056–63.

Ortega L, Jiménez-Heffernan JA, Perna C. Squash cytology of cerebellar haemangioblastoma. Cytopathology. 2002;13:184–5.

Ostrom QT, Gittleman H, Liao P, Rouse C, et al. CBTRUS statistical report: primary brain and central nervous system tumors diagnosed in the United States in 2007–2011. Neuro-Oncology. 2014;16(suppl 4):iv1–iv63. https://doi.org/10.1093/neuonc/nou223.

Patel AJ, Rao VY, Fox BD, Suki D, et al. Radiation-induced osteosarcomas of the calvarium and skull base. Cancer. 2011;117:2120–6.

Perry A, Scheithauer BW, Nascimento AG. The immunophenotypic spectrum of meningeal hemangiopericytoma: a comparison with fibrous meningioma and solitary fibrous tumor of meninges. Am J Surg Pathol. 1997;21:1354–60.

Sangoi AR, Dulai MS, Beck AH, Brat DJ, Vogel H. Distinguishing chordoid meningiomas from their histologic mimics: an immunohistochemical evaluation. Am J Surg Pathol. 2009;33:669–81.

Sangoi AR, Karamchandani J, Lane B, Higgins JP, et al. Specificity of brachyury in the distinction of chordoma from clear cell renal cell carcinoma and germ cell tumors: a study of 305 cases. Mod Pathol. 2011;24:425–9.
Setzer M, Lang J, Turowski B, Marquardt G. Primary meningeal osteosarcoma: case report and review of the literature. Neurosurgery. 2002;51:488–92.
Schweizer L, Koelsche C, Sahm F, Pisa R, et al. Meningeal hemangiopericytoma and solitary fibrous tumors carry the NAB2-STAT6 fusion and can be diagnosed by nuclear expression of STAT6 protein. Acta Neuropathol (Berl). 2013;125:651–8.
Shankar GM, Taylor-Weiner A, Lelic N, Jones RT, et al. Sporadic hemangioblastomas are characterized by cryptic VHL inactivation. Acta Neuropathol Commun. 2014;2:167.
Shinoda J, Kimura T, Funakoshi T, Iwata H, et al. Primary osteosarcoma of the skull –a case report and review of the literature. J Neuro-Oncol. 1993;17:81–8.
Taratuto AL, Molina HA, Diez B, Zúccaro G, Monges J. Primary rhabdomyosarcoma of brain and cerebellum. Report of four cases in infants: an immunohistochemical study. Acta Neuropathol. 1985;66:98–104.
Tresser NJ, Parveen T, Roessmann U. Intracranial lipomas with teratomatous elements. Arch Pathol Lab Med. 1993;117:918–20.
Yilmaz N, Unal O, Kiymaz N, Yilmaz C, Etlik O. Intracranial lipomas-a clinical study. Clin Neurol Neurosurg. 2006;108:363–8.

Chapter 15
Germ Cell Tumors

Intracranial germ cell tumors (iGCTs) presumably arise from primordial germ cells that were trapped within neural tissue during the process of migration at the time of early embryogenesis. Therefore, they are similar to their extraneuraxial counterparts sharing histologic types, immunostaining properties, and, in some aspects, genetic alterations. They commonly affect children and young adults (close to 90% of patients present before age 20 years) and have a marked predilection for males (more than twice as females). In Europe and the USA, the frequency is not high, representing approximately 0.5% of primary intracranial tumors and 3% of tumors affecting children. However, these figures are quadruple in eastern Asia (Taiwan, Japan, China, and Korea) where they represent 2% of all primary intracranial neoplasms and 15% of pediatric cases, being the second most common pediatric brain tumors after astrocytomas. Like other extragonadal germ cell tumors, CNS forms tend to occur in the midline, with only rare cases found laterally. Most arise in the vicinity of the third ventricle involving the pineal or suprasellar regions, but involvement of multiple sites including the basal ganglia or thalamic nuclei is not uncommon (e.g., pineal-suprasellar, pineal-thalamic); very few cases arise in the spinal cord. Extremely large congenital teratomas may occur, either occupying much of the intracranial space or the sacrococcygeal area.

Clinical features are related to the location: pineal region tumors often produce progressive hydrocephalus with intracranial hypertension due to cerebral aqueduct compression. These lesions are also prone to produce paralysis of extraocular movements, especially upward gaze and convergence (Parinaud's syndrome), due to involvement of the tectal plate. Those in a sellar/suprasellar location produce visual field defects, diabetes insipidus, and pituitary failure, resulting from involvement of the optic chiasm and hypothalamo-hypophyseal axis. Neuroimaging features are non-specific and overlap with those of other tumors of this region.

Histologically, they represent a wide array of diseases but can be divided into two highly prognostic groups: pure germinomas and non-germinomatous or "malignant" germ cell tumors (NGGCTs), with teratomas being considered a separate cat-

C. R. Lacruz et al., *Central Nervous System Intraoperative Cytopathology*, Essentials in Cytopathology 13, https://doi.org/10.1007/978-3-319-98491-9_15

Table 15.1 Types of intracranial germ cell tumors

Germinoma
Non-germinomatous or "malignant" germ cell tumors
Embryonal carcinoma
Choriocarcinoma
Yolk sac (endodermal sinus) tumor
Teratoma
Mature teratoma
Immature teratoma
Teratoma with malignant transformation
Mixed germ cell tumor

egory. However, while germinomas occur as pure tumors in 60–65% of cases, NGGCTs more frequently occur as mixed tumors, which most commonly include germinoma and teratoma along with more malignant elements (Table 15.1). CNS GCTs do not carry WHO grade designations.

KIT mutations are the most common alterations found in iGCTs and are more often observed in pure germinomas (25% of cases) than in mixed tumors; *KRAS* and *NRAS* mutations are also identified. *KIT*, *KRAS*, and *NRAS* mutations are mutually exclusive and all together account for about 45% of cases.

Because of their different biological behavior, different prognosis, and their different therapeutic possibilities, it is advisable to differentiate among germinoma, teratoma, and NGGCTs during intraoperative consultation.

Germinoma

Germinoma is the most common iGCT (approximately 2/3 of cases), affecting mainly teenagers and young adults (about 2/3 males). Neuroimaging reveals homogeneous, avidly enhancing masses with occasional enhancing tumor along the ventricular walls due to CSF seeding. Grossly, they are typically homogeneous, soft and friable, tan-white, uni- or multifocal masses. Histologically, germinoma is composed by sheets and lobules of large primordial-like germ cells with clear cytoplasm and prominent nucleoli, admixed with small mature lymphocytes (Fig. 15.1a). Frequently, an intense granulomatous inflammatory reaction resembling sarcoidosis or tuberculosis takes place in the stroma, which may obscure tumor cells (Fig. 15.1b). In 15% of cases, there are giant multinucleated syncytiotrophoblastic cells (germinoma with syncytiotrophoblastic component).

Germinoma has a relatively good prognosis: the 5 and 10 years survival is 95% and 75%, respectively. Because this is a highly radiosensitive and chemosensitive tumor and surgical resection is not necessary, the pathologist needs to consider the diagnosis of germinoma during intraoperative consultation.

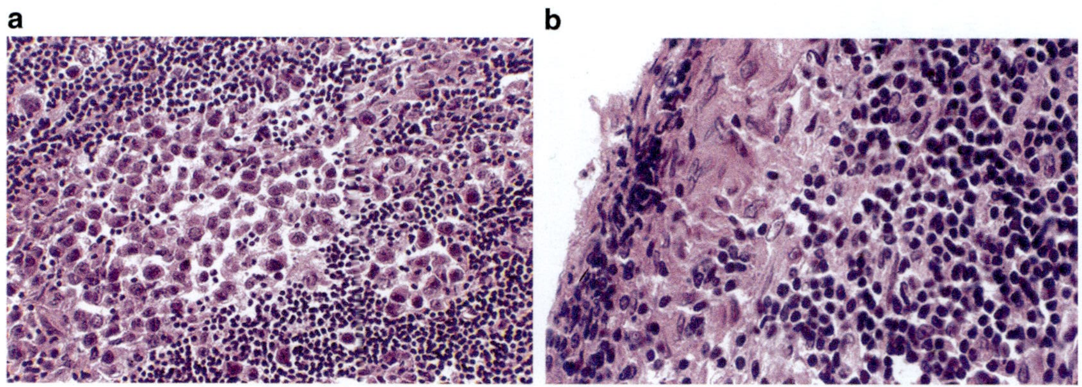

Fig. 15.1 *Germinoma, histology*. (**a**) A classic germinoma is made up of sheets of large tumor cells interrupted by fibrous septae sprinkled with small lymphocytes. (**b**) In this stereotactic biopsy specimen, an intense granulomatous inflammatory reaction overshadows the tumor cells

Cytologic Features

Since the freezing artifact distorts the tumor cells so much that they are not recognizable, the intraoperative diagnosis of germinoma is much easier in smears than in frozen sections. The cytologic picture may be summarized as follows: large germ cells and small lymphocytes in a peculiar granular-vacuolated background, the so-called striped "tigroid" background. The germ cells contain large, spherical nuclei with prominent and characteristically angular nucleoli. The cytoplasm is faint, vacuolated, and lacy due to its high glycogen content. The second cellular component consists of small, mature lymphocytes that are spread out and are occasionally admixed with plasma cells and histiocytes. The third component is the characteristic striped "tigroid" background, resulting from the release of intracytoplasmic glycogen during the squash technique (Fig. 15.2a–c). This background is better revealed by using Romanowsky stains; whereas it does not stand out as well and looks only slightly granular and eosinophilic with H&E or Papanicolaou stains.

Differential Diagnosis Considerations

Because affected sites are difficult to access surgically, specimens often are small stereotactic biopsies and may not be truly representative (not include all components). Thus, the common stromal granulomatous inflammatory reaction may be the only feature that appears on the smears, leading to a misdiagnosis of inflammatory disorder (Fig. 15.3a). On the other hand, stereotactic biopsies showing obvious germinoma features may derive from a mixed germ cell tumor; for example, teratoma with an element of germinoma (Fig. 15.3b). Therefore, it is highly recommended to obtain additional samples in cases showing granulomatous inflammation or displaying only germinoma features in a radiologically heterogeneous lesion. Aside from these two possible pitfalls, the differential diagnosis should include other regional tumors, such as Langerhans cell histiocytosis and pineal parenchymal tumors, as well as other look-alike neoplasms, i.e., metastatic large-cell carcinoma and lymphoma. All these possibilities may cause a serious problem in frozen sections, but in smears the combination of a dual cell population in a striped "tigroid" background allows accurate diagnosis of germinoma (Table 15.2).

Teratoma

Teratomas constitute nearly 20% of all iGCTs, most commonly affect pineal region and may coexist, as previously noted, with other germ cell elements such as germinoma, yolk sac tumor, or embryonal carcinoma (mixed GCTs). In contrast with germinoma, teratomas tend to occur in younger children (may even be congenital

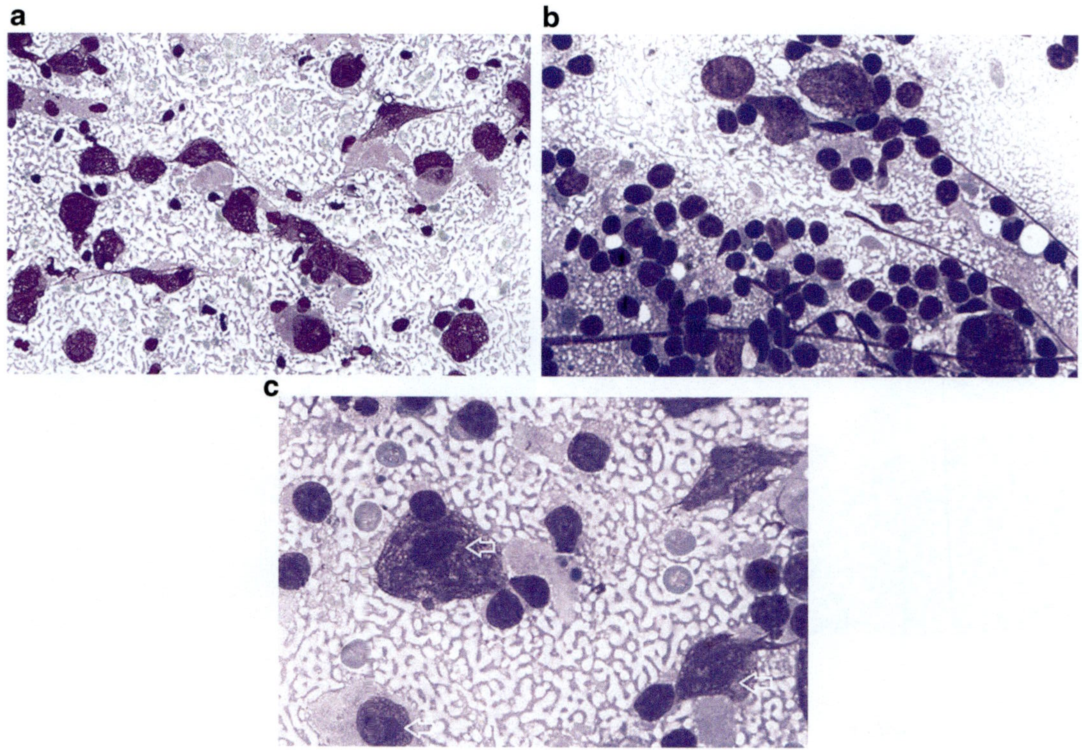

Fig. 15.2 *Germinoma, cytologic features.* (**a**) Distinctive cytomorphologic features include large germ cells, small lymphocytes, and striped "tigroid" background. (**b**) In this case the lymphocytic infiltrates predominate, but large tumor cells with lacy cytoplasm are diagnostic. (**c**) High-power view revealing prominent irregular nucleoli (*arrows*) and characteristic striped "tigroid" background (**a–c**; Smears, Romanowsky)

a b

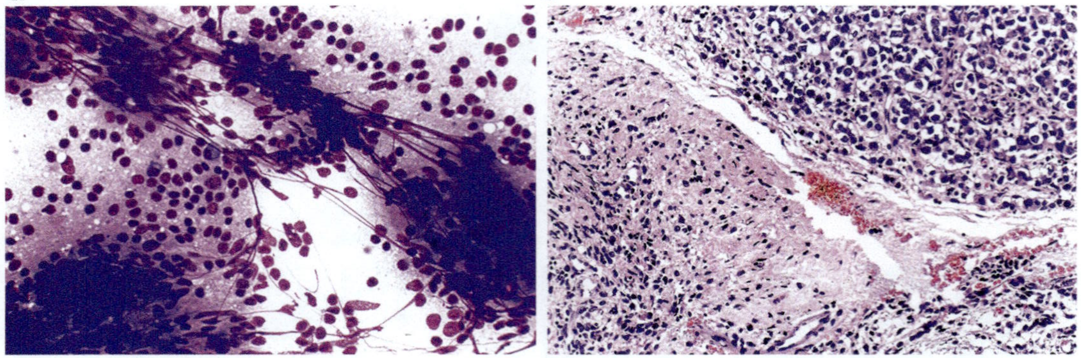

Fig. 15.3 *Germinoma, pitfalls.* (**a**) Preparation from an example with intense granulomatous inflammatory reaction. Tight clusters of epithelioid histiocytes admixed with a heavy chronic inflammatory infiltrate are the only feature that appears in this case (Smear, Romanowsky). (**b**) Immature teratoma showing a germinoma element at the right upper corner (Stereotactic biopsy)

Table 15.2 Characteristics of germinoma

Cytologic features
Dual cell population
Large, primordial germ cells
Small, mature lymphocytes
Striped "tigroid" background (Romanowsky stains)
Frequent granulomatous inflammation
Differential diagnosis and pitfalls
Inflammatory granulomatous processes
Mixed germ cell tumors with an element of germinoma
Langerhans cell histiocytosis
Pineal parenchymal tumors
Metastatic carcinoma
Lymphoma

and diagnosed prenatally). These congenital cases may replace cerebral hemispheres and are usually fatal. In neuroimaging, they are complex, heterogeneous, solid-cystic masses with frequent partial enhancement. On macroscopic inspection, the diagnosis is often suggested by the finding of keratinous- or mucous-filled cysts, cartilaginous nodules, bony spicules, or fat. Histologically, CNS teratomas recapitulate, albeit in disorganized fashion, tissue components of all three germ layers – ectoderm, mesoderm, and endoderm. They are divided into three categories: (1) *mature teratoma*, fully differentiated tissue types (Fig. 15.4a); (2) *immature teratoma*, one or more components are of embryonic or fetal appearance (Fig. 15.4b); and (3) *teratoma with malignant transformation* which includes elements of somatic malignant tumors such as carcinoma, sarcoma, or PNET. Approximately 60% are mature and 25% immature, whereas the remaining 15% shows malignant transformation.

As against other iGCTs, complete gross surgical resection is the treatment of choice for teratomas, a procedure often favored because of their firm texture and good demarcation from the surrounding tissue. Tumors with immature/malignant germ cell elements or with malignant transformation usually require multimodal therapy.

Cytologic Features

The recognition of mature and immature teratomas is usually not problematic when large amounts of tissue are available. The cytologic picture is usually variable, depending on the different tumor tissues and their degree of maturity. *Mature teratomas* are usually cystic, and smears display aggregates of anucleate squames,

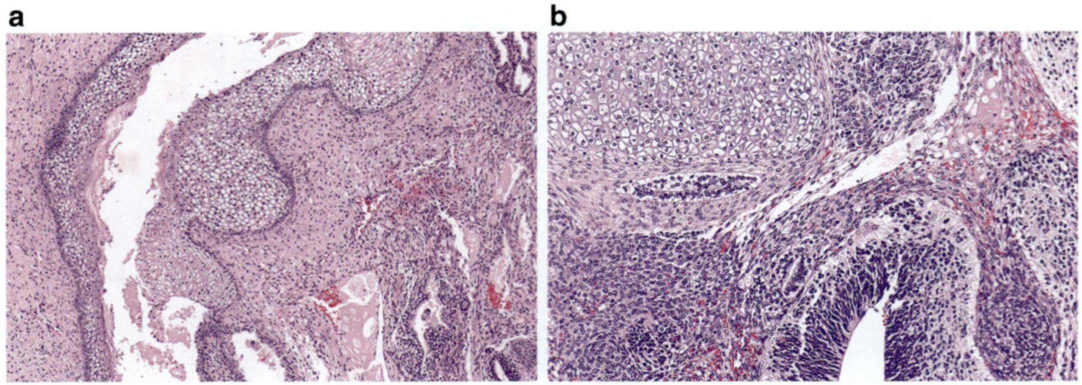

Fig. 15.4 *Teratomas, histology*. (**a**) *Mature teratoma*. This example is composed of squamous epithelium lined cavities (note flaky keratin *inside*) and nests of glandular epithelium in a loose myxoid stroma. (**b**) *Immature teratoma*. Disorganization and lacks of maduration are well seen in this example that combines immature cartilage, glandular epithelium, blastema-like mesenchyma, and island of primitive (embryonic appearing) neuroepithelium including tubules

mucus, and well-differentiated tissue fragments from more than one germinal layer, i.e., the skin, adipose tissue, cartilage, brain (most often choroid plexus), or differentiated glands (Fig. 15.5a, b). On the other hand, preparations from *immature teratomas* often include immature mesenchymal, neuroepithelial, or primitive glandular cellular components with a cytologic appearance similar to that of embryonal or fetal tissues. The more common components are embryonal neuroepithelial elements and primitive, blastema-like mesenchyma (Fig. 15.6a, b). *Teratomas with malignant transformation* can include malignant elements with anaplastic features resembling ordinary carcinoma, sarcoma, or PNET. Most often observed are sarcomatous elements of undifferentiated or rhabdomyosarcomatous appearance.

Differential Diagnosis Considerations

The differential diagnosis of *mature teratoma* ought to include epidermoid/dermoid cysts (only epithelial squames/skin adnexa) and craniopharyngioma ("wet keratin," no mesenchymal or neuroectodermal elements), whereas the *immature variant* should include non-germinomatous "malignant" germ cell tumors (high levels of α-fetoprotein and β-hCG), metastatic carcinoma (elderly patients), and embryonal tumors (monomorphic appearance).

Non-germinomatous (Malignant) Germ Cell Tumors

Non-germinomatous germ cell tumors (NGGCTs) are generally present in older children and adolescents and include GCTs with any malignant germ cell component (*embryonal carcinoma, yolk sac tumor,* or *choriocarcinoma*) or combination of any of them. Clinically, they are aggressive tumors characterized by rapid and bulky growth and extraneural metastases at presentation, most often to the liver and lungs. Assays of serum or CSF α-fetoprotein and serum β-hCG levels are useful in the preoperative evaluation and in monitoring the response to treatment. Neuroimaging is non-specific, showing solid, heterogeneous enhancing masses with frequent local invasion of adjacent structures; hemorrhage suggests the diagnosis of choriocarcinoma.

All NGGCTs (embryonal carcinoma, yolk sac tumor, choriocarcinoma, and mixed GCTs with predominance of one of these histologic subtypes) behave in a highly aggressive manner. Despite multimodal treatment including surgery, craniospinal radiation, and platinum-containing therapy, survival rates are of less than 45%.

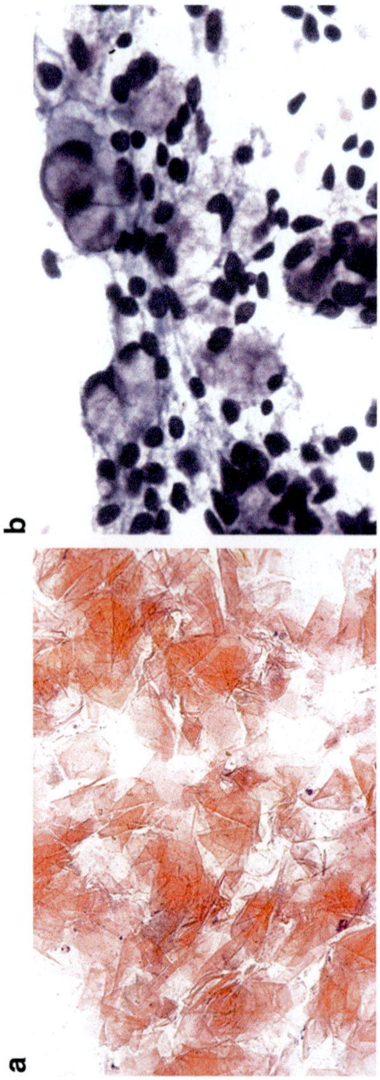

Fig. 15.5 *Mature teratoma, cytologic features.* Sheets of anucleated squamous cells (**a**), and clusters of benign goblet cells (**b**) in this example of mature teratoma (**a**, **b**; Smears, Papanicolaou)

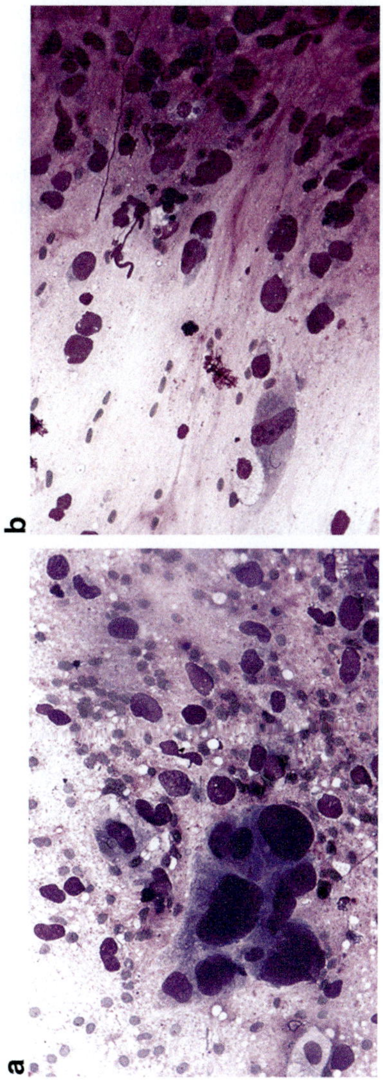

Fig. 15.6 *Immature teratoma, cytologic features*. In cytologic preparations, immature teratomas are often diagnosed by the presence of poorly differentiated neuroepithelial (**a**) and blastema-like components (**b**) in a mesenchymoid metachromatic background (**a, b**; Smears, Romanowsky)

Cytologic Features

The smear features of NGGCTs are similar to those of poorly differentiated adenocarcinoma or large-cell undifferentiated carcinoma, with sheets, three-dimensional groups, or papillae of primitive-looking epithelial cells. Sometimes there are particular cell features depending on the subtype: *choriocarcinoma* may show giant syncytiotrophoblastic cells with multiple dark nuclei (often clustered), admixed with sheets of mononuclear cytotrophoblast cells displaying vesicular nuclei, clear cytoplasm with multiple vacuoles, and well-defined cell boundaries (Fig. 15.7a). *Yolk sac tumor* yield smears very similar to those of a high-grade adenocarcinoma, with three-dimensional and papillary-like epithelial cell clumps. Some cells may display vacuolated cytoplasm and intracytoplasmic hyaline globules of alpha-fetoprotein (Fig. 15.7b). *Embryonal carcinoma* shows a worrisome population of large, polygonal cells resembling those of the embryonic germ disc, with vesicular nuclei, macronucleoli, and a rim of clear to violet-colored cytoplasm. Granular necrotic background also is a common finding (Fig. 15.7c).

Differential Diagnosis Considerations

The differential diagnosis should include metastatic carcinoma, which is not complicated given the age of the patient and the usual location of these tumors, and other regional processes such as pineal parenchymal tumors, meningioma, and craniopharyngioma. Pathologists should also be aware that in the case of "secreting-GCTs" (CSF α-fetoprotein levels $\geq$10 ng/ml and/or β-hCG $\geq$50 IU/l), clinicians may consider treating NGGCTs without a biopsy, and in patients who do not obtain a complete radiographic response after intensive chemotherapy, a subsequent second-look surgery should be considered. In these cases, the residual lesion may be necrosis and fibrosis devoid of tumor or even a mature teratoma, a phenomenon known as *growing teratoma syndrome*. This process should not be misdiagnosed during intraoperative consultation as progressive disease because treatment differs considerably – as for mature teratoma, gross total resection is the treatment of choice in the case of "growing teratoma syndrome."

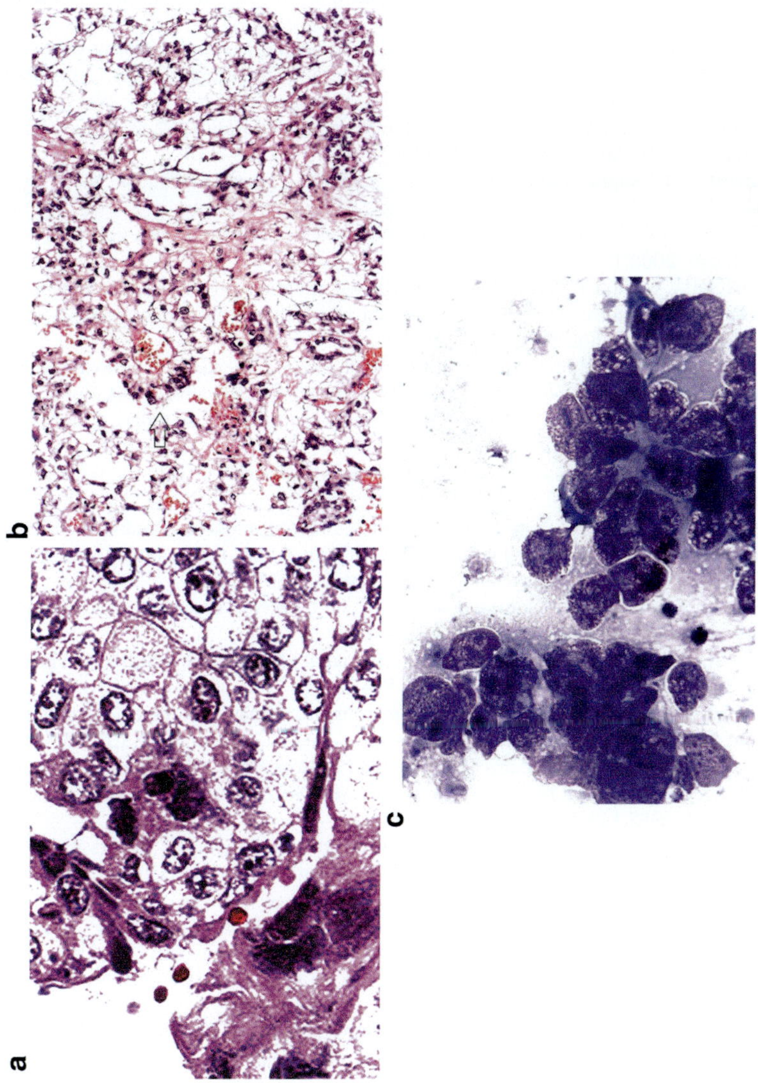

Fig. 15.7 *Non-germinomatous (malignant) germ cell tumors.* (**a**) *Choriocarcinoma.* Typical appearance with a mixture of syncytiotrophoblastic cells (dark nuclei) and cytotrophoblastic cells (vesicular nuclei). Also note the well-defined, clear cytoplasm of cytotrophoblastic cells (Smear, H&E). (**b**) Tissue section from a pineal *yolk sac tumor* sampled by stereotactic technique. Microcystic, glandular-alveolar, and sinusoidal formations can be seen. Also note a distinctive Schiller-Duval body (fibrovascular projection into a sinusoidal space, *arrow*). (**c**) *Embryonal carcinoma.* Clumps of epithelial cells with worrisome features resembling undifferentiated large-cell carcinoma (Smear, Romanowsky)

Suggested Reading

Acharya S, DeWees T, Shinohara ET, Perkins SM. Long-term outcomes and late effects for childhood and young adulthood intracranial germinomas. Neuro-Oncology. 2015;17:741–6.

Akhtar M, Ali A, Huq M, Bakry M. Fine-needle aspiration biopsy of seminoma and dysgerminoma: cytologic, histologic, and electron microscopic correlations. Diagn Cytopathol. 1990a;6:99–105.

Akhtar M, Ali MA, Sackey K, Jackson D, Bakry M. Fine-needle aspiration biopsy diagnosis of endodermal sinus tumor: histologic and ultrastructural correlations. Diagn Cytopathol. 1990b;6:184–92.

Crawford JR, Santi MR, Vezina G, Myseros JS, et al. CNS germ cell tumor (CNSGCT) of childhood: presentation and delayed diagnosis. Neurology. 2007;68:1668–73.

Cuccia V, Alderete D. Suprasellar/pineal bifocal germ cell tumors. Childs Nerv Syst. 2010;26:1043–9.

Echevarría ME, Fangusaro J, Goldman S. Pediatric central nervous system germ cell tumors: a review. Oncologist. 2008;13:690–9.

Fukushima S, Otsuka A, Suzuki T, et al. Mutually exclusive mutations of *KIT* and *RAS* are associated with *KIT* mRNA expression and chromosomal instability in primary intracranial pure germinomas. Acta Neuropathol. 2014;127:911–25.

Gao Y, Jiang J, Liu Q. Clinicopathological and immunohistochemical features of primary central nervous system germ cell tumors: a 24-years experience. Int J Clin Exp Pathol. 2014;7:6965–72.

Gaoyu C, Deyu G, Zhi C, Hua E. Yolk sac tumor in the fourth ventricle: a case report. Clin Neurol Neurosurg. 2009;111:636–7.

Geramizadeh B, Daneshbood Y, Karimi M. Cytology of brain metastasis of yolk sac tumor. Acta Cytol. 2005;49:110–1.

Glass T, Cochrane DD, Rassekh SR, Goddard K, Hukin J. Growing teratoma syndrome in intracranial non-germinomatous germ cell tumors (iNGGCTs): a risk for secondary malignant transformation—a report of two cases. Childs Nerv Syst. 2014;30:953–7.

Goodwin TL, Sainani K, Fisher PG. Incidence patterns of central nervous system germ cell tumors: a SEER Study. J Pediatr Hematol Oncol. 2009;31:541–4.

Goyal N, Kakkar A, Singh PK, Sharma MC, et al. Intracranial teratomas in children: a clinicopathological study. Childs Nerv Syst. 2013;29:2035–42.

Kraichoke S, Cosgrove M, Chandrasoma P. Granulomatous inflammation in pineal germinoma. A cause of diagnostic failure at stereotaxic brain biopsy. Am J Surg Pathol. 1988;12:655–60.

Lacruz CR, Catalina-Fernández I, Bardales RH, Pimentel J, López-Presa D, Sáenz-Santamaría J. Intraoperative consultation on pediatric central nervous system tumors by squash cytology. Cancer Cytopathol. 2015;123:331–46.

Lai IC, Wong TT, Shiau CY, Hu YW, et al. Treatment results and prognostic factors for intracranial nongerminomatous germ cell tumors: single institute experience. Childs Nerv Syst. 2015;31:683–91.

McCarthy BJ, Shibui S, Kayama T, Miyaoka E, et al. Primary CNS germ cell tumors in Japan and the United States: an analysis of 4 tumor registries. Neuro-Oncology. 2012;14:1194–200.

Ng HK. Cytologic diagnosis of intracranial germinomas in smear preparations. Acta Cytol. 1995;39:696–7.

O'Callaghan AM, Katapodis O, Ellison DW, Theaker JM, Mead GM. The growing teratoma syndrome in a nongerminomatous germ cell tumor of the pineal gland: a case report and review. Cancer. 1997;80:942–7.

Plant AS, Chi SN, Frazier L. Pediatric malignant germ cell tumors: a comparison of the neuro-oncology and solid tumor experience. Pediatr Blood Cancer. 2016;63:2086–95.

Sawamura Y, Kato T, Ikeda J, Murata J, et al. Teratomas of the central nervous system: treatment considerations based on 34 cases. J Neurosurg. 1998;89:728–37.

Takami H, Fukushima S, Fukuoka K, Suzuki T, et al. Human chorionic gonadotropin is expressed virtually in all intracranial germ cell tumors. J Neuro-Oncol. 2015;124:23–32.

Wang L, Yamaguchi S, Burstein MD, et al. Novel somatic and germline mutations in intracranial germ cell tumours. Nature. 2014;511:241–5.

Chapter 16
Lymphomas and Histiocytic Tumors

Primary central nervous system lymphomas (PCNLs) and histiocytic tumors are neoplasms that correspond to their nodal or systemic counterparts but are confined to the CNS at presentation. The most common ("typical") types include *diffuse large B cell lymphoma* and *Langerhans cell histiocytosis*, respectively, with the many other subtypes considerably rarer in the CNS.

Primary Central Nervous System Lymphomas

The incidence of PCNLs has increased during the past decades hand-in-hand with AIDS pandemic and iatrogenic immunosuppression (either for the purpose of organ transplantation or due to treatment with drugs such as methotrexate or azathioprine) and also in older (greaterthan60 years) immunocompetent patients. Currently, HIV-associated cases have become relatively rare with the introduction of highly active antiretroviral therapy (HAART), being the overall incidence of PCNSLs about 3–5% of all primary CNS tumors. There are differences in etiology between sporadic and immunodeficiency-associated cases. Nearly all PCNSLs in immunocompromised patients express an Epstein-Barr virus-related genome (EBNA1-6, LMP1, EBER1, EBER2), whereas in immunocompetent patients, the expression is practically nil. On the other hand, PCNSLs can affect all ages and both sexes but also clearly depending on the type: sporadic cases affect the elderly with a peak incidence during the sixth and seventh decades of life (male to female ratio, 3:2), whereas cases associated with immunodeficiency affect adults between 30 and 40 years (almost 95% men among AIDS patients, reflecting the demography of HIV-1 infection). In contrast to secondary CNS lymphomas, whose involvement is nearly always exterior to the pial surface, i.e., meninges, epidural space, and nerve roots, most PCNSLs (approximately 75%) are intraparenchymal masses of the cerebral hemispheres located preferentially periventricularly (deep white matter, corpus

C. R. Lacruz et al., *Central Nervous System Intraoperative Cytopathology*,
Essentials in Cytopathology 13, https://doi.org/10.1007/978-3-319-98491-9_16

callosum, thalamus, and basal ganglia). Most of the remainder involves the cerebellum or brainstem, whereas the spinal cord or craniospinal nerve roots are seldom the primary location. Overall, up to 40% are multiple, with multifocality more common in the immunocompromised patients (85%). T-cell lymphomas appear to arise in the cerebellum more frequently, whereas the rare mucosa-associated lymphoid tissue (MALT) lymphomas are primarily dura-based lesions mimicking meningioma.

The typical clinical presentation of PCNSLs is with focal neurologic deficits (50–80%), followed by cognitive/behavior disturbances (20–30%) and signs of increased intracranial pressure (10–30%). One fifth of patients have ocular involvement (vitreous lymphoma and uveitis) at diagnosis. MRI shows densely enhancing, uni- or multifocal lesions with relatively limited perilesional edema and often evidence of widespread subependymal infiltration. AIDS cases usually are ring-enhancing lesions with central necrosis and marked perilesional edema resembling *Toxoplasma* abscesses. With steroid therapy, lesions may vanish within hours.

The macroscopic features may be very variable, but the most usual one is that of soft, ill-defined masses with "fish-flesh" appearance and slightly darker than gray matter.

Histologically, the vast majority of PCNSLs (almost 98%) are *high-grade lymphoma of the diffuse large B-cell type* (DLBCL) growing as highly cellular, widely infiltrating neoplasms with a perivascular predilection (Fig. 16.1). Additionally, AIDS-related cases frequently show extensive coagulative necrosis. *Low-grade lymphomas* accounts for approximately 3% of all CNS lymphomas, and the majority are of the B-cell lineage.

PCNSLs have a poor prognosis (more aggressive than systemic DLBCL) with 5-year survival rates of 25–45%. Tumors arising in immunocompromised individuals have even a worse prognosis, with median survival of less than 1 year. Current therapy involves chemotherapy (methotrexate), rituximab, and radiotherapy (avoided in some centers as front line treatment), with autologous stem cell transplantation performed in some cases, especially in young patients with relapse.

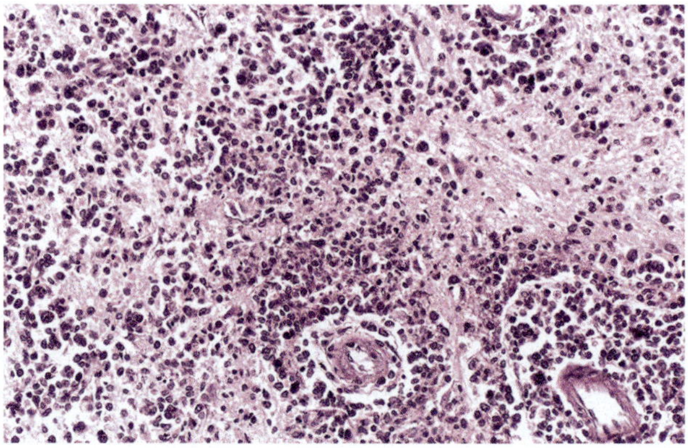

Fig. 16.1 *Diffuse large B-cell lymphoma*. Characteristic histology featuring malignant cells in an angiocentric and diffuse pattern

General Diagnostic Approach

Given the usually deep-seated nature and the fact that PCNSL is not considered a surgical disease, surgery is often restricted to stereotactic biopsy. Smears are recommended for intraoperative procedure because misdiagnosis of lymphoma is one of the most common errors in frozen section evaluation. Likewise, in AIDS patients, contamination of the cryostat and subsequent defrost and sterilization can be avoided.

Cytologic Features

The hematopoietic nature of *DLBCL* is best demonstrated with Romanowsky stains. Stereotactic biopsy tissue spreads easily to yield highly cellular smears with perivascular cuffing and clearly discohesive cells spreading away from vessels. The background often presents a picture similar to demyelination, with granular material, vacuoles from disintegrated neuropil and reactive astrocytes (Fig. 16.2a, b). Individual cells are large, having a small rim of cytoplasm and vesicular nuclei with nucleolar prominence, corresponding to centroblasts or immunoblasts. Apoptotic bodies (small fragments of condensed nuclei), tingible body macrophages (macrophages with phagocytosed nuclear debris), and numerous lymphoglandular bodies (small, membrane-delimited cytoplasmic fragments of lymphoid cells) also are frequent findings (Fig. 16.3a–c). That is to say, the cytologic picture is the usual one for a high-grade, large-cell lymphoma and therefore easily recognizable. However, there are two features that may complicate this comfortable panorama: sparse cellularity following corticosteroid therapy and massive tumor necrosis. In both situations, which are usually related, very little viable tissue may be left for examination and, frequently, only sheets of macrophages and small lymphocytes remain mimicking a benign process. In some cases of these so-called vanishing tumors, it may even be necessary to withdraw steroid therapy for a variable period of time and take another biopsy. With respect to permanent sections, it is advisable to take into account that B-cell immunomarkers, i.e., CD20, are usually positive even in necrotic material. This enables us to confirm the tumoral and lymphoid nature of the process even in such specimens (Fig. 16.4a, b). In the uncommon *low-grade CNS lymphomas*, the cytologic appearance is quite similar to those of an inflammatory/reactive lesion, with a population of small or plasmacytoid lymphocytes without necrosis or apoptosis (Fig. 16.5a, b). In such cases, a preliminary report of "undetermined lymphoid lesion, differential diagnosis includes low-grade lymphoma vs inflammatory/reactive process" is preferable. More definitive and precise classification of such lesions can be done with permanent sections and additional studies. The immunophenotyping and PCR-based molecular techniques (for detection of rearrangements of *IGH* or *TCR* genes) are useful in determining clonality providing further helpful information.

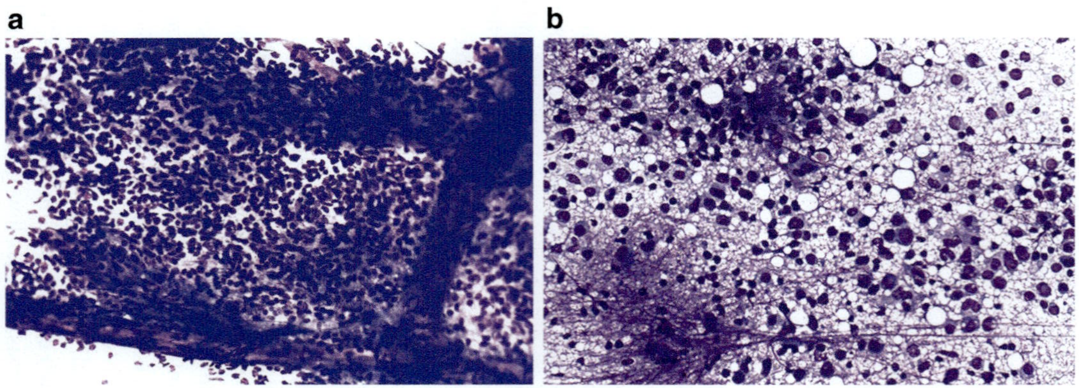

Fig. 16.2 *Diffuse large B-cell lymphoma.* (**a**) A large branching vessel surrounded by atypical cells gives a clue that this is a lymphoma. (**b**) Characteristic single cell pattern of large, atypical lymphoid cells in a granular-vacuolated background of disintegrating neuropil. Note some reactive astrocytes (**a**, **b;** Smears, Romanowsky)

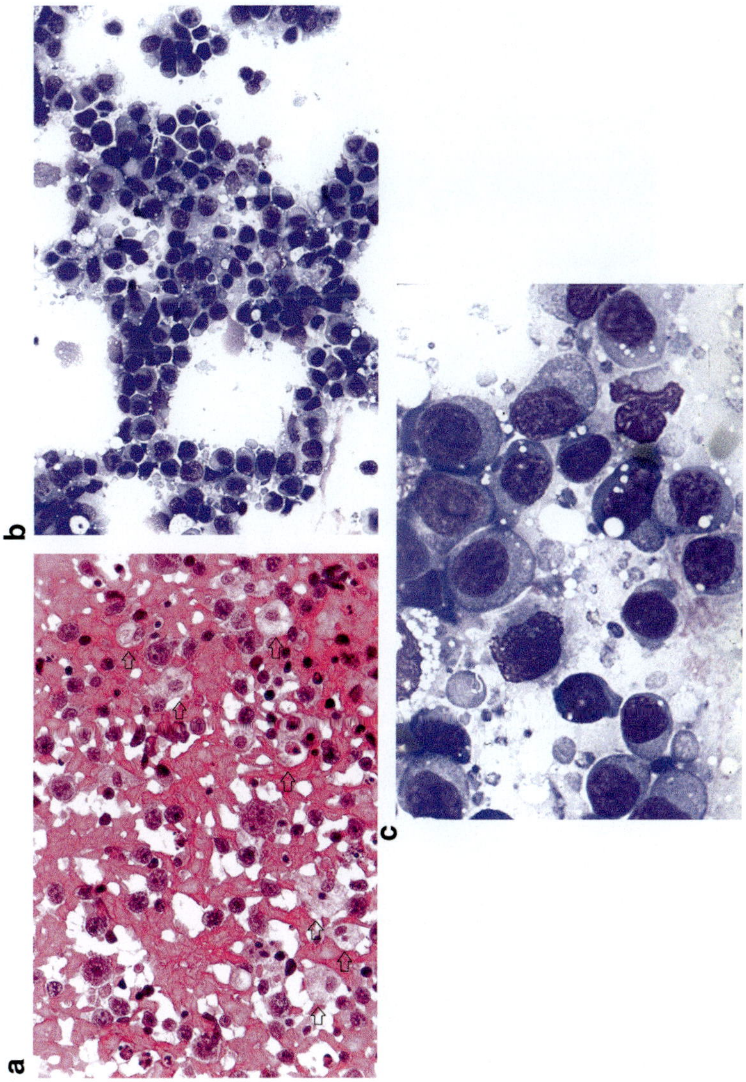

Fig. 16.3 *Diffuse large B-cell lymphoma*. (**a**) The blastic cells are typically characterized by large nuclei with prominent nucleoli. Note background macrophages (*arrows*) and numerous apoptotic bodies (Smear, H&E). (**b**) The lack of cellular cohesion and cytoplasmic processes, respectively, are useful in discriminating this tumor from metastatic carcinoma and glioblastoma, two neoplasms that commonly enter the clinical differential diagnosis. (**c**) Numerous lymphoglandular bodies are typically present in the background. These are best appreciated in Romanowsky-stained preparations (**b, c**; Smears, Romanowsky)

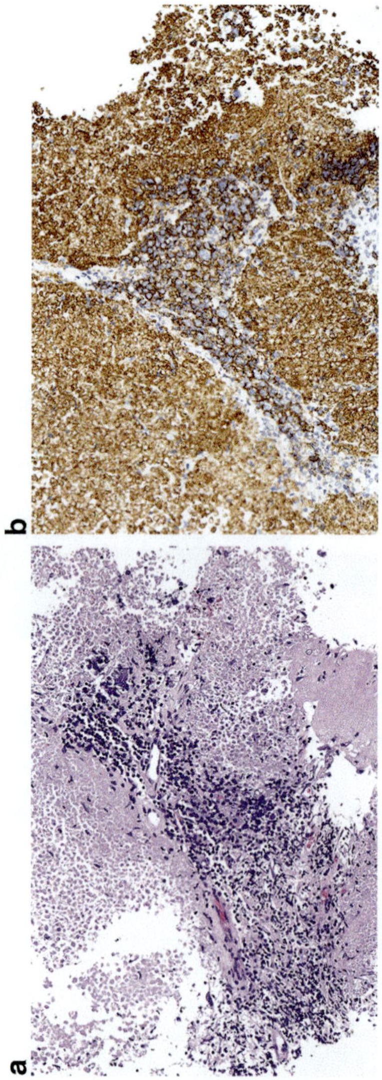

Fig. 16.4 *Diffuse large B-cell lymphoma*, stereotactic biopsy. (**a**) This specimen has extensive necrosis that only spares perivascular infiltrates. (**b**) Preserved and necrotic "ghost" tumor cells show strong expression of the lymphoid immunomarker (CD20 immunostain)

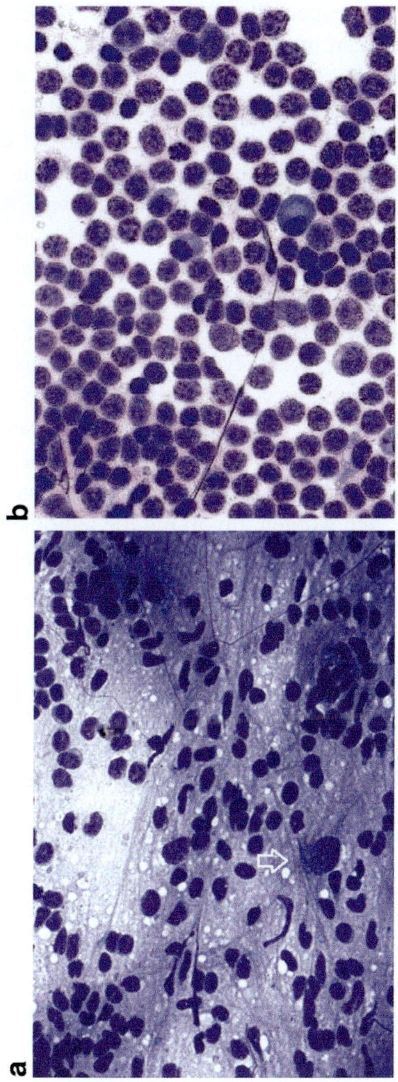

Fig. 16.5 *Low-grade CNS lymphomas*. (**a**) Abundant small lymphoid cells resembling a reactive condition. Note some intermixed neurons (*arrow*). (**b**) This preparation shows a population of small lymphocytes, some bearing irregular nuclei and variable plasmacytic differentiation (**a, b**; Smears, Romanowsky)

Differential Diagnosis Considerations

DLBCL must be differentiated from glioblastoma, metastatic carcinoma, and germinoma, but cells of lymphoma lack the cell processes of glioblastoma, the cohesiveness of metastatic carcinoma, and the clear (glycogen-rich) cytoplasm of germinoma. Small-cell carcinoma presents an especially difficult case; to be diagnostic of lymphoma and exclude small-cell carcinoma, the rim of cytoplasm should show no adherence to neighboring cells, nor should this envelope allow their nuclei to mold into each other. Some authors include embryonal tumors in the differential diagnosis, but these neoplasms have smaller and more compact nuclei than do most CNS lymphomas, whereas their background lacks the characteristic lymphoglandular bodies of lymphoid lesions. Pathologists should also be aware that sampling artifacts, especially when the tissue is at the inflammatory edge of a lymphoma, can lead to a false impression of a primary inflammatory lesion (i.e., demyelination or viral encephalitis) rather than neoplasia. Careful correlation of clinical, radiologic, and surgical information with the cytologic features may facilitate adequate sampling and the correct diagnosis. *Low-grade lymphomas*, as we have seen, can easily be misinterpreted as being inflammatory or reactive in nature, which is why the definitive diagnosis should be made by deferred immunohistochemical and molecular ancillary tests. On the other hand, *MALT-lymphoma of the dura* may closely mimic, both clinically and cytomorphologically, lymphoplasmacytic-rich meningioma: usually afflicting middle-age women, involving the leptomeninges and dura, it is composed by a population of small (histiocytoid or plasmacytoid) lymphocytes and follows a rather indolent course (Table 16.1).

Histiocytic Tumors

Histiocytic tumors affecting the CNS are a heterogeneous group of tumors or tumor-like lesions composed primarily of histiocytes (either macrophage type or dendritic Langerhans cell type) that are totally homologous to those of an extraneuraxial location. The presence or absence of Langerhans cells (CD1a, CD207 [langerin] IHC +) determines their separation into two groups: Langerhans cell histiocytosis (LCH) and non-Langerhans cell histiocytosis (Table 16.2).

General Features of Histiocytic Disorders

As a group, these lesions are relatively infrequent, with LCH being the most common. Most of them occur in children and young people, and often the behavior is relatively benign, except in the very rare histiocytic sarcoma, 40–50% of patients with Erdheim-Chester disease, and systemic LCH disease. Aside from these

Table 16.1 Characteristics of primary central nervous system lymphomas

Cytologic features
Highly cellular smears
Perivascular cuffing and clearly discohesive cells
Large, pleomorphic nuclei with prominent nucleoli
Scant cytoplasm without processes
Apoptotic bodies and tingible body macrophages
Granular-vacuolated or necrotic background with LGBs
Beware of sparse viable cellularity following:
Corticosteroid therapy
Massive tumor necrosis
Differential diagnosis and pitfalls
Glioblastoma
Metastatic carcinoma
Germinoma
Embryonal tumors
Encephalitis (edge of the tumor)
Low-grade lymphomas
Inflammatory/reactive processes
Lymphoplasmacytic-rich meningioma

LBGs lymphoglandular bodies

Table 16.2 Types of CNS histiocytic disorders

Langerhans cell histiocytosis
This term substitute former:
Eosinophilic granuloma of bone
Abt-Letterer-Siwe disease
Hand-Schüller-Christian disease
Hashimoto-Pritzker disease
Non-Langerhans cell histiocytosis
Rosai-Dorfman disease
Erdheim-Chester disease
Juvenile xanthogranuloma
Histiocytic sarcoma

common features of the group, there are particular characteristics of each type, particularly with respect to location. *LCH* typically occurs as a solitary lytic lesion in the skull or spine and often invade the CNS or scalp secondarily; brain infiltrates may also occur, especially in axial locations (hypothalamus, pituitary gland, optic chiasm). The preferential intracranial or intraspinal involvement of *Rosai-Dorfman disease* is in the form of dura-based masses that mimic meningioma (often involving both sides of the dura); parenchymal or intrasellar lesions may also occur. *Erdheim-Chester disease* has special tropism for the hypothalamus, pituitary gland, and posterior fossa, especially the dentate nucleus of cerebellum and brainstem. In *juvenile xanthogranuloma*, CNS involvement is characterized by uni- or multifocal infiltrations of the brain, nerve roots, and meninges.

From the molecular point of view, both LCH and Erdheim-Chester disease have a *BRAF* V600E mutation (BRAF VE1 IHC +) in more than a half of cases. Patients with *BRAF* mutations may benefit from the *BRAF* inhibitor *vemurafenib*. Likewise, histiocytic sarcoma may also express *BRAF* V600E mutation and respond to inhibitors.

Cytologic Features

As a general rule, a mixture of histiocytes and chronic inflammatory cells (eosinophils, lymphocytes, plasma cells) in a smear from a cranial/intracranial mass should raise the consideration of some type of histiocytosis, especially in children and young adults. A more specific diagnosis may be supported by the clinico-radiologic findings (particular to each type) and by the following morphologic features.

Cytology and histology of *LCH* are similar, being characterized by abundant Langerhans cells in addition to a variable cell infiltrate of nonneoplastic reactive elements, such as eosinophils, neutrophils, macrophages, small lymphocytes, and occasional multinucleated cells. Langerhans-type histiocytes have grooved and folded nuclei with tiny nucleoli and pale to lightly eosinophilic cytoplasm (Fig. 16.6a–c).

In *Rosai-Dorfman disease*, smears show a mixture of macrophage-type histiocytes, lymphocytes, and plasma cells. Histiocytic cells often are large, multinucleated, and engage in emperipolesis (well-preserved lymphocytes and plasma cells inside phagocytic cytoplasmic vacuoles). These features are more visible in smears than in frozen sections (Fig. 16.7).

Histiocytic sarcoma, an extremely rare malignant tumor, is characterized by a discohesive pattern of large, atypical histiocytes with abundant cytoplasm and folded nuclei with pleomorphic shapes and often prominent nucleoli. Frequent mitotic figures and inflammatory background also are common findings (Fig. 16.8).

In the remainder histiocytic lesions (*Erdheim-Chester disease* and *juvenile xanthogranuloma*), the cytomorphologic appearance is similar: cellularity consists mostly of bland, foamy to spindled histiocytes with nonreniform nuclei. Scattered Touton multinucleated giant cells, eosinophils, and lymphocytes may be seen.

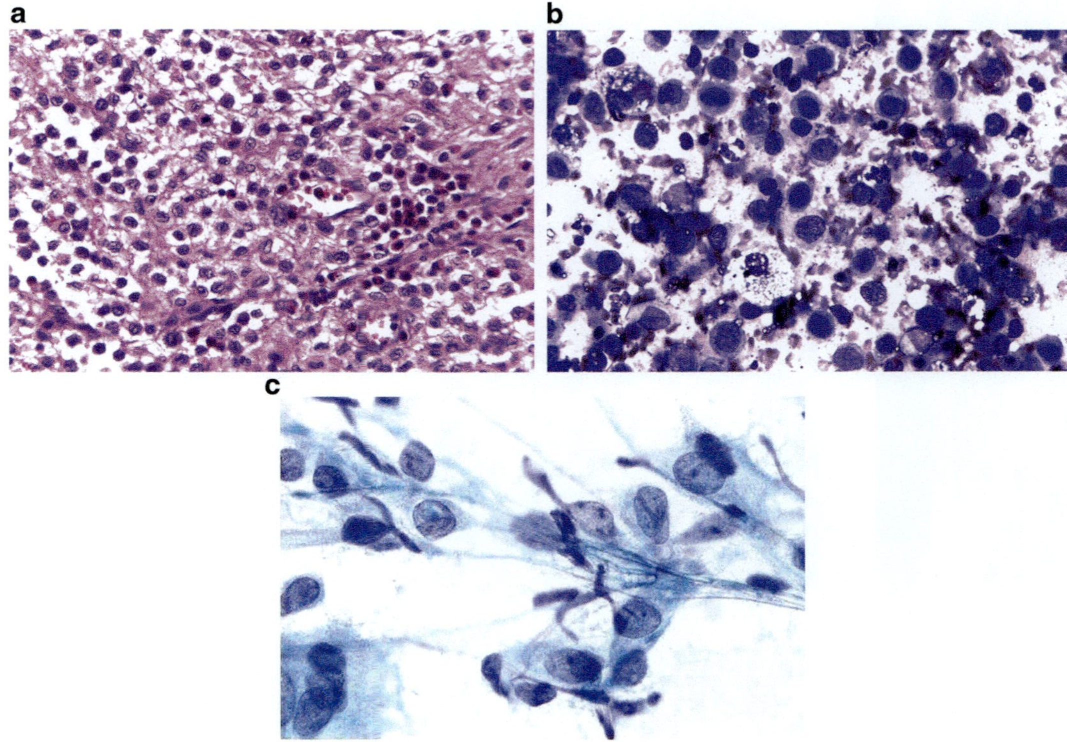

Fig. 16.6 *Langerhans cell histiocytosis*. (**a**) Typical histology includes histiocytic cells with nuclear grooves in the setting of a variable inflammatory infiltrate rich in eosinophils. (**b**) Cytologic preparation showing distinctive Langerhans cells with rounded or reniform, clefted nuclei, and discrete amount of pale cytoplasm (Smear, Romanowsky). (**c**) The characteristic nuclear deep grooves are better seen in alcohol-fixed preparations (Smear, Papanicolaou)

Fig. 16.7 *Rosai-Dorfman disease*. Large histiocytic cells with well-preserved lymphocytes and plasma cells inside phagocytic vacuoles (*emperipolesis*) are distinctive (Smear, Papanicolaou)

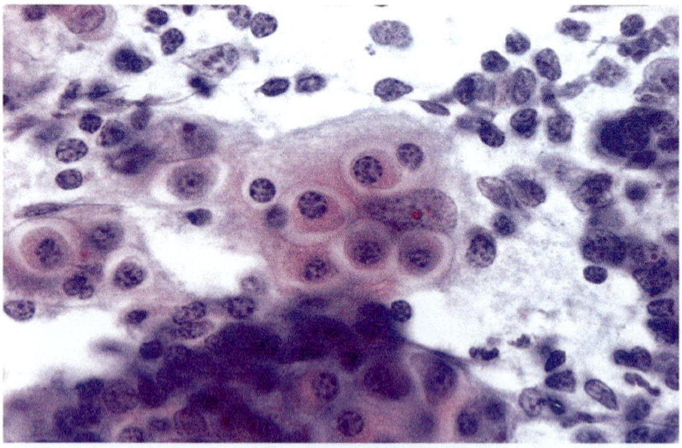

Fig. 16.8 *Histiocytic sarcoma*. Single cell pattern of large histiocytes with abundant vacuolated cytoplasm and irregular, folded nuclei. Also note frequent binucleation, mitotic figures (*arrows*) and scattered lymphocytes in the background (Smear; Romanowsky)

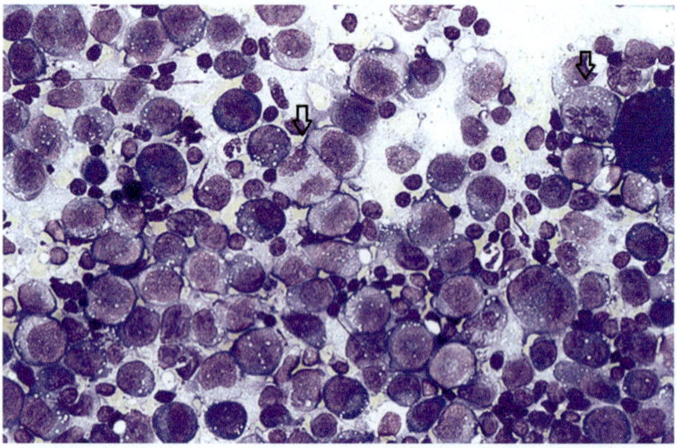

Suggested Reading

Batchelor T, Loeffler JS. Primary CNS lymphoma. J Clin Oncol. 2006;24:1281–8.

Bubolz AM, Weissinger SE, Stenzinger A, Arndt A, et al. Potential clinical implications of BRAF mutations in histiocytic proliferations. Oncotarget. 2014;5:4060–70.

Chen KTK. Crush cytology of Rosai-Dorfman disease of the central nervous system. A report of 2 cases. Acta Cytol. 2003;47:1111–5.

Demellawy DE, Young JL, de Nanassy J, Chernetsova E, Nasr A. Langerhans cell histiocytosis: a comprehensive review. Pathology. 2015;47:294–301.

Dubuisson A, Kaschten B, Lénelle J, Martin D, et al. Primary central nervous system lymphoma: report of 32 cases and review of the literature. Clin Neurol Neurosurg. 2004;107:55–6.

Estupiñán-Díaz B, Salazar-Rodríguez S, Jiménez-Galainena J, García-Maeso N, et al. Primary histiocytic sarcoma of the central nervous system. A case report and review of the literature. Rev Esp Patol. 2015;48:222–30.

Giannini C, Dogan A, Salomão DR. CNS lymphoma: a practical diagnostic approach. J Neuropathol Exp Neurol. 2014;73:478–94.

Haroche J, Charlotte F, Arnaud L, von Deimling A, et al. High prevalence of BRAF V600E mutations in Erdheim-Chester disease but not in other non-Langerhans cell histiocytoses. Blood. 2012;120:2700–3.

Hung YP, Lovitch SB, Qian X. Histiocytic sarcoma: new insights into FNA cytomorphology and molecular characteristics. Cancer Cytopathol. 2017;125(8):604–14.

Idbaih A, Mokhtari K, Emile JF, et al. Dramatic response of a BRAF V600E-mutated primary CNS histiocytic sarcoma to vemurafenib. Neurology. 2014;83:1478–80.

Nahm JH, Yoon G, Do SI, Kim HS. Squash smear cytology of Langerhans cell histiocytosis. Int J Clin Exp Pathol. 2015;8:7998–8007.

Namiki TS, Nichols P, Young T, Martin SE, Chandrasoma P. Stereotaxic biopsy diagnosis of central nervous system lymphoma. Am J Clin Path. 1988;90:40–5.

Plasswilm L, Herrlinger U, Korfel A, Weller M, et al. Primary central nervous system (CNS) lymphoma in immunocompetent patients. Ann Hematol. 2002;81:415–23.

Purav P, Ganapathy K, Mallikarjuna VS, Balamuguram M. Rosai-Dorfman disease of the central nervous system. J Clin Neurosci. 2005;12:656–9.

Rodríguez-Pereira C, Borrás-Moreno JM, Pesudo-Martínez JV, Vera-Román JM. Cerebral solitary Langerhans cell histiocytosis: report of two cases and review of the literature. Br J Neurosurg. 2005;19:192–7.

Rushing EJ, Kaplan KJ, Mena H, Sandberg GD, Koeller K, Bouffard JP. Erdheim-Chester disease of the brain: cytological features and differential diagnosis of a challenging case. Diagn Cytopathol. 2004;31:420–2.

Scott BJ, Douglas VC, Tihan T, Rubenstein JL, Josephson SA. A systematic approach to the diagnosis of suspected central nervous system lymphoma. JAMA Neurol. 2013;70:311–9.

Sherman ME, Erozan YS, Mann RB, Kumar AJ, et al. Stereotactic brain biopsy in the diagnosis of malignant lymphoma. Am J Clin Pathol. 1991;95:878–83.

Sun W, Nordberg ML, Fowler MR. Histiocytic sarcoma involving the central nervous system: clinical, immunohistochemical, and molecular genetic studies of a case with review of the literature. Am J Surg Pathol. 2003;27:258–65.

Tian Y, Wang J, Li M, Lin S, et al. Rosai-Dorfman disease involving the central nervous system: seven cases from one institute. Acta Neurochir. 2015;157:1565–71.

Tu PH, Giannini C, Judkins AR, Schwalb JM, et al. Clinicopathologic and genetic profile of intracranial marginal zone lymphoma: a primary low-grade CNS lymphoma that mimics meningioma. J Clin Oncol. 2005;23:5718–27.

Weidauer S, von Stuckrad-Barre S, Dettmann E, Zanella FE, Lanfermann H. Cerebral Erdheim-Chester disease: case report and review of the literature. Neuroradiology. 2003;45:241–5.

Yu GH, Montone KT, Frias-Hidvegi D, Cajulis RS, Brody BA, Levy RM. Cytomorphology of primary CNS lymphoma: review of 23 cases and evidence for the role of EBV. Diagn Cytopathol. 1996;14:114–20.

Chapter 17
Nerve Sheath Tumors of the Craniospinal Axis

A large number of neurosurgical specimens originate outside of the central neuraxis proper from the nerve sheath cells of the cranial and spinal nerve roots, the vast majority of which are schwannomas.

Schwannoma

Schwannomas are benign (WHO grade I) nerve sheath tumors composed entirely of well-differentiated Schwann cells. They account for about 10% of intracranial tumors, 85% of cerebellopontine angle masses, and almost one-third of spinal nerve root tumors. Outside the setting of *neurofibromatosis type 2* (bilateral vestibular examples are the hallmark of *NF2*), almost all schwannomas are solitary. Inactivating mutations of the *NF2* gene are identified in about 60% of schwannomas, and loss of the immunohistochemical expression of the *NF2* gene product (merlin) is identified in the vast majority of schwannomas, regardless of their *NF2* gene mutations or allelic status. Multifocal, non-vestibular schwannomas without other manifestations of NF2 (i.e., spinal ependymomas) constitute a syndrome known as *schwannomatosis*. Schwannomas affect individuals of all ages, with a peak incidence in the fourth to sixth decade of life, and both sexes equally. In the CNS, schwannomas may develop in most cranial nerves, except I and II, which do not have Schwann cells, but show a strong predilection for sensory nerves, particularly for the vestibular branch of cranial nerve VIII (vestibular schwannoma), and the dorsal, sensory spinal nerve roots (spinal schwannomas). Tumors in the later location often assume a "dumbbell" configuration by squeezing through adjacent intervertebral foramina into the paravertebral soft tissues. The rare primary intra-axial (cerebral or intramedullary) schwannomas arise from peripheral nerve fibers accompanying blood vessels into the parenchyma.

C. R. Lacruz et al., *Central Nervous System Intraoperative Cytopathology*, Essentials in Cytopathology 13, https://doi.org/10.1007/978-3-319-98491-9_17

The most common symptoms are hearing loss, facial paresthesia, and tinnitus (vestibular tumors) and radicular pain and spinal cord compression (spinal tumors). In neuroimaging, appear as well-circumscribed, often cystic, heterogeneous enhancing masses. Vestibular examples frequently show a nipple-like extension into the internal auditory canal with enlargement of the internal auditory meatus.

Macroscopically, schwannomas are truly encapsulated and globoid masses. The cut surface reveals a light tan, glistening aspect with bright yellow patches due to lipid deposition. Cystic degeneration is a common finding, particularly in large tumors.

Histologically, two main types of schwannomas are recognized: conventional schwannoma (more than 90% of cases) and cellular schwannoma (5–10% of cases). Melanotic schwannoma is now considered as a distinct entity rather than as a variant. *Conventional schwannoma's* histologic features often include a biphasic Antoni A and B structure, infiltration by foamy macrophages, and vascular hyalinization. The compact regions comprise the Antoni A component, in which tumor cells and processes are arranged in compact fascicles with occasional Verocay bodies (Fig. 17.1a) or whorls (Fig. 17.1b), whereas a looser cell disposition with indistinct cell processes and delicate vacuolization characterizes the Antoni B component (Fig. 17.1c). Nuclear, degenerative-type atypia (pleomorphism and hyperchromatism) is a frequent feature in long-standing "ancient" tumors (Fig. 17.2). *Cellular Schwannoma* is a densely populated spindle cell tumor, typically devoid of Antoni B areas and Verocay bodies. Mitotic figures may be frequent, although lessthan10/10HPF (Fig. 17.3). Unlike conventional schwannoma, the cellular type has a predilection for the paraspinal areas of the pelvis, retroperitoneum, and mediastinum, whereas intracranial examples are rare.

Immunohistochemical stains demonstrate consistent expression of tumoral Schwann cell markers –CD57, S100 protein, and SOX10.

Schwannomas are slow-growing tumors that infrequently recur and only rarely undergo malignant transformation (WHO grade I). Recurrences are more common (30–40%) for cellular schwannomas.

Cytologic Features

Schwannomas in general tend to be very resistant to disaggregation and difficult to crush. Even forceful attempts produce only cohesive tissue fragments with very few, if any, single cells separating out from the clusters. In smears from Antoni A areas, tissue remains as thick fragments with sharp borders (Fig. 17.4a). Clusters are composed of interanastomosing fascicles of tightly packed spindle cells without visible cytoplasmic boundaries (Fig. 17.4b). The nuclei have a distinctive long, club-shaped feature with pointed or rounded tips (Fig. 17.4c). Antoni B tissue smears more easily, with interstitial matrix separating cells into strands. Within these cells there are less regular ones, with round to oval nuclei and somewhat stellate processes. Foamy histiocytes may be present among the neoplastic cells (Fig. 17.5). While *"ancient"*

a b c
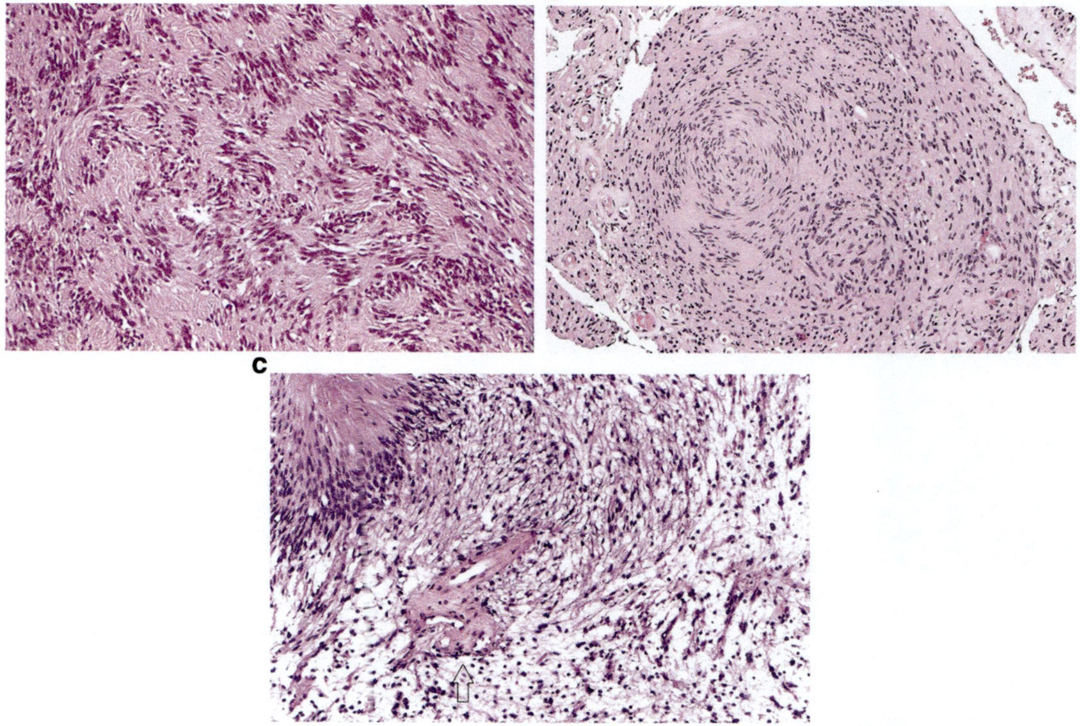

Fig. 17.1 *Schwannoma, histology.* (**a**) *Antoni A zone* displaying compact parallel rows with nuclear palisades or Verocay bodies. These are a highly useful but sometimes unapparent feature of schwannomas, particularly those of the eighth cranial nerve. (**b**) Like meningioma, schwannoma may harbor whorl formation. (**c**) *Antoni B zone* characteristic appearance with tumor cells separated by edematous fluid and thickened vascular walls with hyaline sclerosis (*arrow*). Also note an Antoni A zone in the left upper corner

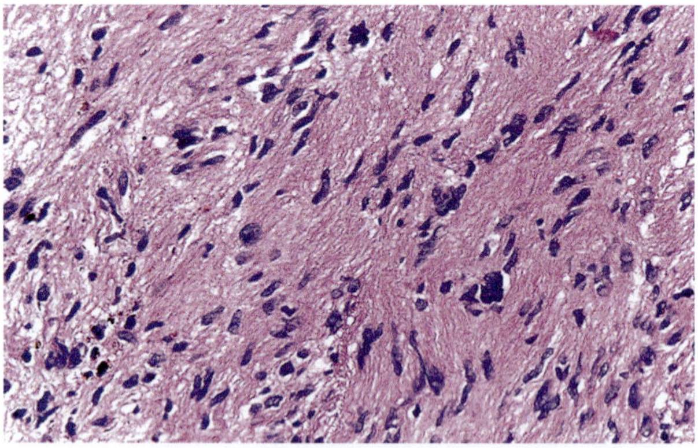

Fig. 17.2 *Long-standing "ancient" schwannoma* displaying prominent degenerative nuclear atypia

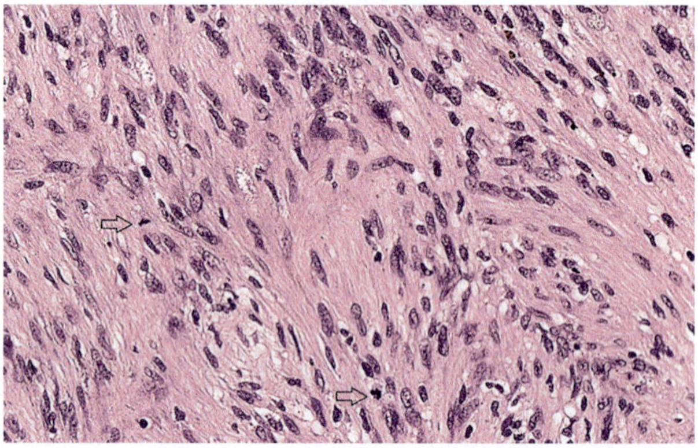

Fig. 17.3 *Cellular schwannomas* are, by definition, mitotically active. Mitosis (*arrows*) up to 4/10 HPFs are common

schwannomas are benign tumors, they can display a significant degree of both nuclear hyperchromasia and pleomorphism, and smears often show numerous bizarre-appearing nuclei (Fig. 17.6). In c*ellular schwannoma,* smears show a monotonous aspect of cohesive, highly cellular groups of spindle cells containing oval to elongated hyperchromatic nuclei. Mitotic figures can be present, but conspicuous Antoni B type areas and anaplastic features are absent (Fig. 17.7).

Differential Diagnosis Considerations

Schwannomas may share some clinical-radiologic data and morphologic features with pilocytic astrocytoma and fibrous meningioma. The tightly cohesive nature of smeared fragments is by far the more distinctive feature in distinguishing schwannoma from those other tumors and can be recognized at low power magnification. On the other hand, schwannoma lacks the fibrillary background of astrocytoma and the characteristic nuclear features of meningioma. In *cellular schwannoma,* the

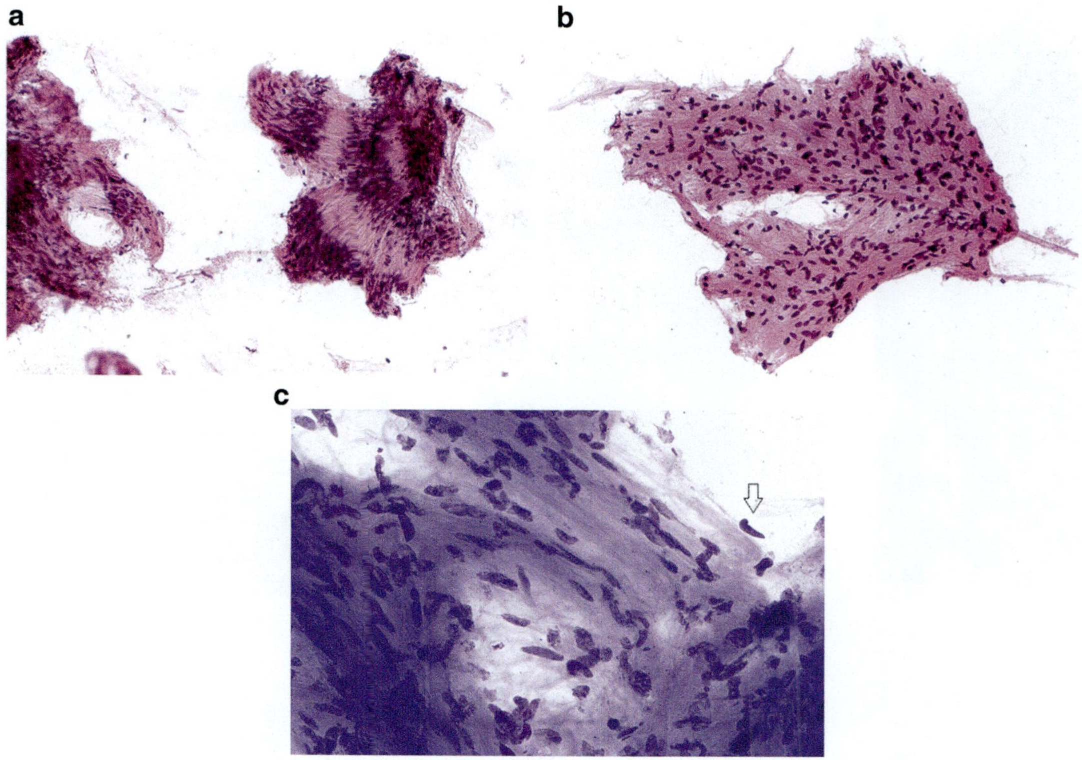

Fig. 17.4 *Schwannoma (Antoni A zone), cytologic features.* (**a**) Thick fragments with sharp borders. There are no single cells (Smear, H&E). (**b**) Cluster composed of tightly packed spindle cells without visible cytoplasmic borders (Smear, H&E). (**c**) Higher magnification showing characteristic club-shaped nuclei with tapering or curved (*arrow*) ends (Smear, Romanowsky)

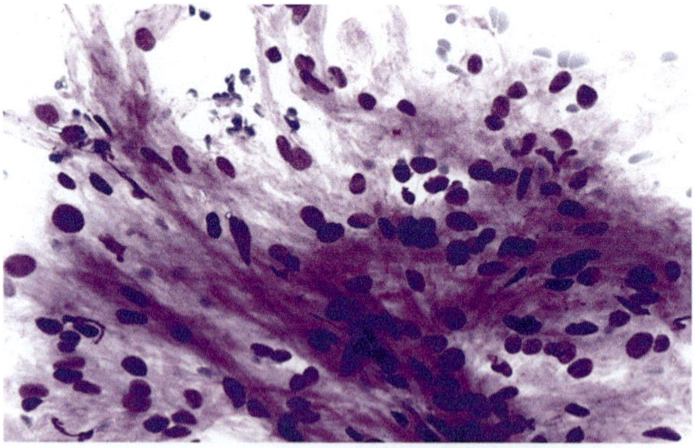

Fig. 17.5 *Schwannoma (Antoni B zone), cytologic features.* Loose cluster composed by less regular cells exhibiting round to oval nuclei (Smear, Romanowsky)

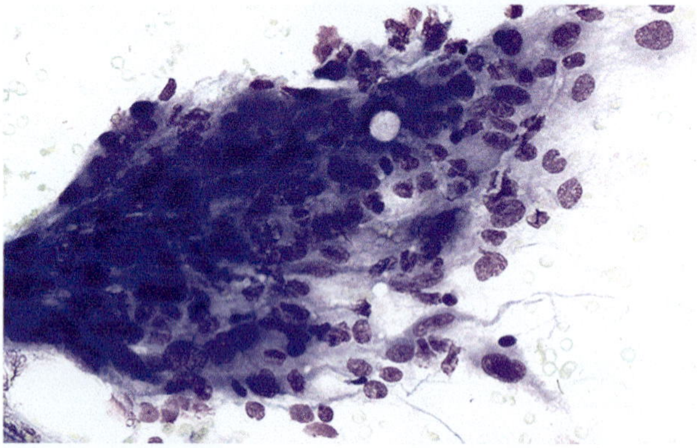

Fig. 17.6 *"Ancient" schwannoma, cytologic features.* This compact cellular sheet displays numerous pleomorphic, bizarre-appearing nuclei (Smear, Romanowsky).

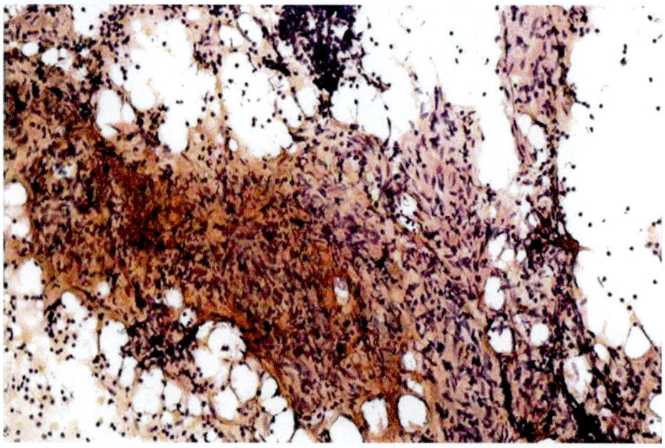

Fig. 17.7 *Cellular schwannoma, cytologic features.* This preparation from a paraspinal mass shows highly cellular tissue fragments of spindle cells. Note that cells are more crowded as opposed to those in conventional schwannomas. Despite hypercellularity, nuclear uniformity is typical (Smear, H&E)

differential diagnosis is more difficult based on the high percentage of cases that are mistaken for sarcomas. The main problematic neoplasms are low-grade fusiform sarcomas, particularly malignant peripheral nerve sheath tumor (MPNST). However, in cellular schwannoma, tumor cells are more uniform with less nuclear

Table 17.1 Characteristics of schwannoma

Conventional schwannoma
Cytologic features
Specimens very difficult to smear
Antoni A areas:
Cohesive tissue fragments without single cells
Spindle cells with club-shaped nuclei
Antoni B areas:
Loosely cellular sheets
Round to oval nuclei and stellate processes
Cellular schwannoma
Only highly cellular Antoni A-type groups
Mild to moderate hyperchromatism
Absence of anaplastic features
Differential diagnosis and pitfalls
Conventional schwannoma
Pilocytic astrocytoma
Fibrous meningioma
Neurofibroma
Cellular schwannoma
Low-grade fusiform sarcomas

pleomorphism and hyperchromatism, whereas smeared tissue fragments are tightly cohesive essentially without single cells separating out from the clusters (Table 17.1).

Melanotic Schwannoma

Melanotic schwannoma (*MS*) is a rare, circumscribed but unencapsulated, grossly pigmented tumor composed of melanin-producing Schwann cells (S100 protein, SOX10, HMB-45, Melan-A, and tyrosinase IHC +). The peak age incidence of this tumor is a decade younger than that of conventional schwannoma, and more than 10% of cases follow a malignant course with distant metastases. Melanotic schwannoma most commonly occur in the paraspinal region, arising in spinal nerve roots and paraspinal ganglia, particularly at the cervical and thoracic levels. Given the frequent loss-of-function germline mutations of the *PRKAR1A* tumor suppressor gene (rather that involvement of the *NF2* gene), the alternative term of *malignant melanotic schwannian tumor* has been advocated. Grossly, they are usually solitary and ovoid with a variable gray to pitch-black cut surface. Histologically, this tumor occurs in both non-psammomatous and psammomatous varieties. *Melanotic schwannomas* (MS) are composed of spindle-shaped and epithelioid cells, arranged in lobules and fascicles, with variable patchy pigmentation. Nuclei are round to oval and contain delicate chromatin and small distinct nucleoli (Fig. 17.8a). Additionally, in *psammomatous melanotic schwannoma* (PMS) laminated psammoma bodies can be found (Fig. 17.8b). Distinguishing between these two varieties is important, because approximately 50% of patients with PMS have *Carney complex*, an autosomal dominant disorder characterized by cardiac myxomas, spotty facial pigmentation, and endocrine overactivity manifested as Cushing's syndrome associated with adrenal hyperplasia and acromegaly due to pituitary adenoma.

Cytologic Features

Smears from *MS* are composed of loosely cohesive sheets and single cells. The cellular morphology is either epithelioid- or spindle-shaped, whereas nuclei are round to oval with finely granular chromatin, small nucleoli, and occasional pseudoinclusions. Some tumor cells contain fine or coarse cytoplasmic brown pigment, which are easier to discern in crush smear preparations than in frozen sections (Fig. 17.9a). In addition, the presence of laminated calcospherites is the hallmark of *PMS* (Fig. 17.9b). Indeed, except for the presence of cytoplasmic pigment or melanophages, the smears of both tumors resemble the smears of meningioma more than those of a conventional schwannoma.

Differential Diagnosis Considerations

MS should primarily be differentiated from melanocytoma and melanoma (primary or secondary), because all these tumors share many morphologic and immunohistochemical features. Correlation with surgical and clinico-radiologic data is necessary – consider the possibility of *MS*, no melanocytoma/melanoma, if tumor involves spinal nerve roots or dorsal root ganglia. On the other hand, if we do not pay attention to the presence of abundant cytoplasmic pigment or melanophages, smears from *PMS* and psammomatous meningioma may be indistinguishable.

Neurofibroma

Neurofibroma is a benign (WHO grade I) nerve sheath tumor, which is composed of all the constituents of the normal nerve (Schwann cells, fibroblasts, perineurial-like cells, and axons). All ages and both sexes are affected, being most cases sporadic

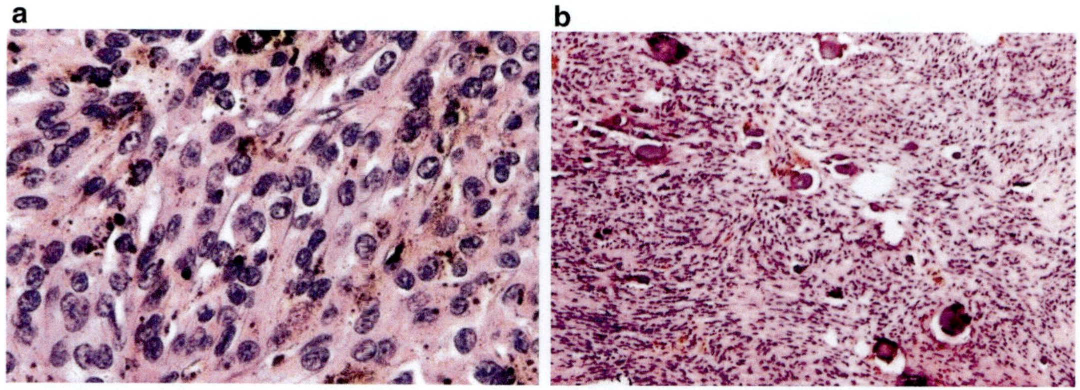

Fig. 17.8 *Melanotic schwannoma, histology*. (**a**) Typical features include spindle and epithelioid, heavily pigmented tumor cells. (**b**) Additionally, the *psammomatous variant* has calcified psammoma bodies

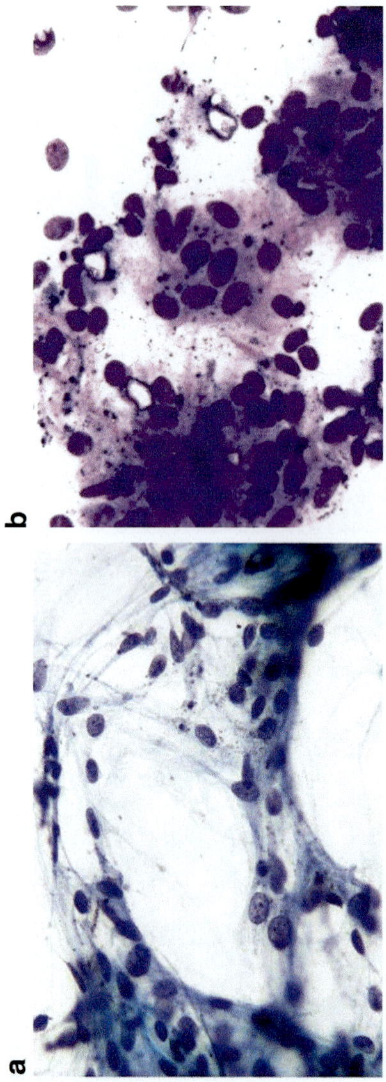

Fig. 17.9 *Melanotic schwannoma, cytologic features*. (**a**) Loosely cohesive sheet of spindle-shaped cells with uniform oval nuclei and pigment-laden bipolar processes (Smear, Papanicolaou). (**b**) *Psammomatous variant* displaying epithelioid cells with heavy black pigmentation and colorless crystals corresponding to fragmented psammoma bodies (Smear, Romanowsky)

and solitary nodules, whereas multiple nerve involvement is typical of *neurofibromatosis type 1* (NF1). NF1 results from germline inactivation of the *NF1* tumor suppressor gene, encoding a large, ubiquitous cytoplasmic protein – neurofibromin – which functions in part to decrease cell proliferation by promoting inactivation of the p21-ras proto-oncogene. Unlike schwannomas, neurofibromas are uncommon in the cranial and spinal nerves, at least within the confines of the dura. Thus, they are most often found in the extradural prolongation of the spinal nerve roots, giving rise to paraspinal masses.

Clinically, tumors present as a rarely painful mass, whereas multiple nerve involvement is the hallmark of NF1. An increased incidence of transformation to malignant peripheral nerve sheath tumor (MPNST) is seen in the setting of NF1.

Macroscopically, these are well-delimited, nodular to fusiform expansions of a nerve. On being cut, neurofibromas are soft to firm, showing glistening and grayish tan cut surfaces. Unlike schwannoma, cysts, yellow patches, and hemorrhage are absent (useful features for differential diagnosis).

Microscopically, neurofibromas are composed in large part of spindle cells arrayed in wavy bundles in a variably myxoid and collagenous matrix. Occasional axons pass through the tumor tissue, whereas blood vessels lack hyalinization (Fig. 17.10a). *Ancient neurofibroma* is defined by degenerative nuclear atypia (pleomorphism, smudgy chromatin, nuclear pseudoinclusions) but lacks any other features of malignancy (analogous to ancient schwannoma). *Atypical neurofibroma* is a variant defined by worrisome features (loss of architecture, high cellularity, cytological atypia, mitotic figures) and is notoriously difficult to distinguish from low-grade MPNST, being considered a premalignant tumor.

Cytologic Features

Neurofibroma tends to smear more easily than schwannoma, with abundant interstitial matrix separating cells into strands. The tissue fragments show a relatively low cellularity of spindle-shaped cells embedded in a variably myxoid background. Nuclei are thin, with tapered or curved features and have considerable smaller size than those of schwannomas. The loose myxoid background is better seen in Romanowsky-stained preparations (Fig. 17.10b).

Differential Diagnosis Considerations

In extradural spinal cord tumors, it is important to distinguish between schwannoma and neurofibroma, because the decision to open the dura sometimes hinges on this distinction. Relatively low cellularity, abundant metachromatic myxoid matrix,

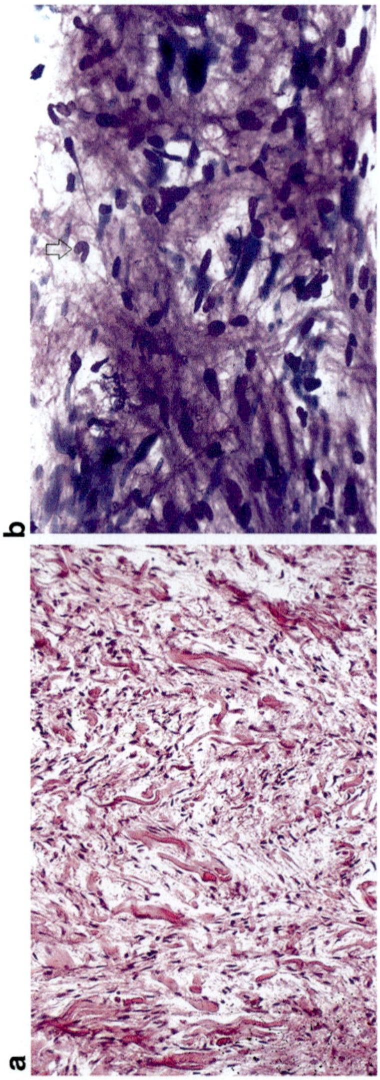

Fig. 17.10 *Neurofibroma*. (**a**) Typical histoarchitecture with wavy bundles of spindle cells arrayed in a myxoid-collagenous matrix. (**b**) Cytologic preparations are typically hypocellular with scattered spindle cells embedded in abundant myxoid stroma. Note nuclear curved feature (*arrow*; Smear, Romanowsky)

considerable smaller nuclei, and the absence of biphasic pattern (Antoni A and B areas) favor neurofibroma. *Atypical neurofibromas* may be mistaken for low-grade MPNST, and a preliminary intraoperative report of "spindle cell neoplasm with atypical features, grading deferred" is preferable.

Malignant Peripheral Nerve Sheath Tumors

Malignant peripheral nerve sheath tumors (MPNSTs) represent malignant neoplasms originating from, or demonstrating differentiation toward, nerve sheath elements. In about 50% of cases correspond to a transformed plexiform neurofibroma associated with NF1 but may also be associated with radiation therapy (about 10%) or arise de novo. They primarily affect young to middle-aged adults (peak incidence between the ages of 30 and 50 years) being deep-seated large nerves (sciatic nerve, brachial plexus, and sacral plexus) the most commonly involved; although well documented, MPNSTs originating in cranial nerves (most often vagus and vestibular) or spinal nerve roots have been reported. Histologically, the majority of cases (about 80%) resemble *spindle cell sarcomas*, with interlacing fascicles of tightly packed spindle-shaped cells (Fig. 17.11a). The remaining 20% of cases show unusual histologic features, including *epithelioid* (5%) and *heterologous mesenchymal or glandular differentiation* (15%). MPNSTs are highly aggressive tumors with tendency to recur and metastasize, more often to the lung, with an overall 5-year survival rate of around 50%. Inactivating mutations in genes encoding polycomb repressive complex (PRC2) components (*EED* or *SUZ 12)* are found in a majority of MPNSTs. These alterations are recognizing by loss of the histone H3 lysine 27 trimethylation (H3K27me3), which is mediated normally by PRC2 and may be detected by immunohistochemistry in tumor tissue (complete loss of H3K27me3 immunoreactivity in tumor cells, with staining present only in nonneoplastic cells providing a positive internal control).

Cytologic Features

Smears show dispersed or clustered spindle-shaped cells with oval to elongated hyperchromatic nuclei (the contrast between the dark hyperchromatic nuclei and the light cytoplasm is typical of MPNST). Tumor nuclei have, at least, triple size of neurofibroma nuclei and are smooth contoured with tapered or curved ends (Fig. 17.11b, c). The *epithelioid* (round or polygonal cells) and *anaplastic* (giant and polymorphous cells including heterologous elements) MPNSTs share cytomorphologic features with other types of pleomorphic sarcomas.

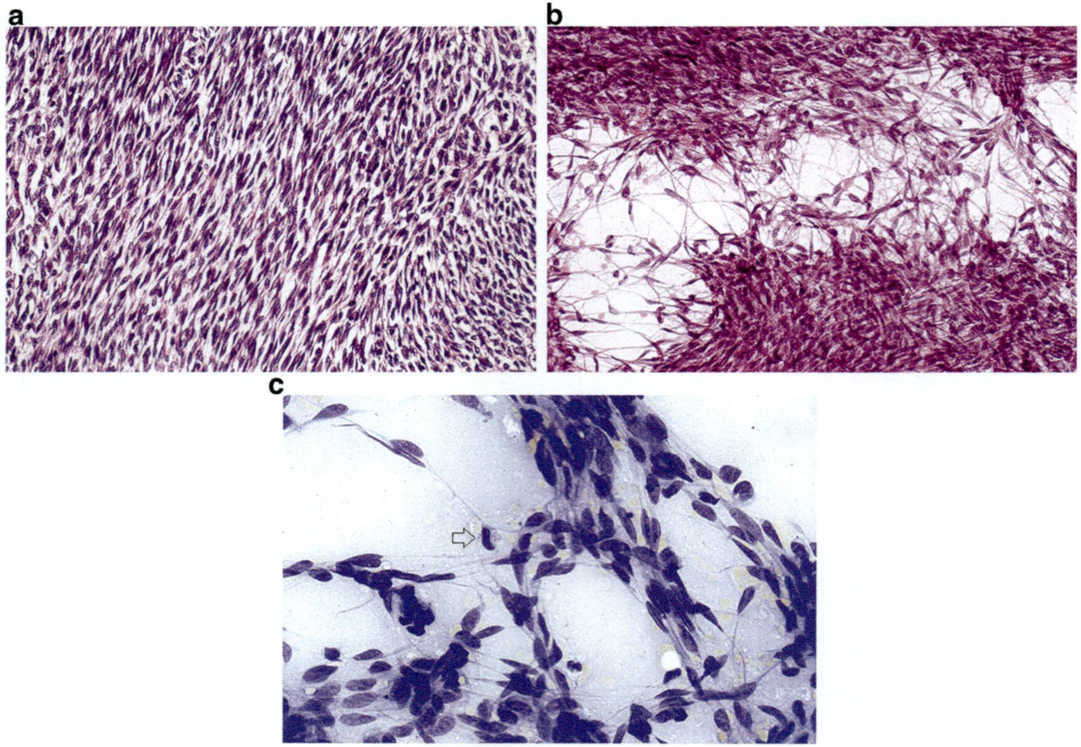

Fig. 17.11 *Malignant peripheral nerve sheath tumor (MPNST)*. (**a**) Histology. Interwoven fascicles of tightly packed hyperchromatic spindle cells characterize this tumor. (**b**) Highly cellular preparation displaying large, hyperchromatic nuclei and conspicuous cellular dissociation (Smear, H&E). (**c**) Spindle-shaped cells with oval to elongated nuclei and tapering or curved (*arrow*) ends. In contrast to cellular schwannoma, MPNST displays increased number of dispersed cells in cytologic preparations (Smear, Romanowsky)

Differential Diagnosis Considerations

In *conventional spindle cell variant*, the main differential diagnosis is cellular schwannoma. Both are highly cellular, and both may lack specific architectural features in frozen sections. Cytologic preparations showing MPNST distinctive nuclear size and increased number of dispersed cells are especially valuable and combined with the clinico-radiologic setting (origin of the tumor from a nerve trunk, patients with known history of NF1) allow an accurate preliminary diagnosis in many cases. In *high-grade*, *anaplastic tumors*, the diagnosis of malignancy is simple, what is complicate is to determine the neurogenic nature of the tumor. Presence of elongated nuclei with tapered or curved ends and, less commonly, a fibrillary metachromatic background are features suggestive of neurogenic differentiation. But, in a majority of cases, only a preliminary report of "pleomorphic malignant tumor" can be rendered.

Ganglioneuroma

Ganglioneuromas are benign tumors arising from the autonomous nervous system. These can arise at any age but more often affect older children and young adults (10–20 years) and show a characteristic female predilection. The association of ganglioneuroma with NF1 is well established. The most common locations include posterior mediastinum, retroperitoneum, and adrenal gland, but they have been identified in a variety of other locations. On imaging, most cases are solitary and discrete masses, some associated with expansion of the spinal foramen or even intraspinal extension. Histologically, ganglioneuroma consists of mature ganglion cells and axonal processes accompanied by satellite cells and Schwann cells, respectively (Fig. 17.12a). A correct evaluation of this lesion is of crucial importance, as there are some malignant neoplasms (neuroblastoma, ganglioneuroblastoma) that may have similar clinical presentations. The diagnostic approach can be a CT or endoscopic ultrasound-guided needle aspiration biopsy or an intraoperative consultation in the course of excisional surgery. In both diagnostic procedures, cytologic preparations reveal large, rotund ganglion cells and cohesive tissue fragments of spindle-shaped elements. Ganglion cells can display "neuromelanin" accumulation as a brown pigment, which has histochemical and electron microscopic properties resembling both melanin and lipofuscin (Fig. 17.12b, c).

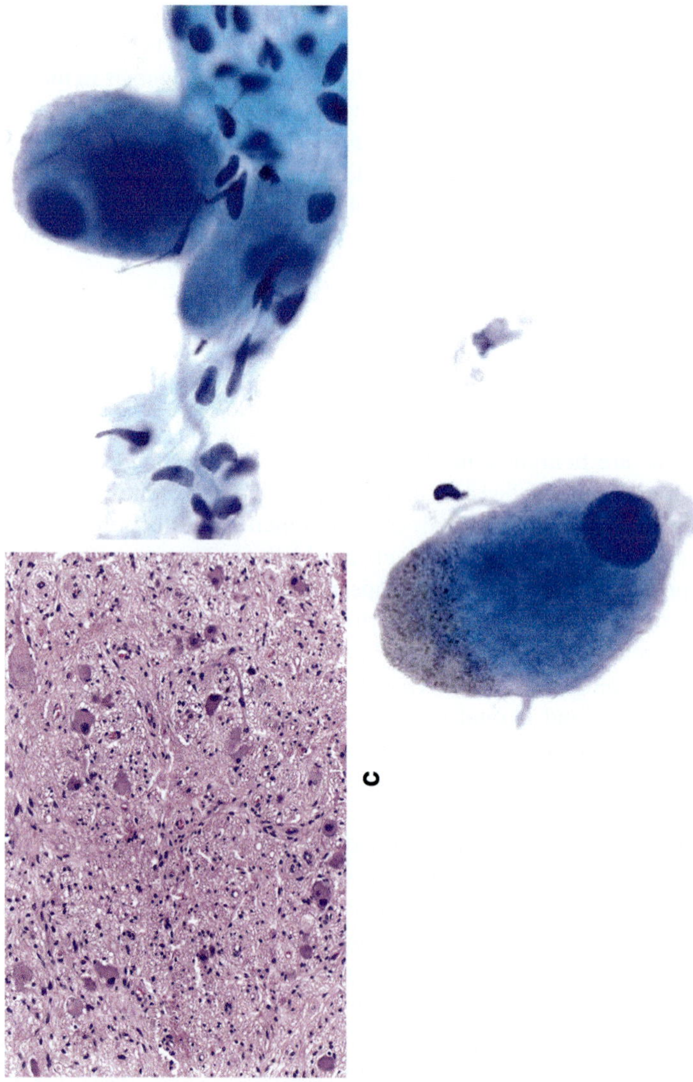

Fig. 17.12 *Ganglioneuroma.* (**a**) Characteristic histologic features include haphazardly arranged ganglion cells in a loose stroma of spindle-shaped elements. (**b**) Rotund ganglion cell and cohesive tissue fragment of spindle-shaped elements. (**c**) This ganglion cell has "neuromelanin" accumulation, a characteristic metabolic by-product in dopaminergic neurons (**b**, **c**; Preparations from an imaging-guided needle aspiration biopsy; Thin Prep; Papanicolaou)

Suggested Reading

Azarpira N, Torabineghad S, Sepidbakht S, Rakei M, Bagheri MH. Cytologic findings in pigmented melanotic schwannoma. A case report. Acta Cytol. 2009;53:113–5.

Carney JA. Psammomatous melanotic schwannoma. A distinctive heritable tumor with special associations, including cardiac myxoma and the Cushing syndrome. Am J Surg Pathol. 1990;14:206–22.

Cleven AH, Al Sannaa GA, Briaire-de Bruijn I, Ingram DR, et al. Loss of H3K27 tri-methylation is a diagnostic marker for malignant peripheral nerve sheath tumors and an indicator for an inferior survival. Mod Pathol. 2016;29:582–90.

Dim DC, Nugent SL, Peng HQ. Ganglioneuroma presenting as a paraesophageal mass lesion diagnosed by endoscopic ultrasound-guided fine needle aspiration cytology: a case report. Acta Cytol. 2010;54:321–4.

Dodd LG, Marom EM, Dash RC, McLendom RE. Fine-needle aspiration cytology of "ancient" schwannoma. Diagn Cytopathol. 1999;20:307–11.

Domanski HA. Fine-needle aspiration of ganglioneuroma. Diagn Cytopathol. 2005;32:363–6.

Gandolfi A, Tedeschi F, Brizzi R. The squash-smear technique in the diagnosis of spinal cord neurinomas. Report of three cases. Acta Cytol. 1983;27:273–6.

Jiménez-Heffernan JA, López-Ferrer P, Vicandi B, Hardisson D, Gamallo C, Viguer JM. Cytologic features of malignant peripheral nerve sheath tumor. Acta Cytol. 1999;43:175–83.

Karamchandani JR, Nielsen TO, van de Rijn M, West RB. Sox10 and S100 in the diagnosis of soft-tissue neoplasms. Appl Immunohistochem Mol Morphol. 2012;20:445–50.

Klijanienko J, Caillaud JM, Legacé R. Cytohistologic correlations in schwannomas (neurilemmomas) including "ancient", cellular, and epithelioid variants. Diagn Cytopathol. 2006;34:517–22.

Klijanienko J, Caillaud JM, Lagacé R, Vielh P. Cytohistologic correlations of 24 malignant peripheral nerve sheath tumor (MPNST) in 17 patients: the Institut Curie experience. Diagn Cytopathol. 2002;27:103–8.

Kobayashi S. Meningioma, neurilemmoma and astrocytoma specimens obtained with the squash method for diagnosis. Acta Cytol. 1993;37:913–22.

Laforga JB. Cellular schwannoma: report of a case diagnosed intraoperatively with the aid of cytologic imprints. Diagn Cytopathol. 2003;29:95–100.

Lee W, Teckie S, Wiesner T, Ran L, et al. PRC2 is recurrently inactivated through EED or SUZ12 loss in malignant peripheral nerve sheath tumors. Nat Genet. 2014;46:1227–32.

Martinez-Izquierdo MA, Lopez-Soto MV, Saenz-Santamaria J, Lacruz CR. Intraoperative cytological findings in two cases of psammomatous melanotic schwannoma. Cytopathology. 2011;22:60–2.

Marton E, Feletti A, Orvieto E, Longatti P. Dumbbell-shaped C-2 psammomatous melanotic malignant schwannoma. Case report and review of the literature. J Neurosurg Spine. 2007;6:591–9.

Miettinen MM, Antonescu CR, Fletcher CDM, Kim A, et al. Histopathologic evaluation of atypical neurofibromatous tumors and their transformation into malignant peripheral nerve sheath tumor in patients with neurofibromatosis 1-a consensus overview. Hum Pathol. 2017;67:1–10.

Mosunjac MB, Johnston EI, Mosunjac MI. Fine-needle aspiration cytologic diagnosis of metastatic melanotic schwannoma: familial case of a mother and daughter with Carney's complex and literature review. Diagn Cytopathol. 2007;35:130–4.

Nguyen GK, Johnson ES, Mielke BW. Cytology of meningiomas and neurilemomas in crush preparations. A useful adjunct to frozen sections. Acta Cytol. 1988;32:362–5.

Pekmezci M, Reuss DE, Hirbe AC, Dahiya S, et al. Morphologic and immunohistochemical features of malignant peripheral nerve sheath tumors and cellular schwannomas. Mod Pathol. 2015;28:187–200.

Prieto-Granada CN, Wiesner T, Messina JL, Jungbluth AA, Chi P, Antonescu CR. Loss of H3K27me3 expression is highly sensitive marker for sporadic and radiation-induced MPNST. Am J Surg Pathol. 2016;40:479–89.

Sola-Pérez J, Pérez-Guillermo M, Bas-Bernal A, Giménez-Bascuñana A, Montes-Clavero C. Melanocytic schwannoma: the cytologic aspect in fine-needle aspiration cytology; report of a case located in the spinal cord. Diagn Cytopathol. 1994;11:291–6.

Torres-Mora J, Dry S, Li X, Binder S, Amin M, Folpe AL. Malignant melanotic schwannian tumor: a clinicopathologic, immunohistochemical, and gene expression profiling study of 40 cases, with a proposal for the reclassification of "melanotic schwannoma". Am J Surg Pathol. 2014;38:94–105.

White W, Shiu MH, Rosenblum MK, Erlandson RA, Woodruff JM. Cellular schwannoma. A clinicopathologic study of 57 patients and 58 tumors. Cancer. 1990;66:1266–75.

Chapter 18
Metastatic Tumors

Brain metastases from systemic malignancies are the most common intracranial tumors, which account for approximately 30% of clinically significant CNS tumors in adults and about 2% in children, and their incidence is rising. It is estimated that 40% of cancer patients will develop brain metastases, usually late in disease (especially renal cell carcinoma and ocular melanoma). While most cancers spread to the brain hematogenously, regional malignancies from the head and face can spread by direct local invasion along cranial nerves or through the foramina of the skull base. Direct spread from the adjacent bones of the craniospinal vault may also occur. Due to the secondary nature of the process, age, gender, and prevalence are those of the original tumor. In adults, up to 90% of cases arise from five organs that, in order of the frequency, are the lung, breast, skin (melanoma), kidney, and the gastrointestinal tract, whereas metastases from malignant bone or mesenchymal neoplasms are very uncommon. In children, the most common tumors to exhibit CNS metastasis are of kidney/adrenal origin (i.e., Wilms tumor, neuroblastoma), followed by those from bone/soft tissue (i.e., Ewing sarcoma, osteogenic sarcoma, pleomorphic undifferentiated sarcoma). Lymphomas are considered systemic diseases, therefore not metastatic when involving the brain. From the topographic point of view, metastases to the CNS may affect both the parenchyma and its coverings (Table 18.1). On the basis of their parenchymal distribution, about 80% of brain metastases are located in the cerebral hemispheres (most often frontoparietal lobes), 15% in the cerebellum, and 5% in the brainstem, whereas very few cases are localized in the spinal cord.

It is also worth noting, for reasons that are not clear, the predilection of certain tumors for certain regions of the CNS (Table 18.2). All of this information is of the greatest interest for the intraoperative diagnosis, because the statistical and topographic data may help the physician to make a correct assessment.

Clinical symptoms are related to the mass effect (increased intracranial pressure) and local neurologic deficits, but some patients present acutely with seizure or stroke due to hemorrhage. Patients with meningeal carcinomatosis may have mul-

C. R. Lacruz et al., *Central Nervous System Intraoperative Cytopathology*,
Essentials in Cytopathology 13, https://doi.org/10.1007/978-3-319-98491-9_18

Table 18.1 Topography of central nervous system metastatic tumors

Parenchymal metastasis
Solitary or multiple nodular masses
Diffuse perivascular invasion ("carcinomatous encephalitis")
Meningeal metastasis
Dural involvement
Leptomeningeal involvement
Meningeal carcinomatosis/ melanomatosis
CSF spread from primary CNS malignancies
Craniospinal bone metastasis
With secondary involvement of the brain
With secondary involvement of the spinal chord

Table 18.2 Predilection of different CNS metastatic tumors types by site

Leptomeninges	*Dura*
Lung carcinoma	Prostatic carcinoma
Breast carcinoma	Lung carcinoma
Melanoma	Breast carcinoma
Spinal epidural space	*Posterior fossa*
Myeloma	Renal cell carcinoma
Lung carcinoma	Colorectal carcinoma
Breast carcinoma	*Choroid plexus*
Prostatic carcinoma	Renal cell carcinoma
Pancreatic carcinoma	*Spinal cord (intramedullary)*
Colorectal carcinoma	Small-cell lung carcinoma

tiple neurologic deficits, mental disturbances, ataxia, and radiculopathy, being the diagnosis usually established by the demonstration of malignant cells on cytologic inspection of the CSF (Fig. 18.1). In neuroimaging, in contrast to common glial neoplasms, metastatic tumors tend to be circumscribed masses, which show either a diffuse or ringlike pattern of contrast enhancement with a surrounding zone of vasogenic edema. Most cerebral metastases are superficially located in arterial watershed zones at gray-white matter junction (Fig. 18.2). Because of the paramagnetic qualities of melanin, intrinsic, bright T1 signal is characteristic of pigmented metastatic melanomas. In carcinomatosis, contrast-enhanced MRI will reveal diffuse thickening or nodular enhancement of the leptomeninges or dura.

Grossly, in contrast to the common glial neoplasms of adulthood, intraparenchymal metastases usually appear as either single or multiple sharply circumscribed nodules with "pushing" margins, surrounded by an edematous-looking rim. Multicentricity is more common in lung carcinoma (especially small cell), breast

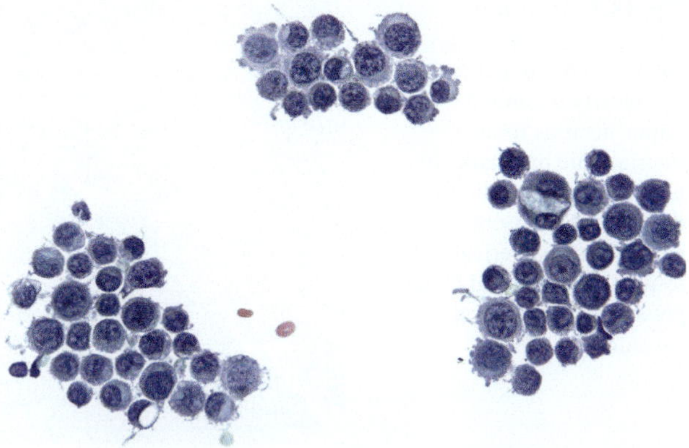

Fig. 18.1 *Meningeal carcinomatosis in CSF.* The malignant cells of this Bloom-Richardson grade III ductal breast carcinoma are large, round, and variable in size. Note typical clustering (Thin Prep, Papanicolaou)

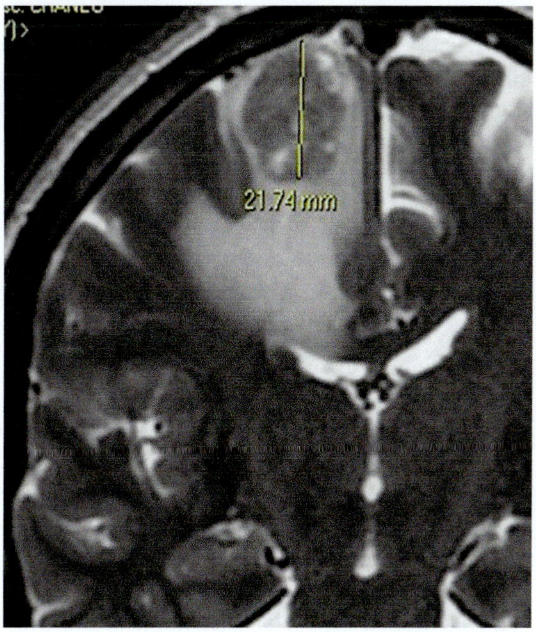

Fig. 18.2 *Metastatic tumors, typical imaging features.* A coronal T2 MR image shows sharp demarcation, intense peritumoral edema, and the typical location at the gray-white matter junction

carcinoma, and melanoma. Their interior may show necrotic and hemorrhagic zones, with hemorrhagic zones particularly frequent in choriocarcinoma, melanoma, and renal cell carcinoma (search for these metastatic tumors in intracranial hemorrhages). Dural involvement usually takes the form of globoid or in-plaque dura-based mass(es), whereas in leptomeningeal involvement the membranes appear cloudy or opaque.

Histologically, most intraparenchymal metastases displace rather than infiltrate the brain parenchyma evoking a rim of edema, reactive gliosis, and chronic inflammation (Fig. 18.3); variable perivascular growth in the adjacent CNS tissue (so-called

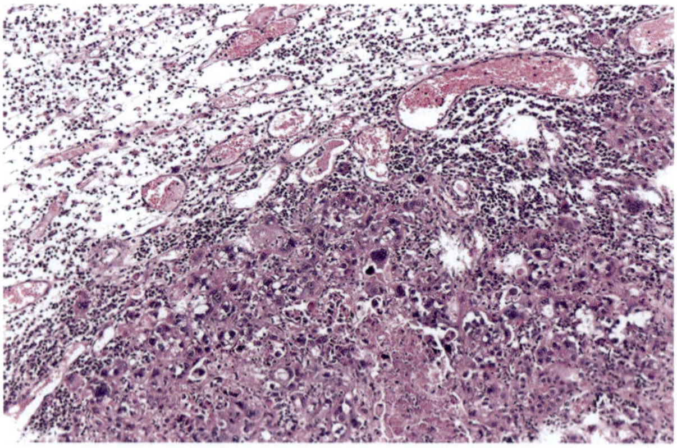

Fig. 18.3 *Metastatic tumors, typical histology.* A cohesive growth pattern and clearly delimited tumor-nervous tissue interface are hallmarks of neoplasms metastatic to the brain. The discrete nature of the spherical lesion is accentuated by the presence of considerable surrounding edema

vascular co-option) also is common. Necrosis is frequent and often extensive, particularly in colonic carcinoma. On the other hand, leptomeningeal metastases extend through the Virchow-Robin spaces, from which they can infiltrate the adjacent parenchyma. As a rule of thumb, the diverse microscopic appearances retain primary features but may be poorly differentiated.

General Diagnostic Approach

Recent advances in the management of patients with CNS metastases have made accurate diagnosis of these tumors of paramount importance. Due to metastases in most cases take on the radiologic aspect of either single or multiple circumscribed masses, the method of choice for obtaining diagnostic material is a CT-guided stereotactic biopsy. In 80–90% of cases, the presence of such brain masses occurs in a patient with a known primary neoplasm; therefore, stereotactic biopsy is used for confirmation of this diagnostic suspicion. However, in as many as 10–20% of patients with brain metastases, no primary tumor is found at presentation ("metastasis of unknown primary"). Notably lung and kidney cancers and melanoma often present clinically as metastases to the brain, which is why the lesion must be distinguished from a primary tumor and may constitute a diagnostic challenge. In both situations, the smear technique has great diagnostic value.

Cytologic Features

Smears from metastatic cancers usually show abundant exfoliation of hyperchromatic cells with a high nuclear-to-cytoplasmic ratio. In contrast to glial tumors, metastatic tumors are present in a nonfibrillary background, and large clusters, small groups, and single cells may be present in the same smear. In some tumor types, the cell discohesive tendency may be striking, particularly in melanoma and lobular breast carcinoma. Both cell clusters and individual cells show smooth boundaries without processes, whereas molding of adjacent cells is a helpful feature often present. On the other hand, the background is clear; however, in the presence of extensive necrosis, the background shows granular debris (Fig. 18.4a, b). Often, preparations reveal the same features as those of the primary neoplasm, including specialized differentiation – papillae, extra- or intracellular mucin, keratinization, neuroendocrine features, melanin, etc. – which allows the recognition of some tumor types. *Adenocarcinoma* may be recognized by the presence of papillary structures, three-dimensional groups (cell balls), and intra- or extracellular mucin; whereas the individual cells generally have delicate, finely vacuolated cytoplasm, open or vesicular chromatin pattern, and conspicuous or prominent nucleoli (Fig. 18.5a, b). *Squamous cell carcinoma* usually forms broad sheets of cells and may show whorls; whereas the individual cells have dense cytoplasm and coarse chromatin with inconspicuous nucleoli (Fig. 18.6a, b). *Small-cell carcinoma* shows small cell size, inconspicuous cytoplasm, nuclear molding, stippled chromatin, and crush artifact (Fig. 18.7a, b). *Breast carcinoma* may have many cytologic patterns, but the presence of cytoplasmic vacuoles containing mucin secretion is very characteristic (Fig. 18.8a, b). *Renal cell carcinoma* often displays sheets of large cells with clear "foamy" cytoplasm and prominent nucleoli (Fig. 18.9a, b). *Urothelial cell carcinoma* show flattened sheets of cells with homogeneous cytoplasm and isolated "cercariform" cells, which display elongated unipolar cytoplasmic processes and a blunt pole that contains the nucleus (Fig. 18.10a, b). *Colonic carcinoma* usually has columnar cells with elongated "cigar-shaped" nuclei forming palisades (Fig. 18.11a, b). *Melanoma*, the "great mimicker," occasionally poses a problem as a result its myriad morphologic patterns. However, most cases typically smear out as individual cells with round, epithelioid, or fusiform features and anaplastic nuclei with prominent nucleoli. Binucleated or multinucleated forms and nuclear pseudoinclusions also are frequent Likewise, melanoma cells typically have abundant cytoplasm that remains sharply demarcated; only the most poorly differentiated melanomas lose their cytoplasm. Dark-brown (H&E and Papanicolaou stains) or black (Romanowsky stain) granular cytoplasmic pigment is extremely helpful if present, but it is absent in about a half of cases (Fig. 18.12a, b).

Differential Diagnosis Considerations

Perhaps the most commonly encountered differential diagnostic dilemma is metastatic carcinoma versus glioblastoma in adult patients with a single ring-enhancing lesion. In such a circumstance, cytological preparations are, by far, more useful than frozen sections for differentiation between the two. Carcinoma cells tend to cluster in a nonfibrillary background, while glial tumors will reveal a dispersed cell pattern within a fibrillary background. Also, since metastasis from small-cell carcinoma is treated with radiation therapy or chemotherapy (or both) rather than aggressive

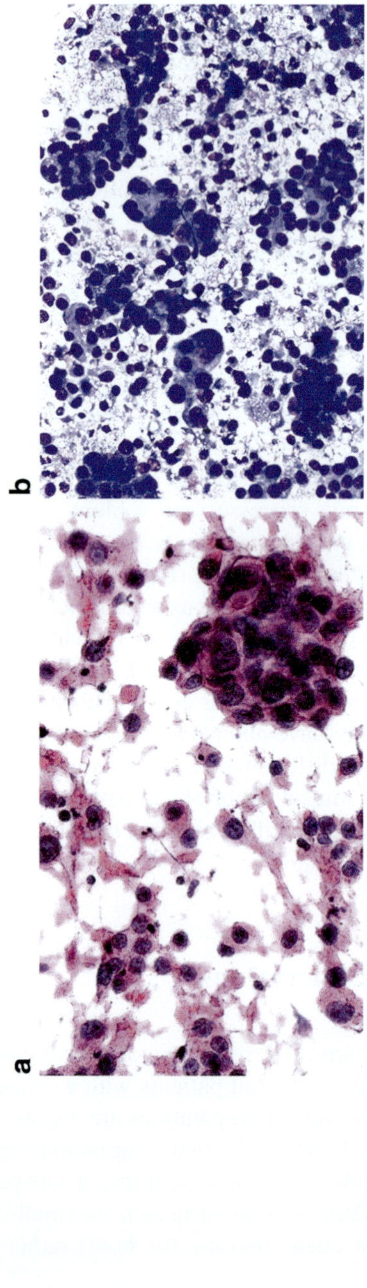

Fig. 18.4 *Metastatic carcinoma, cytologic features.* (**a**) Ductal carcinoma from a mammary primary. This preparation shows clusters or dispersed malignant cells with well-defined cytoplasmic boundaries (Smear, H&E). (**b**) Adenocarcinoma from a lung primary. This preparation displays large and small cell groups and isolated malignant cells (Smear, Romanowsky). In both preparations, the cellular cohesion characteristic of most epithelial neoplasms and foreign to gliomas and lymphomas is maintained facilitating rapid intraoperative diagnosis. Also note the absence of fibrillary (glial) background

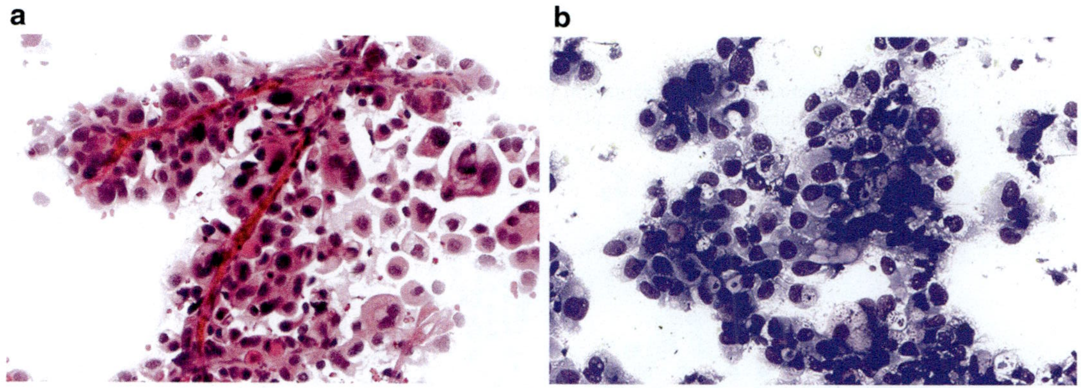

Fig. 18.5 *Metastatic adenocarcinoma*. (**a**) Metastasis from a lung primary. Papillary fragments with vascular core help identify the lesion as adenocarcinoma (Smear, H&E). (**b**) Metastasis from a lung primary. Intracytoplasmic vacuoles containing the secretory product help in the identification of the tumor as adenocarcinoma (Smear, Romanowsky)

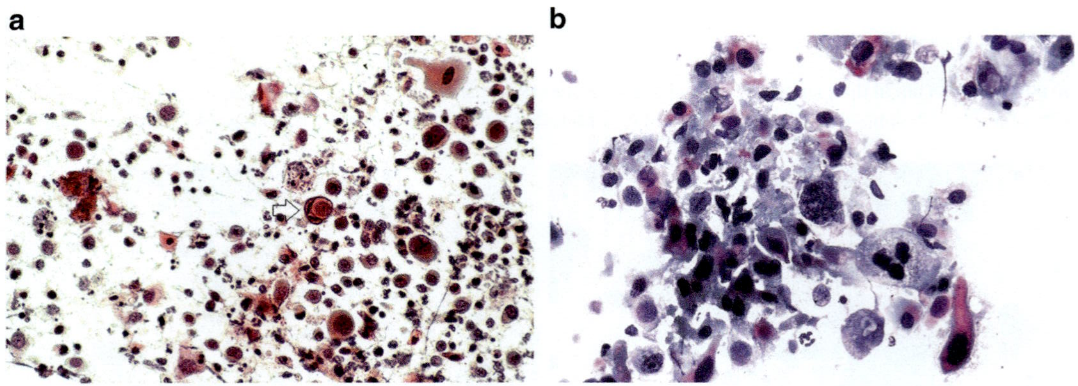

Fig. 18.6 *Metastatic squamous carcinoma*. (**a**) Metastasis from a lung primary. Atypical keratinized squamous cells with orange, dense cytoplasm and a small cell whorl (*arrow*) help identify the tumor as squamous carcinoma. (**b**) A high magnification shows characteristic pleomorphism, dense cytoplasm, coarse chromatin, and inconspicuous nucleoli (**a**, **b**; Smears, Papanicolaou)

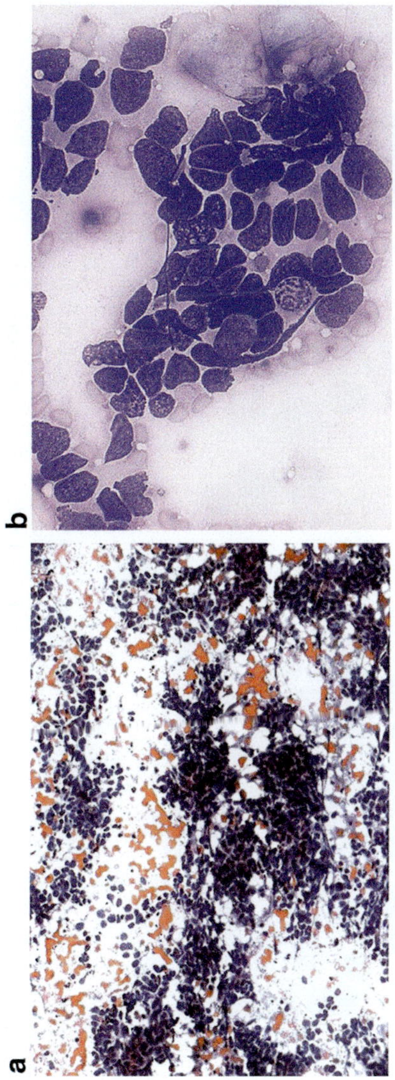

Fig. 18.7 *Metastatic small-cell carcinoma of the lung*. **(a)** Small, undifferentiated cells with very high N/C ratio showing characteristic crush artifact. Also note some lining up of cells (Smear, Papanicolaou). **(b)** High-magnification view showing scant cytoplasm, speckled chromatin, and conspicuous nuclear moldings (Smear, Romanowsky)

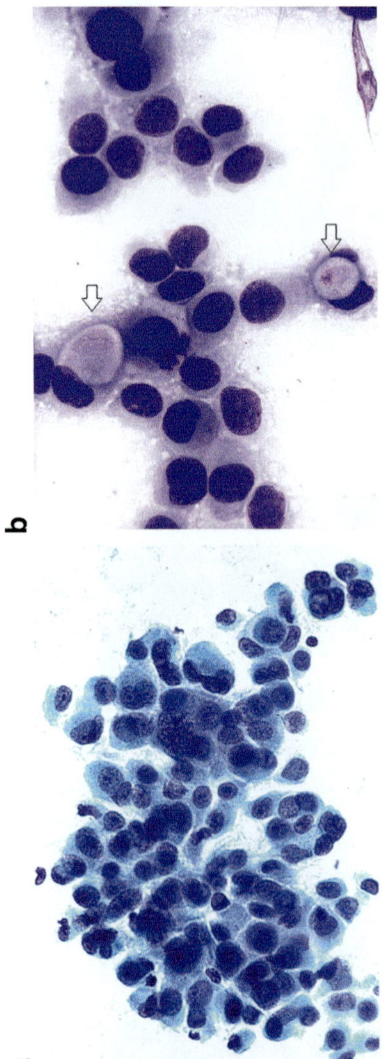

Fig. 18.8 *Metastatic breast carcinoma*. (**a**) This high-grade, ductal carcinoma displays cohesive clusters and individual cells. Note the well-demarcated cell boundaries without processes (Smear, Papanicolaou). (**b**) Lobular carcinomas are often less cohesive than their ductal counterparts and spread more easily in the smear. Note intracytoplasmic mucin droplets (*arrows*) and discohesive cell pattern (Smear, Romanowsky)

a b
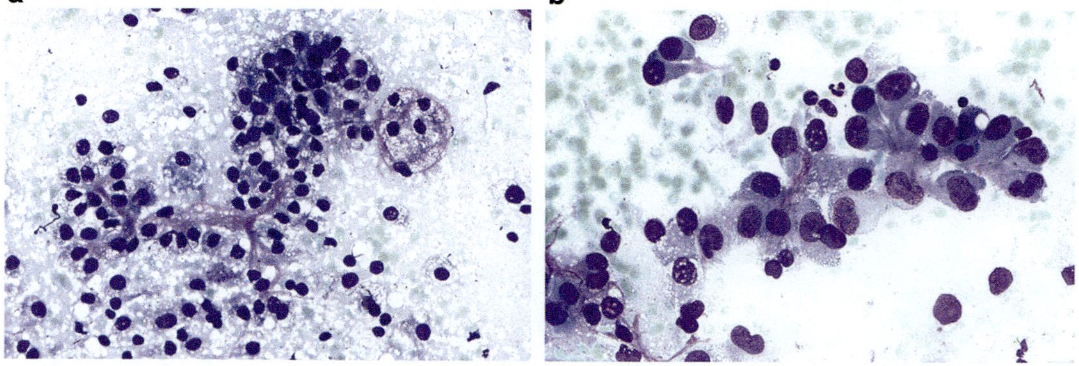

Fig. 18.9 *Metastatic renal cell carcinoma.* (**a**) Clear cell type. This preparation displays stromal core sheets of clear cells with finely vacuolated cytoplasm. (**b**) Papillary type. In this case the tumor cells are arranged in a papillary structure (**a**, **b**; Smears, Romanowsky)

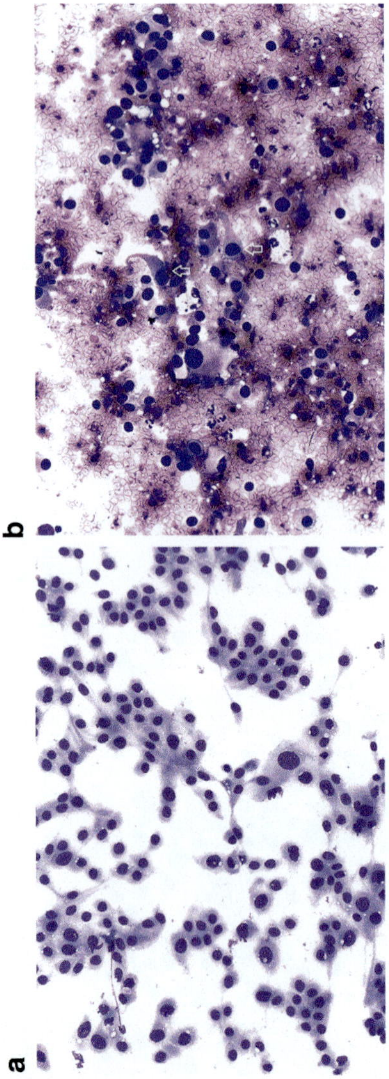

Fig. 18.10 *Metastatic urothelial cell carcinoma.* (**a**) Flattened sheets of cells with homogeneous cytoplasm and large, hyperchromatic nuclei. (**b**) This preparation shows two "cercariform" tumor cells (*arrows*) with elongated, unipolar cytoplasmic processes and a blunt pole that contains the nucleus (**a**, **b**; Smears, Romanowsky)

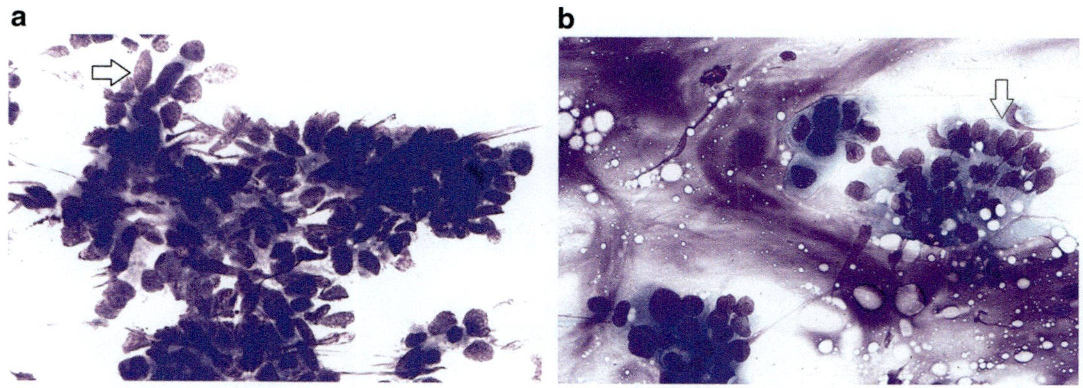

Fig. 18.11 *Metastatic colonic adenocarcinoma.* (**a**) Conventional type, displaying tissue fragments consisting of palisaded malignant columnar cells with elongated "cigar-shaped" nuclei (*arrow*). (**b**) This mucinous variant shows columnar cells with nuclear stratification (*arrow*) and abundant thick mucoid material in the background (**a**, **b**; Smears, Romanowsky)

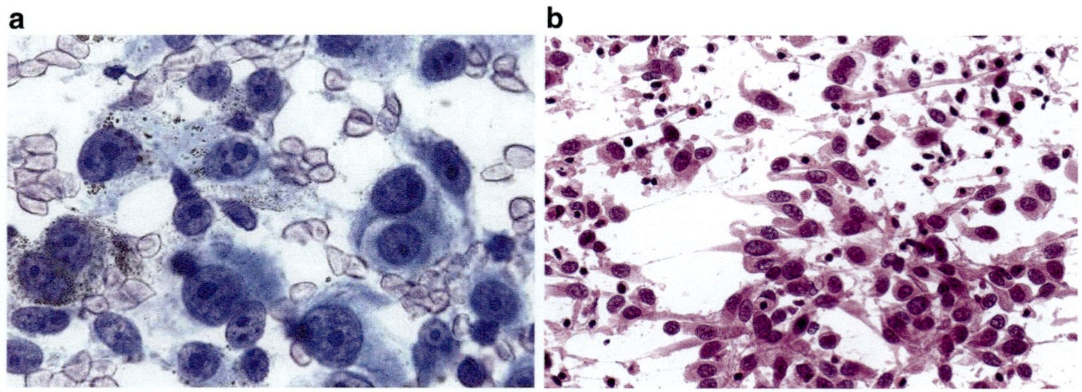

Fig. 18.12 *Metastatic melanoma.* (**a**) Round, epithelioid, or fusiform cells exhibiting large nuclei and prominent nucleoli. Some of them display intracytoplasmic brow pigment (Smear, Papanicolaou). (**b**) Amelanotic type. This is the characteristic appearance of melanoma: predominantly single cells with an epithelioid or fusiform morphology and anaplastic nuclei, but melanin pigment is absent (Smear, H&E)

Table 18.3 Characteristics of central nervous system metastases

Cytologic features
Highly cellular smears
Cohesive clumps of cells
High nuclear/cytoplasmic ratio
Distinct cell outlines without processes
Nonfibrillary background
Features of differentiation
Glandular, squamous, melanocytic, neuroendocrine, etc.
Differential diagnosis and pitfalls
Glioblastoma
Anaplastic oligodendroglioma
Meningioma
CNS lymphoma
Small-cell carcinoma vs embryonal tumors
Papillary adenocarcinoma vs choroid plexus tumors
Renal cell carcinoma vs hemangioblastoma
Metastatic carcinoma to the sella vs pituitary adenoma

surgery, distinction between small-cell carcinoma and non-small-cell carcinoma should be made when possible. On the other hand, metastatic cancer versus meningioma, anaplastic oligodendroglioma, and primary CNS lymphoma; renal cell carcinoma versus hemangioblastoma; small-cell lung carcinoma versus embryonal tumors; metastatic papillary carcinomas versus choroid plexus tumors; and metastatic carcinoma to the sella versus pituitary adenoma are covered in the corresponding chapters. In difficult cases, correlation with clinical and radiologic findings is invaluable in arriving at an accurate diagnosis (Table 18.3).

Suggested Reading

Aragon-Ching JB, Zujewski JA. CNS metastasis: an old problem in a new guise. Clin Cancer Res. 2007;13:1644–7.

Berghoff AS, Schur S, Füreder LM, Gatterbauer B, et al. Descriptive statistical analysis of a real life cohort of 2419 patients with brain metastases of solid cancers. ESMO Open. 2016;1(2):e000024.

Chamberlain MC. Leptomeningeal metastasis. Curr Opin Neurol. 2009;22:665–74.

Gavrilovic IT, Posner JB. Brain metastases: epidemiology and pathophysiology. J Neuro-Oncol. 2005;75:5–14.

Giordana MT, Cordera S, Boghi A. Cerebral metastases as first symptom of cancer: a clinico-pathologic study. J Neuro-Oncol. 2000;50:265–73.

Girgis S, Ramzy J, Baer SC, Schwartz MR. Fine needle aspiration diagnosis of transitional cell carcinoma metastatic to the brain. Acta Cytol. 1999;43:235–8.

Kapusta LR, Taylor M, Ang LC, Schwartz M. Cytologic diagnosis of a solitary brain metastasis from papillary carcinoma of the thyroid. A case report. Acta Cytol. 1999;43:432–4.

Monabati A, Kumar PV, Kamkarpour A. Intraoperative cytodiagnosis of metastatic brain tumors confused clinically with brain abscess. A report of three cases. Acta Cytol. 2000;44:437–41.

Preusser M, Capper D, Ilhan-Mutlu A, Berghoff AS, et al. Brain metastases: pathobiology and emerging targeted therapies. Acta Neuropathol. 2012;123:205–22.

Reyes CV, Thompson KS, Jensen JD. Cytopathologic evaluation of lung carcinomas presenting as brain metastasis. Diagn Cytopathol. 1999;20:325–7.

Schouten LJ, Rutten J, Huveneers HA, Twijnstra A. Incidence of brain metastases in a cohort of patients with carcinoma of the breast, colon, kidney, and lung and melanoma. Cancer. 2002;94:2698–705.

Soffietti R, Abacioglu U, Baumert B, Combs SE, et al. Diagnosis and treatment of brain metastases from solid tumors: guidelines from the European Association of Neuro-Oncology (EANO). Neuro-Oncology. 2017;19:162–74.

Suki D, Abdulla RK, Ding M, Khatua S, et al. Brain metastases in patients diagnosed with a solid primary cancer during childhood: experience from a single referral cancer center. J Neurosurg Pediatr. 2014;14:372–85.

Taillibert S, Laigle-Donadey F, Chodkiewicz C, Sanson M, Hoang-Xuan K, Delattre JY. Leptomeningeal metastases from solid malignancy: a review. J Neuro-Oncol. 2005;75:85–99.

Wiens AL, Hattab EM. The pathological spectrum of solid CNS metastases in the pediatric population. J Neurosurg Pediatr. 2014;14:129–35.

Part III
Nonneoplastic

Chapter 19
Benign Cystic Lesions

A variety of benign cysts – most of developmental origin – can arise in the parenchymal, ventricular, or subarachnoid spaces throughout the cranial and spinal cavities. They can be classified according to their cell lining into epithelial-lining cysts (squamous and columnar-to-cuboidal) and nonepithelial-lining cysts (arachnoid membrane and astrocytic gliosis). Cyst puncture and aspiration under direct vision with a stereotactic neuroendoscopic instrument allows for a potentially safe and practical therapeutic approach in some cases. The specimens that are usually submitted for diagnosis are cyst contents and biopsies of the cyst wall, yielding a variety of fluids and cell types depending on the cyst origin. The differential diagnosis depends largely on their location, as well as on the lining cells (when intact) and cyst contents (Table 19.1).

Squamous Epithelium-Lined Cysts

Epidermoid Cyst

Epidermoid cyst accounts for approximately 1% of all intracranial masses and is most often present in middle age, with a peak incidence in the sixth decade. The histogenesis is related to ectodermal displacements in the developing brain. The cyst is filled with a lamellated "flaky" type of keratin (dry keratin) and is lined by keratinizing stratified squamous epithelium (Fig. 19.1a). Because epidermoid cysts are thin-walled, not well encapsulated lesions, they may extend quite widely within the subarachnoid space. MRI shows a lobular and discrete extra-axial mass with a radiologic signal of keratinaceous material (hyperintensity [bright] on diffusion-weighted sequences). Lesions become clinically apparent through mass effect. Occasionally, leakage of their contents into cerebrospinal fluid results in sterile

C. R. Lacruz et al., *Central Nervous System Intraoperative Cytopathology*,
Essentials in Cytopathology 13, https://doi.org/10.1007/978-3-319-98491-9_19

Table 19.1 Benign cystic lesions of the neuraxis

Type	Common locations	Content	Lining
Epidermoid	Cerebellopontine angles	Keratinous	Squamous
	Suprasellar/parasellar		
	Ventricular system		
	Calvarian bones		
Dermoid	Fontanels	Cheesy	Squamous
	Posterior fossa		
	Skull base		
	Spinal		
Colloid	Third ventricle	Mucinous	Columnar/cuboidal
Rathke cleft	Sellar/suprasellar	Mucinous	Columnar/cuboidal
Endodermal	Anterior to spinal cord	Mucinous	Columnar/cuboidal
	Anterior to brainstem		
Ependymal	Paraventricular	Watery	Columnar/cuboidal
	Over the convexities		
	Intramedullary		
Choroid plexus	Lateral ventricles	Watery	Columnar/cuboidal
Arachnoid	Sylvian fissures	Watery	Meningothelial
	Cisterna magna		
	Cerebellopontine angles		
	Spinal		
Glial	Cerebellum	Watery	Astrocytic gliosis
Pineal	Pineal gland	Watery	Astrocytic gliosis

chemical meningitis, and repeated episodes of this spillage of keratinous debris into the subarachnoid space can evoke a xanthogranulomatous inflammation with a proliferative fibrous reaction (*cholesteatoma*), making total removal difficult.

Dermoid Cyst

Dermoid cysts are less common and occur in the midline, and most cases occur in children or adolescents. There is a frequent association with bone and dermal defects, especially in a spinal location (spina bifida and dermal sinuses). The wall of the dermoid cyst is thick, lined by keratinizing squamous epithelium and endowed with cutaneous adnexal structures including pilosebaceous units, eccrine, and, occasionally, apocrine glands (Fig. 19.1b). The presence of such adnexal structures determines the more heterogeneous MRI signal of the dermoid cyst as well as the typical keratinous/sebaceous (cheesy) and matted hair contents.

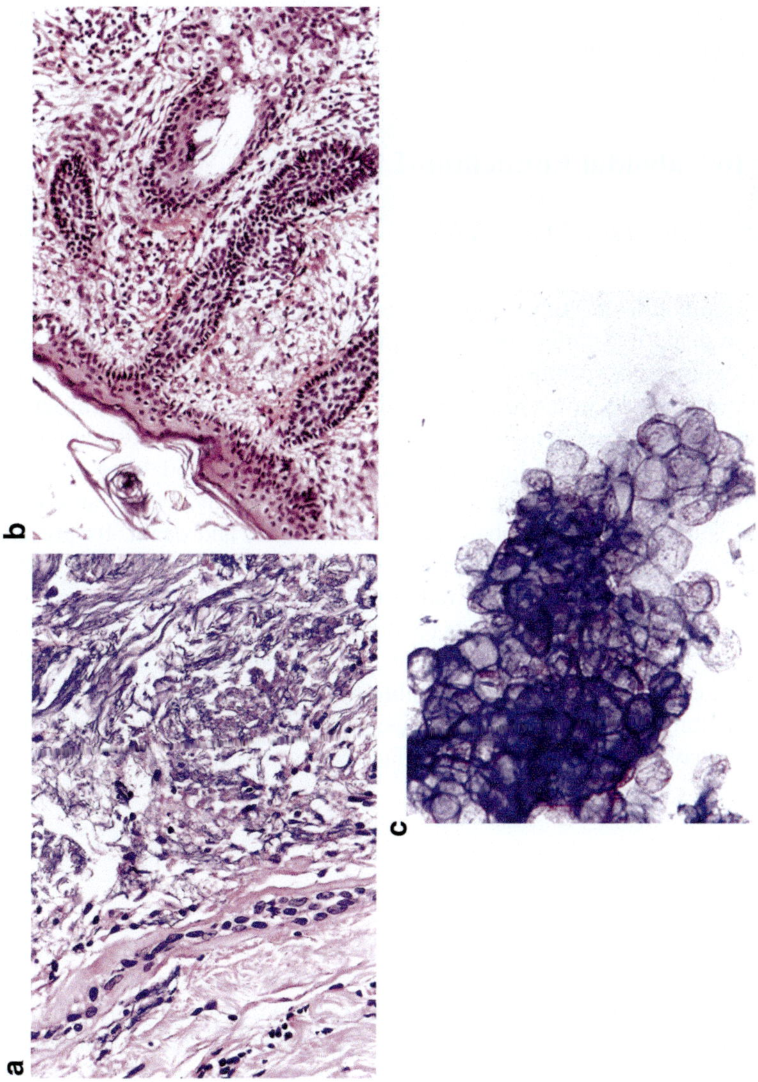

Fig. 19.1 *Squamous epithelium-lined cysts.* (**a**) *Epidermoid cyst*, histology. Cyst lined by squamous epithelium and filled with lamellated “dry” keratin. Unlike the skin, there is no equivalent of the dermis and its adnexa. (**b**) *Dermoid cyst*, histology. In this case the cyst is also lined by squamous epithelium, but the capsule is endowed with pilosebaceous units. (**c**) Detached anucleated squames or “cell ghosts” are typical of both epidermoid and dermoid cysts in cytologic preparations (Smear, Romanowsky)

Cytologic Features and Differential Diagnosis

Smears from the cyst content of both lesions show numerous anuclear "flaky" squamous cells piled up in large clusters and amorphous debris (Fig. 19.1c). Additionally, dermoid cysts may have hair and waxy debris.

The *differential diagnosis* includes other cystic lesions with squamous cells, such as craniopharyngioma and mature cystic teratoma.

Columnar to Cuboidal Epithelium-Lined Cysts

Colloid Cyst of the Third Ventricle

This is an uncommon lesion most often present in adults (20–50 years). Colloid cysts have been noted in familiar clusters, typically in females, but it is not clear whether this represents a specific genetic defect or coincidence. Because of the characteristic cyst location in the anterior third ventricle, near the interventricular foramen of Monro, it causes symptoms related to the intermittent obstruction of CSF flow (ball valve effect) including headaches, incontinence, and "drop attacks" (sudden transient paralysis of the lower extremities); occasionally, it may cause sudden impaction with acute hydrocephalus, brain herniation, and death. Its precise location, together with its grape-like appearance (bright on T1, T2, and FLAIR sequences), allows us to make a certain radiologic diagnosis. Microscopy shows a simple cyst filled with liquid to mucinous (colloid) PAS-positive content and a distinctive epithelial lining of ciliated columnar cells and interspersed goblet cells (Fig. 19.2). Cyst expansion may be responsible for the progressive attenuation of the lining epithelium, and in long-standing lesions, a proliferative xanthogranulomatous reaction may fill the cyst with total effacement of the epithelial lining.

Rathke Cleft Cyst

Rathke cleft cyst presumably derives from stomodeum remnants and accounts for approximately 5–10% of patients who have sellar/suprasellar masses. Symptomatic lesions cause galactorrhea, hypopituitarism, and/or visual disturbances. Radiologic findings are variable, according to the lining and cyst contents, and may on occasion be confused with craniopharyngioma or pituitary adenoma. Rathke cleft cyst is also a mucinous cyst lined by columnar-to-cuboidal ciliated and goblet cells, but *nonkeratinizing squamous metaplasia* may be extensive making differentiation with papillary craniopharyngioma challenging. In this respect, the presence of BRAF VE1

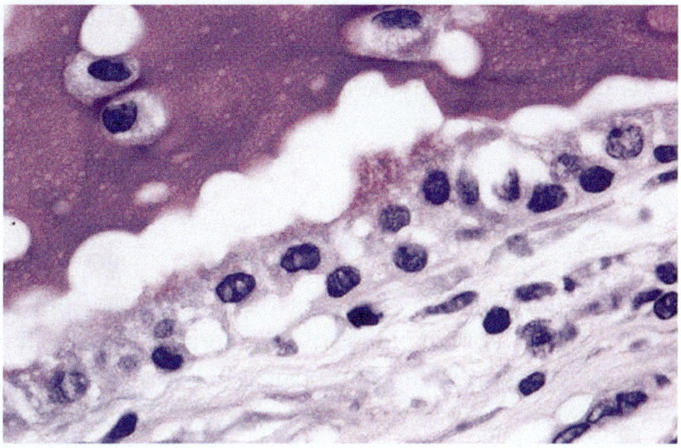

Fig. 19.2 *Colloid cyst of the third ventricle,* histology. Thin fibrous capsule lined by a layer of ciliated prismatic epithelium and filled with a mucinous (colloid) content (PAS-Alcian blue)

positivity by IHC is a suitable diagnostic marker for papillary craniopharyngioma. Like in colloid cyst of the third ventricle, in long-standing lesions a proliferative xanthogranulomatous reaction may fill the cyst with total effacement of the epithelial lining.

Endodermal (Enterogenous) Cyst

This is another mucinous cyst of endodermal origin, typically located anterior to the spinal cord in the subarachnoid space (most commonly in the cervical region). Occasionally, it may occur in the posterior fossa (anterior to the brainstem) and third ventricle. All ages, including infants, children, and adults, are affected. Like the colloid and Rathke cleft cysts, the enterogenous cyst is lined by a prismatic-to-cuboidal ciliated epithelium with goblet cells that may be predominant.

Ependymal Cyst

Ependymal cysts are thought to be of ependymal origin from developmentally displaced ventricular lining and are rarely seen in surgical practice. These may occur in diverse extraventricular locations including over the convexities, within the brain parenchyma, or near the midbrain and may also occur intramedullary in the spinal cord, most commonly in the thoracic segments. On imaging studies, ependymal cysts are well-circumscribed, fluid-filled masses, with the same signal characteristics of the cyst contents as CSF. Cases affecting cerebral hemispheres are typically large and often contain septations. As their name implies, they are lined by a simple columnar-to-cuboidal epithelium (resembling mature ependymocytes) resting on a glial stroma with little, if any, surrounding gliosis. The lining cells may occasionally be ciliated, but do not exhibit goblet cell differentiation.

Choroid Plexus Cyst

This is an extremely common, often multiple, and usually asymptomatic lesion involving the choroid plexus of the lateral ventricles. It is encountered as an incidental finding in up to half of autopsies. Fetal cysts may be associated with trisomies of chromosomes 18 or 21 and *Aicardi syndrome* (an X-linked dominant sporadic syndrome occurring almost exclusively in females). It is lined by a scalloped profile of choroid plexus cells that may be cuboidal or flattened by chronic pressure.

Cytologic Features and Differential Diagnosis

With the exception of the ependymal and choroid plexus types, smears from simple columnar-to-cuboidal epithelium-lined cysts will contain a dense colloid-like or amorphous proteinaceous background and a few prismatic ciliated or mucus-secreting cells. Nuclei are uniformly round and basally located (Fig. 19.3). The presence of metaplastic squamous cells is not infrequent in long-standing Rathke cleft cysts (Fig. 19.4). The radiographic characteristics and the typical location prevent mistakes in differential *diagnosis*, but extensive squamous metaplasia and/or xanthogranulomatous inflammation may complicate the diagnosis because of their confusion with craniopharyngioma or squamous-lined cysts. In samples with

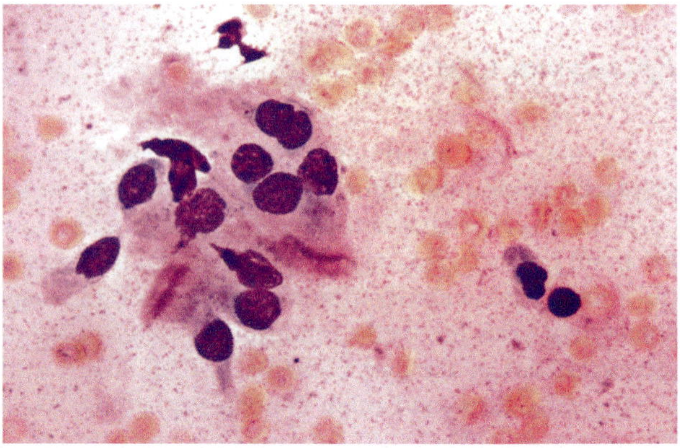

Fig. 19.3 *Colloid cyst of the third ventricle.* Smear from the cystic content showing a small group of columnar ciliated cells in a mucinous metachromatic background (Romanowsky)

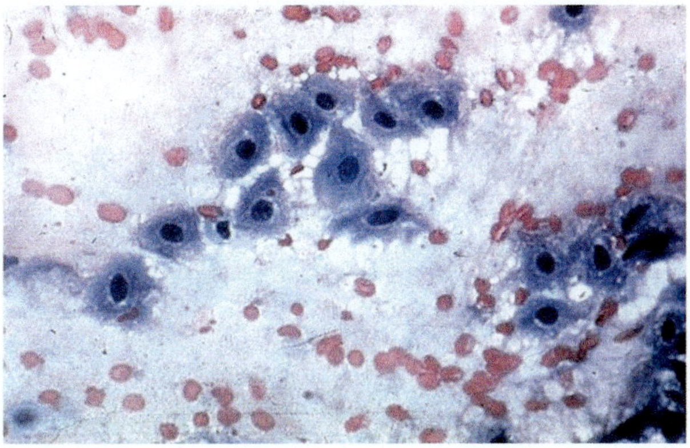

Fig. 19.4 *Rathke cleft cyst*. Presence of metaplastic squamous cells is a frequent finding in the fluid content of long-standing lesions. Note characteristic intercellular bridges (spines) of the squamous epithelium (Smear, Papanicolaou)

insufficient lining, a descriptive diagnosis of "benign epithelial cyst" may be rendered.

Nonepithelial-Lining Cysts

Arachnoid Cyst

They are focal collections of cerebrospinal fluid within both cranial and spinal meninges, accounting for approximately 1% of all intracranial masses. Germline abnormalities at 16q and 11p15 have been described in familial cases of arachnoid cysts. They may arise throughout the neuraxis, but favored locations include middle fossa (near the temporal lobe), cerebellopontine angle and cisterna magna in the posterior fossa, and in association with the thoracic spine. An osmotic and/or valve mechanism allowing entry of CSF into the cyst enables these watery collections to reach a large size and expand at expense of the brain or spinal cord. MRI shows a bright expansion of the subarachnoid space with characteristic CSF signal. Lesions of this type are lined by a collapsible, translucent to thick fibrovascular membranes covered, diffusely or focally, by mature meningothelial cells. Endoscopic or open fenestration and cystoperitoneal shunting are the main treatments in symptomatic cases (asymptomatic cysts do not require treatment). Occasionally, *intraoperative smears* can be prepared from the cyst wall that show delicate sheets of flattened arachnoid cells (Fig. 19.5).

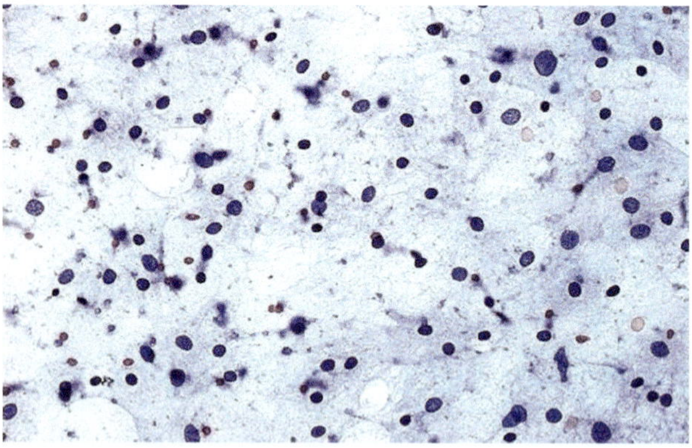

Fig. 19.5 *Arachnoid cyst*. Preparation from the cyst wall displaying a delicate loosely cohesive sheet of flattened arachnoid cells (Smear, toluidine blue)

Glial Cyst

The simple glial cyst most often arises in the cerebellar hemispheric white matter of middle-aged or elderly adults and usually represents "burnt-out" pilocytic astrocytoma. No communication with the ventricle and no enhancement after contrast injection are noted. The wall is lined by chronic astrocytic gliosis with Rosenthal fibers (pilocytic gliosis) and variable hemosiderin.

Pineal Cyst

The pineal cyst is a glial cyst within the pineal gland, and most often it is an incidental radiologic finding, with cysts larger than 5 mm in 2–4% of healthy individuals. T2/FLAIR MRI shows a hyperintense, unilocular, round intrapineal cavity. A minority of cases – usually young adults – are large enough (> 1 cm) to compress aqueduct and cause symptoms due to CSF obstruction. In such cases, a stereotactic approach is used for diagnosis and treatment. The material sent to the Pathology Department may be only proteinaceous fluid content, but in some cases the cyst wall is biopsied. *Intraoperative smears* from these specimens show chronic reactive gliosis with Rosenthal fibers (pilocytic gliosis) and occasionally a population of isomorphic, normal-looking pinealocytes (Fig. 19.6a, b). These findings confirm the non-tumoral nature of the process, and they must not be confused with the findings in pilocytic astrocytoma or pineocytoma.

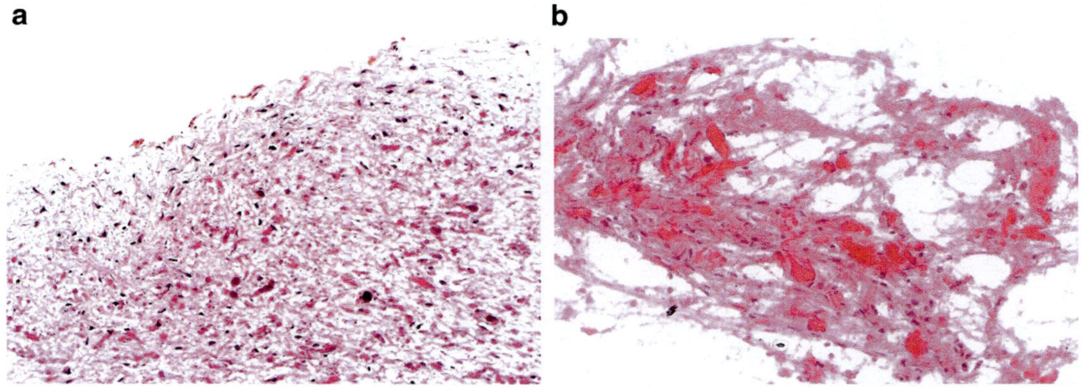

Fig. 19.6 *Pineal cyst*. (**a**) Tissue section displaying the wall of a pineal cyst with "piloid" gliosis lining. Note abundant Rosenthal fibers. (**b**) This preparation displays a dense fibrillary tissue fragment with numerous Rosenthal fibers, which may lead to a mistaken diagnosis of pilocytic astrocytoma (Smear, H&E)

Suggested Reading

Akhaddar A, Mahi M, Amarti A, el Quessar A, et al. Simple cyst of the cerebellum. Report of a case. J Neuropathol. 2001;28:209–14.

Arriola G, de Castro P, Verdú A. Familial arachnoid cysts. Pediatr Neurol. 2005;33:146–8.

Barlas O, Karadereler S. Stereotactically guided microsurgical removal of colloid cyst. Acta Neurochir. 2004;146:1199–204.

Berhouma M, Ni H, Delabar V, Tahhan N, et al. Update on the management of pineal cysts: case series and a review of the literature. Neurochirurgie. 2015;61:201–7.

Bilguvar K, Ozturk AK, Bayrakli F, Guzel A, et al. The syndrome of pachygyria, mental retardation, and arachnoid cysts maps to 11p15. Am J Med Genet. 2009;149:2369–572.

Boogaarts J, Decq P, Grotenhuis JA, Beems T. Long-term results of the neuroendoscopic management of colloid cysts of the third ventricle: a series of 90 cases. Neurosurgery. 2011;68:179–87.

Burger PC, Scheithauer BW. Benign cystic lesions. In: Tumors of the central nervous system. AFIP atlas of tumor pathology. Series 4. Washington DC: ARP Press; 2007. p. 471–90.

Caldas JG, Gilbert D, Comoy J, Lacroix C, Doyon D. Simple intraparenchymal cysts of the cerebellum. Apropos of 2 cases. J Neuroradiol. 1995;22:48–53.

Fuller GN, Ballester LY, Perry A. Cysts of the central nervous system. In: Perry A, Brat DJ, editors. Practical surgical neuropathology. A diagnostic approach. Philadelphia: Elsevier; 2018. p. 393–404.

Kim JH, Paulus W, Heim S. BRAF V600E mutation is a useful marker for differentiating Rathke's cleft cyst with squamous metaplasia from papillary craniopharyngioma. J Neuro-Oncol. 2015;123:189–91.

Mena H, Armonda RA, Ribas JL, Ondra SL, Rushing EJ. Nonneoplastic pineal cysts: a clinicopathologic study of twenty-one cases. Ann Diagn Pathol. 1997;1:11–8.

Mohanty A, Venkatrama SK, Rao BR, Chandramouli BA, Jayakumar PN, Das BS. Experience with cerebellopontine angle epidermoids. Neurosurgery. 1997;40:24–9.

Naylor MF, Scheithauer BW, Forbes GS, Tomlinson FH, Young WF. Rathke cleft cyst: CT, MR, and pathology of 23 cases. J Comput Assist Tomogr. 1995;19:853–9.

Oprişan A, Popescu BO. Intracranial cysts: an imagery diagnostic challenge. Scientific World J. 2013;2:172154.

Osborn AG, Preece MT. Intracranial cysts: radiologic-pathologic correlation and imaging approach. Radiology. 2006;293:650–64.

Parwani AV, Fatani IY, Burger PC, Erozan YS, Ali SZ. Colloid cyst of the third ventricle: cytomorphologic features on stereotactic fine-needle aspiration. Diagn Cytopathol. 2002;27:27–31.

Parwani AV, Taylor DC, Burger PC, Erozan YS, Olivi A, Ali SZ. Keratinized squamous cells in fine needle aspiration of the brain. Cytopathologic correlates and differential diagnosis. Acta Cytol. 2003;47:325–31.

Schelper RL, Ramzy I, Durr N. Ependymal cyst of the subarachnoid space. Cytologic diagnosis and developmental considerations. Acta Cytol. 1985;29:44–7.

Schweizer L, Capper D, Hölsken A, Fahlbusch R, et al. BRAF V600E analysis for the differentiation of papillary craniopharyngiomas and Rathke's cleft cysts. Neuropathol Appl Neurobiol. 2015;41:733–42.

Shim KW, Lee YH, Park EK, Park YS, Choi JU, Kim DS. Treatment option for arachnoid cysts. Childs Nerv Syst. 2009;25:1459–66.

Silverman JF, Timmons R, Harris LS. Fine needle aspiration cytology of primary epidermoid cyst of the brain. Acta Cytol. 1985;29:989–93.

Smith AR, Elsheikh TM, Silverman JF. Intraoperative cytologic diagnosis of suprasellar and sellar cystic lesions. Diagn Cytopathol. 1999;20:137–47.

Socin HV, Born J, Wallemacq C, Betea D, Legros JJ, Beckers A. Familial colloid cyst of the third ventricle: Neuroendocrinological follow-up and review of the literature. Clin Neurol Neurosurg. 2002;104:367–70.

Taillibert S, Le Rhun E, Chamberlain MC. Intracranial cystic lesions: a review. Curr Neurol Neurosci Rep. 2014;14:481.

Wang Y, Wang F, Yu M, Wang W. Clinical and radiological outcomes of surgical treatment for symptomatic arachnoid cysts in adults. J Clin Neurosci. 2015;22:1456–61.

Zada G, Lin N, Ojerholm E, Ramkissoon S, Laws ER. Craniopharyngioma and other cystic epithelial lesions of the sellar region: a review of clinical, imaging, and histopathological relationships. Neurosurg Focus. 2010;28:E4.

Chapter 20
Infectious, Inflammatory, and Reactive Lesions

There is a large number of infectious, inflammatory, and reactive processes affecting the CNS, but here we will only cover those that lend themselves to intraoperative consultation. According to the predominant cellular component, these processes may be grouped together – along with benign cystic lesions – into the five categories that we listed in the algorithm for nonneoplastic disorders (Box 20.1). Benign cystic lesions were covered in the previous chapter, which is why we will cover the four remaining ones together with an independent section on inflammatory/infectious lesions in AIDS patients because of their special features.

Box 20.1 Nonneoplastic disorders of the CNS: algorithmic approach

Benign cystic lesions

Predominance of acute inflammatory cells (brain abscess, subdural empyema, epidural abscess)

Predominance of perivascular chronic inflammatory cells (encephalitis, vasculitis)

Predominance of epithelioid macrophages (granulomatous inflammation)

Predominance of macrophages (resolving infarction, demyelinating disorder)

General Diagnostic Approach

One of the most difficult issues in surgical neuropathology is differentiating inflammatory and reactive processes from neoplasms. Indeed, brain lesions with predominance of inflammatory cells and/or macrophages may suggest neoplasm, both clinically and pathologically. To complicate more this scenario, inflammatory and reactive lesions are often more challenging than neoplastic lesions at frozen sections evaluation, being the source of considerable confusion and anxiety. In this compromising situation, the cytologic method can be the best ally, because the characteristic features of inflammatory cells and macrophages, often obscured in frozen

C. R. Lacruz et al., *Central Nervous System Intraoperative Cytopathology*,
Essentials in Cytopathology 13, https://doi.org/10.1007/978-3-319-98491-9_20

sections, are nicely preserved and evident in smears. Thus, the unequivocal identification of large numbers of inflammatory cells and/or macrophages in cytological preparations virtually rules out the possibility of neoplasia and leads to the diagnosis of an inflammatory lesion, a nonneoplastic necrotizing process, or a demyelinating disorder.

Acute Inflammatory-Cell-Rich Lesions

The presence of polymorphonuclear leukocytes raises two possibilities: acute tissue destruction or acute bacterial infection, but a sea of polys strongly suggests a bacterial infection. Focal suppurative bacterial infections in the CNS include brain abscess, subdural empyema, and epidural abscess.

Brain Abscess

Bacterial brain abscesses represent the second most common infection of the nervous system after meningitis. They can form anywhere within the brain and spare no age group. Hematogenous dissemination of bacteria (usually from pulmonary source) and direct extension from sinusitis, otitis, mastoiditis, or recent dental work are the most common causes. Infection starts as a focus of *cerebritis*, corresponding to an ill-defined area of parenchyma with collections of neutrophils associated with necrosis, edema, and extravasated erythrocytes. Without effective treatment, liquefactive necrosis follows and turns into a purulent content (basically pus and necrotic brain), surrounded by a granulation tissue-like zone of fibroblastic and angioblastic activity that ultimately evolves into a firm, fibrous capsule (i.e., *pyogenic abscess*); this, in turn, is bordered by edematous, chronically inflamed, and gliotic brain tissue (Fig. 20.1a). At this stage, after approximately 2 weeks, the lesion has the distinctive ring enhancement by imaging studies and may be approached surgically to be drained or biopsied if the radiologic image was mistaken with that of a ring-enhancing malignancy (i.e., glioblastoma, metastasis). Smears from the purulent content show abundant hypersegmented neutrophils, broken-down nuclei, and acellular debris (Fig. 20.1b); this smear pattern can be reported as "abscess content, favor bacterial." If the biopsy specimen is taken from the organizing edge of the lesion, one may encounter plump fibroblasts, proliferating vessels, and prominent gliosis; beware of mistaking it for a neoplasm (an untreated brain abscess may cause cerebral herniation or rupture into the ventricles causing severe fatal meningitis). In this respect, just smelling the specimen may be a diagnostic clue (biopsies from brain abscesses often stink due to anaerobic bacteria metabolites). Triaging tissue

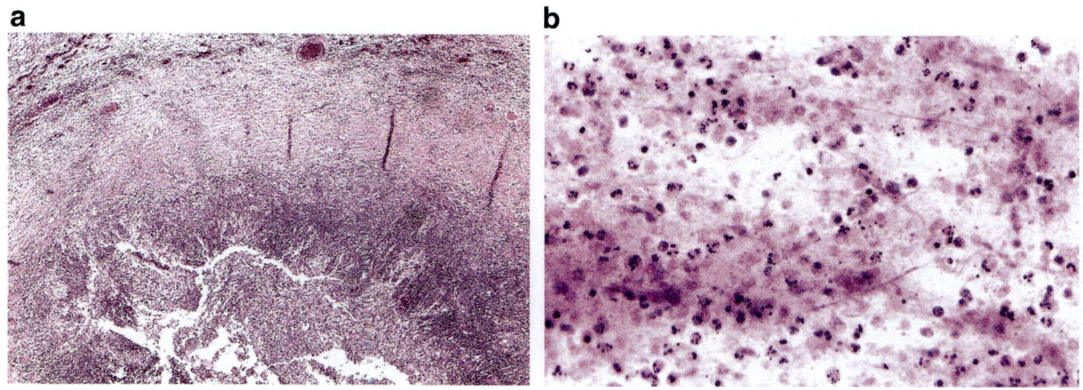

Fig. 20.1 *Pyogenic abscess.* (**a**) Characteristic histology, displaying a well-developed collagen capsule with prominent vessels and chronic inflammatory cells surrounding the purulent content. (**b**) Smeared purulent content includes many hypersegmented neutrophils (pyocytes) and associated cellular breakdown products (*Smear*, H&E)

from the sterile operating field to document organisms is essential. The most commonly identified are *Staphylococcus aureus*, *Streptococcus cocci*, anaerobic and microaerophilic organisms (*Bacteroides*, *S.milleri*), and aerobic gram-negative bacilli (*Proteus*, *Escherichia coli*, *Klebsiella-Enterobacter*, and *Haemophilus* species), but polymicrobial infections are common. Opportunistic organisms (*Mycobacterium*, *Nocardia*, and fungi) are more prevalent in immunocompromised patients.

Subdural Empyema

Subdural empyema is a suppurative infection located between the arachnoid and overlying dura and typically arises from extension of local ear or sinus frontal infection (it has been estimated that it may complicate up to 1–2% of cases of frontal sinusitis). Patients with subdural empyema usually appear acutely ill with fever, headache, and obtundation and may rapidly develop focal neurologic signs. MRI shows location of the infection, degree of associated edema or mass effect, and, if present, associated primary infection (e.g., sinusitis, mastoiditis). Identification of specific organisms requires CT-guided needle aspiration, and smears show similar features to those observed in the purulent content of brain abscesses.

Epidural Abscess

Since 90% of cases are situated at spinal levels, we discuss epidural abscess – suppurative infections between the dura and the overlying bone – in the chapter of the spine and epidural space.

Perivascular Chronic Inflammatory Cell-Rich Lesions

Aside from indicating chronicity, a predominantly perivascular lymphocytic infiltrate is less specific. A wide variety of stimuli can recruit these immune cells and cause vascular-based, chronic inflammation, although the most common is infectious encephalitis (Table 20.1).

Table 20.1 CNS perivascular chronic inflammatory cell-rich lesions

Encephalitis
Infectious encephalitis
Rasmussen's encephalitis (single cerebral hemisphere)
Paraneoplastic encephalitis (limbic)
Lymphocytic primary angiitis of the CNS (PACNS)
Lymphocytic systemic vasculitis involving the CNS
Secondary to active demyelination
Secondary to neoplasms (neuroepithelial tumors, metastases)
Immune reconstitution inflammatory syndrome (IRIS)

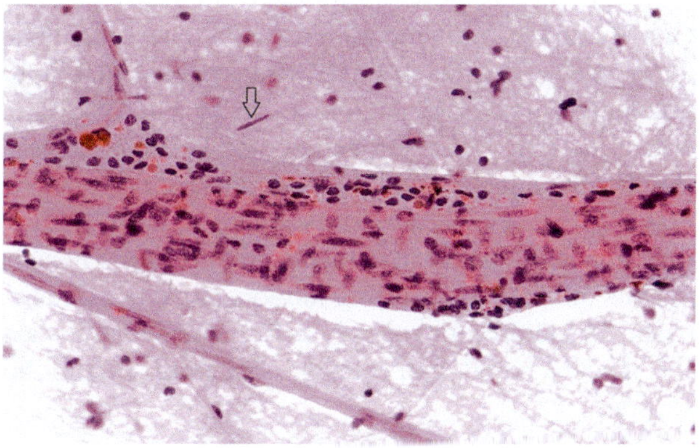

Fig. 20.2 *Encephalitis.* Perivascular cuffing by lymphocytes is often more conspicuous in smears than in tissue sections. Also note perivascular hemosiderin deposits from focal microhemorrhage and activate microglia (*arrow*). The final diagnosis on this case was herpes simplex virus encephalitis (Smear, H&E)

Infectious Encephalitis

Most cases of infectious encephalitis are caused by virus, either epidemic (arbovirus, enterovirus) or sporadic (herpes simplex virus, varicella-zoster virus, Epstein-Barr virus). Non-viral forms include Rocky Mountain spotted fever (*Rickettsia*) and encephalitis due to *Mycoplasma* and *Leptospira*. Diagnosis largely depends on recognizing clinical features (fever, headache, seizures, focal neurological signs, and altered mental status) in conjunction with laboratory studies (molecular diagnostic methods for most viruses can be performed on CSF). However, in equivocal cases, i.e., atypical or mild forms of the disease, a stereotactic brain biopsy should be considered, and if the biopsy has been taken from an appropriate site (i.e., the temporal lobe in a case of herpes simplex virus encephalitis), perivascular lymphocytic cuffing is readily apparent in smears (Fig. 20.2).

Noninfectious Perivascular Chronic Inflammation

As already mentioned, perivascular cuffing by lymphocytes is not diagnostic of encephalitis, since it is also seen in vasculitis, active demyelination, immune reconstitution inflammatory syndrome (IRIS), and occasionally adjacent to metastases or neuroepithelial tumors (most often low grade, including pilocytic astrocytoma, ganglioglioma, and pleomorphic xanthoastrocytoma). Thus, a correct diagnosis requires correlation of the pathologic findings with the clinical presentation and imaging features. Likewise, careful examination looking for evidence of cytologic atypia of the lymphoid cells present in such infiltrates is important. The presence of an atypical lymphoid population raises the possibility of a lymphoproliferative process.

Epithelioid-Cell-Rich Lesions (Granulomatous Inflammation)

Granulomatous inflammation is a chronic inflammatory response comprised of aggregates of epithelioid cells (transformed macrophages) with or without other inflammatory cells. Granulomas can be classified into necrotizing (with caseating central necrosis) and non-necrotizing (without central necrosis). Even though we should take into account all processes that can cause granulomatous inflammation (Table 20.2), in most instances granulomatous disease is a result of sarcoidosis or infection, particularly mycobacterial infection. Thus, the identification of a granulomatous inflammation during intraoperative consultation should prompt triaging of tissue for cultures and/or polymerase chain reaction assay (PCR). Additional stains for mycobacterial and fungal organisms should be performed on permanent sections.

Table 20.2 CNS granulomatous inflammatory lesions

Sarcoidosis
Infections (mycobacterial, fungal)
Parasites (i.e., neuroschistosomiasis)
Granulomatous angiitis
Primary granulomatous angiitis of the nervous sytem (GANS)
Granulomatous arteritis caused by varicella-zoster virus
Granulomatous arteritis associated with amyloid angiopathy
Secondary to germinoma
Secondary to foreign body
Suture material
Textiloma (muslinoma, gauzoma, gossypiboma)

Neurosarcoidosis

CNS involvement occurs in approximately 5–15% of sarcoidosis patients and typically manifest as a cranial neuropathy, more often involving the optic nerves; but pituitary gland, brainstem, spinal cord, or cerebellar disease may also occur. Intraoperative smears show noncaseating epithelioid granulomas – the foot prints of sarcoidosis – often accompanied by chronic inflammatory infiltrate and occasional multinucleated giant cells, but necrosis is absent (Fig. 20.3a, b) (pattern reported as "non-necrotizing granulomatous inflammation"). Microorganisms should be ruled out subsequently by special techniques, even if their absence does not mean with absolute certainty that this is a case of sarcoidosis. Clinical and laboratory information must be coupled with negative testing for infectious agents, including mycobacterial, parasitic, and fungal organisms

Mycobacterial Infections

CNS tuberculous mycobacterial infection is common in immunocompromised patients – particularly in HIV-seropositive individuals – and in developing countries. In addition to *chronic meningitis*, with its classic location in the basal cisterns, tuberculosis may cause one or more mass lesions in the brain and spinal cord (tuberculomas) or epidural, subdural, or cerebral abscesses. *Tuberculoma* is by far the most common variant of neuroparenchymal tuberculosis and may comprise 10–30% of brain masses in endemic areas (e.g., India, Pakistan), being cerebellum and pons commonly affected. Histologically, they are discrete, expansile, and bosselated lesions with central caseous necrosis and an outer rim of granulomatous inflammation (Fig. 20.4a, b). Depending on biopsied zone, cytologic preparations may be purely necrotic or display loosely formed granulomas with admixed granular necrotic debris and inflammatory cells, including multinucleated giant cells (Fig. 20.5a, b) (pattern reported as "necrotizing granulomatous inflammation"). Smears from *tuberculous abscesses* are similar to those of pyogenic abscess and typically lack epithelioid granulomas and giant cells. Thus, in such cases, the definitive diagnosis must be performed with the aid of ancillary techniques such as PCR assay, immunoperoxidase stains, or acid-fast bacilli stains (Fig. 20.6).

Immunosuppression also predisposes to disease with less virulent, atypical mycobacteria (*M. avium-intracellulare*, *M. kansasii*, *M. bovis*, and others). Atypical Mycobacteria infection does not elicit a vigorous granulomatous reaction, but sheets of foamy macrophages are packed with acid-fast microorganisms (*mycobacterial pseudotumor*), and intraoperative smears may demonstrate only a nonspecific pattern of dispersed foamy macrophages. In such cases, a grayish tinge is helpful when

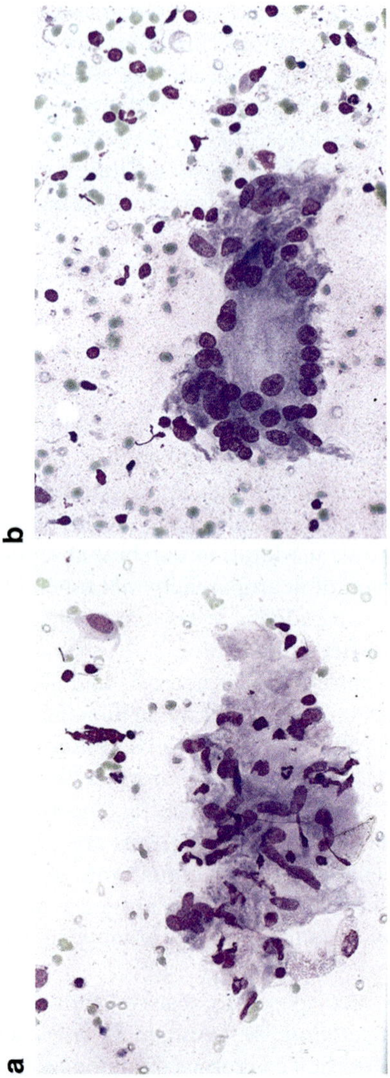

Fig. 20.3 *Sarcoidosis*. Granulomas with tightly packed epithelioid macrophages (**a**), multinucleated giant cells, chronic inflammatory infiltrate, and absence of necrosis (**b**) are characteristic features in sarcoidosis. Note distinctive epithelioid macrophages with kidney bean or boomerang-shaped nuclei and abundant ill-defined cytoplasm (**a, b**; Smears, Romanowsky)

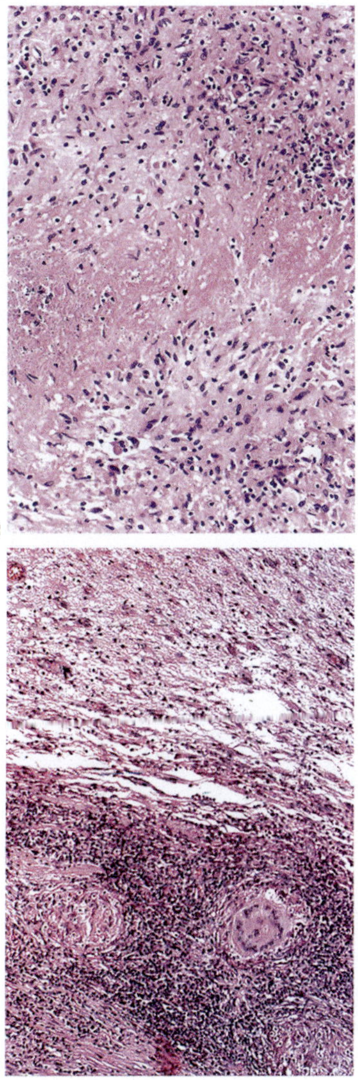

Fig. 20.4 *Tuberculoma, histology.* (**a**) Well-demarcated cerebral tuberculoma with an outer rim of chronically inflamed fibrous tissue, scattered islands of lymphoid cells, tubercles, and giant cells. (**b**) High-power view showing characteristic caseous necrosis surrounded by epithelioid and inflammatory cells

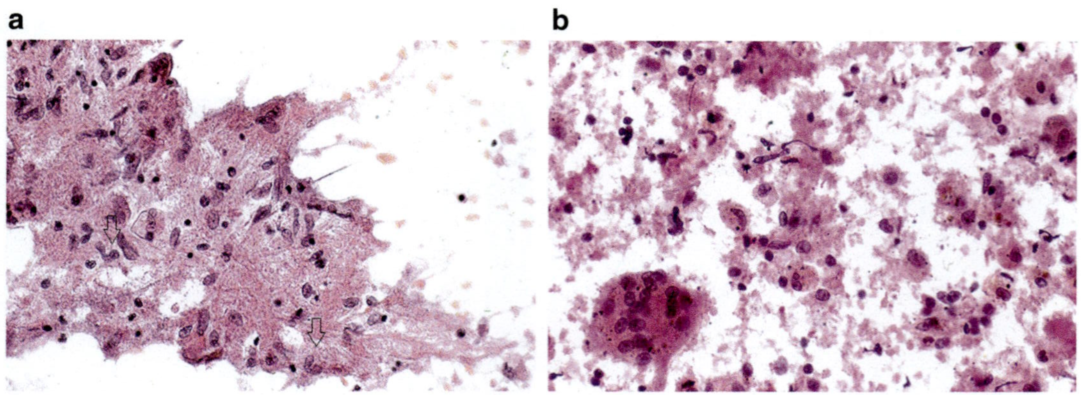

Fig. 20.5 *Tuberculoma, cytologic features.* (**a**) Loose cluster of epithelioid cells (granuloma) displaying characteristic kidney bean or boomerang-shaped (*arrows*) nuclei. (**b**) This preparation shows a multinucleated giant cell, epithelioid macrophages, and inflammatory cells in a granular necrotic background (**a, b**; Smears, H&E)

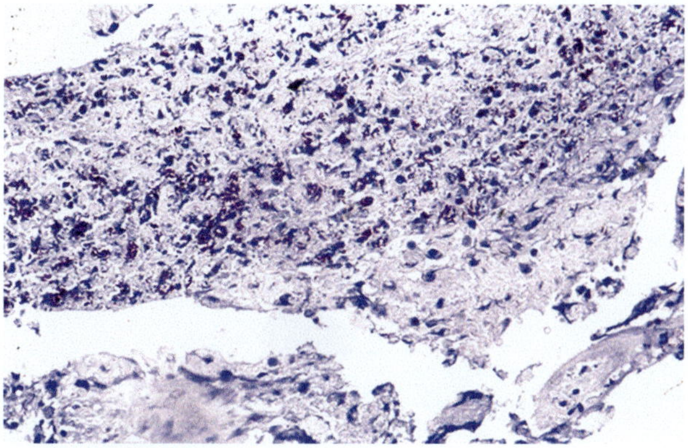

Fig. 20.6 *Tuberculous abscess*. This tissue section from the wall of a tuberculous abscess has abundant acid-fast mycobacterial organisms (Zhiel-Neelsen)

suspecting that the cytoplasm of macrophages is stuffed with myriads of organisms rather than generic phagocytized debris (Fig. 20.7a, b).

Macrophage-Rich Lesions

Although macrophages may be seen on treated malignant tumors, particularly in lymphoma, their presence is a strong indicator of a nonneoplastic disorder and leads to reconsider the diagnosis of tumor. There are numerous CNS lesions, of very different nature, that share a conspicuous component of lipid-laden or foamy macrophages, and some are authentic rarities. Table 20.3 lists only those lesions amenable to occasional neurosurgical intervention to harvest material for a definitive diagnosis.

Atypical mycobacterial infection, histiocytosis, and xanthogranulomatous reaction in cysts have already been covered. We discuss progressive multifocal leukoencephalopathy in the special section of infectious-inflammatory lesions found in AIDS.

Tumorlike Demyelinating Lesion "A Potential Litigation Diagnosis"

The multicentric foci of demyelination of classic multiple sclerosis (MS) usually does not present a diagnostic problem. However, isolated lesions, which can be correlated with the initial phase of MS or some other demyelinating variant, may present as space-occupying lesions associated with considerably mass effect, edema, and evidence of disruption of the blood-brain barrier on neuroimaging, which is why they may be mistaken for aggressive neoplasms (i.e., high-grade gliomas). These so-called tumorlike demyelinating lesions (TLDLs) may involve any region

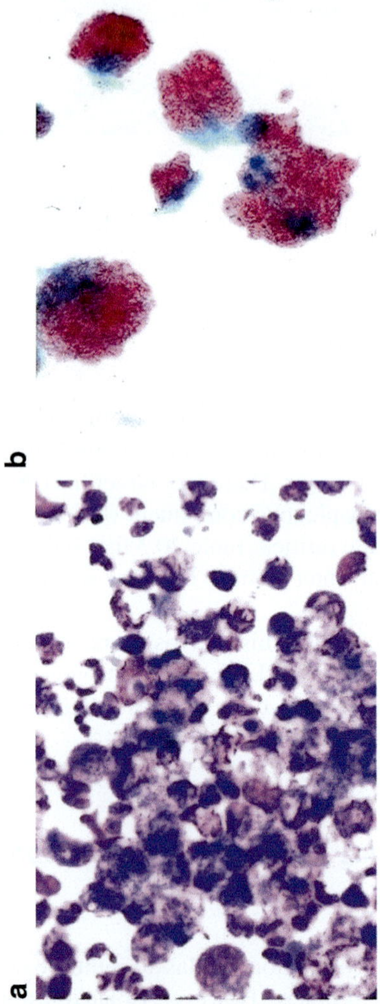

Fig. 20.7 *Atypical mycobacterial infection*. (**a**) Intraoperative smear demonstrating foamy macrophages with a grayish tinge of the cytoplasm (Romanowsky). (**b**) They are packed with myriads of acid-fast microorganisms (Zhiel-Neelsen)

Table 20.3 CNS macrophage-rich lesions

Tumorlike demyelinating lesion (tumefactive demyelination)
Resolving infarction
Progressive multifocal leukoencephalopaty
Histiocytosis
Xanthogranulomatous reaction in cysts
Atypical mycobacterial infection
Whipple's disease (macrophages stuffed with PAS + bacilli)

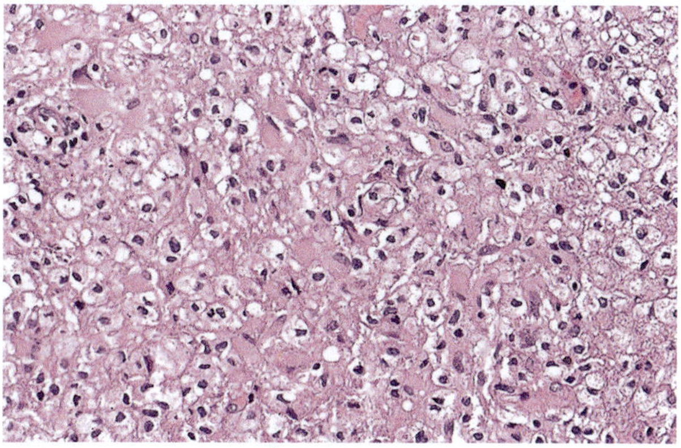

Fig. 20.8 *Tumorlike demyelinating lesion, histology*. The admixture of reactive astrocytes and the cellularity of the process may result in the mistaken diagnosis of glioma, typically a high-grade astrocytoma, oligodendroglioma, or mixed oligoastrocytoma

of the central nervous system, the spinal cord included, but most are located in the subcortical or periventricular white matter. Due to their tumorlike presentation, TLDLs often lead to biopsy, which gives rise to a serious diagnostic challenge, because the abundant macrophages and reactive astrocytes – characteristics of this process – can appear shockingly similar to neoplastic oligodendrocytes and astrocytes in frozen sections and even in permanent sections (Fig. 20.8). In fact, it has been suggested that the misdiagnosis of this process as a malignant glioma represents the most common type of malpractice case in surgical neuropathology, which results in patients being subjected to subsequent often devastating cerebral irradiation. In such compromising situation, the use of squash/smear cytology can be the best ally in intraoperative consultation. Cytologic preparations show well-defined foamy macrophages and distinctive reactive astrocytes in a finely granular-vacuolated (no fibrillary) background. Macrophages appear isolated with sharp borders, foamy or granular cytoplasm, and bland eccentrically placed nuclei (Fig. 20.9a), whereas reactive astrocytes typically display fine, radiating, fibrillary processes, and little, if any, nuclear atypia (Fig. 20.9b). Some astrocytes may have fragment nuclear material that either resembles scattered chromosomes (*granular mitosis*) or multiple micronuclei (*Creutzfeldt cells*), which, while nonspecific, are quite characteristic of TLDLs (Fig. 20.9c). A chronic inflammatory cell component of small

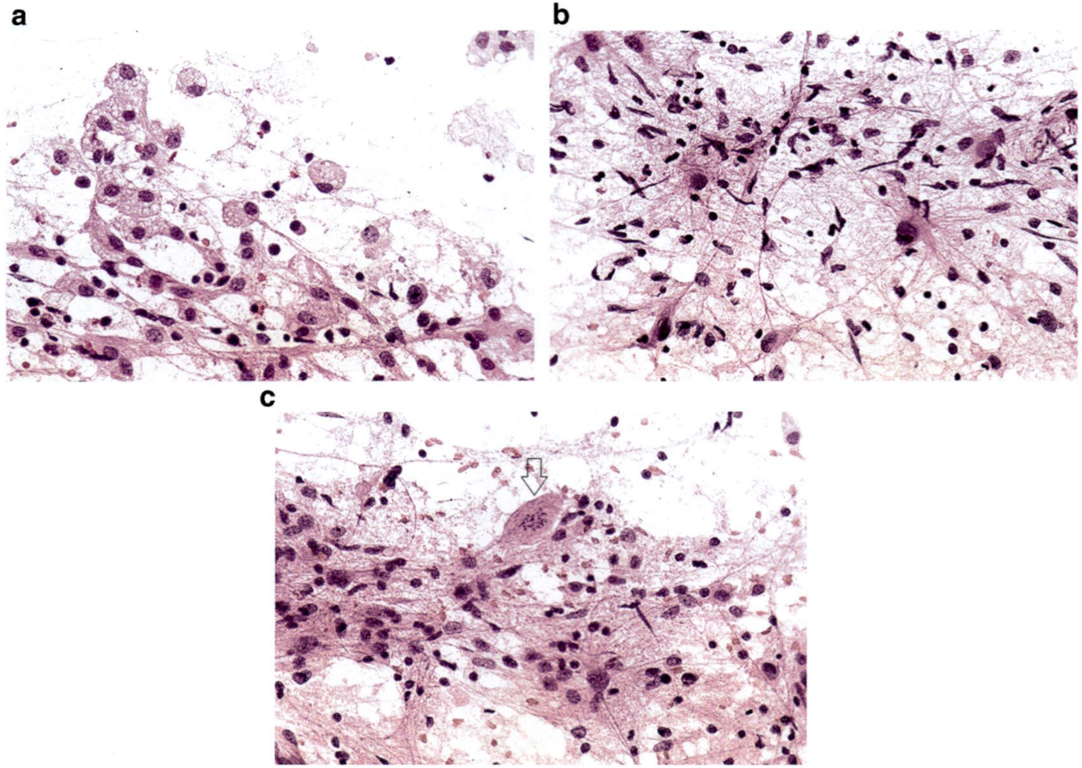

Fig. 20.9 *Tumorlike demyelinating lesion*, *cytologic features*. Preparations exhibit numerous well-defined foamy macrophages (**a**), admixed with mature lymphocytes and stellate reactive astrocytes (**b**), some displaying granular mitosis (*arrow*; **c**). This type of mitosis can be seen in a variety of pathologic conditions but are particularly characteristic of demyelinating diseases (**a–c**; Smears, H&E)

lymphocytes is often present, but a fibrillary background with neoplastic astrocytes (diffuse astrocytoma) or round oligodendrocytes with scant and wispy cytoplasm (oligodendroglioma) are lacking. Because some patients never developed subsequent lesions and some were temporally associated with recent vaccination or possible infections, it was speculated that this form of tumefactive demyelination may in some instances be a postinfectious phenomenon.

Cerebral Infarction

Biopsies of infarcts are very uncommon, arising only when the clinical picture does not point to a stroke (young patient age, atypical vascular distribution, no sudden onset). The range of cytomorphologic changes is variable depending on the severity of tissue injury and evolving time, but cases that do eventually undergo biopsy often display well-developed and noticeable findings during an intraoperative consultation. After an initial phase of edema, degenerative cell changes and acute inflammatory infiltrate occur; at about the 5th to 7th days, the changes progress to obvious tissue necrosis with infiltration by foamy or lipid-laden macrophages (subacute state). This macrophage infiltration is joined progressively by a proliferation of reactive astrocytes and neoformed vessels that can be misinterpreted as a glial neoplasm in frozen section evaluation (Fig. 20.10a). However, smears reveal a picture very different from that of a glioma, with abundant, well-defined macrophages in a granular-vacuolated (not fibrillary) background. Proliferating vessels and reactive astrocytes may be observed, but, unlike active demyelinating lesions, cerebral infarction usually lacks conspicuous lymphocytic infiltration (Fig. 20.10b, c). Report this pattern as "necrotizing lesion" or "necrotic and gliotic tissue."

Infectious-Inflammatory Lesions in AIDS

A subset of AIDS patients (about 10%) develop neurologic symptoms related to the presence of solitary or multifocal cerebral round mass/es on neuroimaging. In such cases, the most common causes are toxoplasmosis and lymphoma, even though other etiologies cannot be ruled out clinically or by conventional neuroimaging. In centers without positron emission tomography or single photon emission computed tomography, stereotactic biopsies offer the best hope of rapid diagnosis, although lesions are often treated empirically as toxoplasmosis with pyrimethamine-sulfadiazine, reserving biopsy for cases that fail to respond. Other AIDS-related infectious processes occasionally biopsied by stereotactic procedures and sent for intraoperative consultation are progressive multifocal leukoencephalopathy and cytomegalovirus encephalitis.

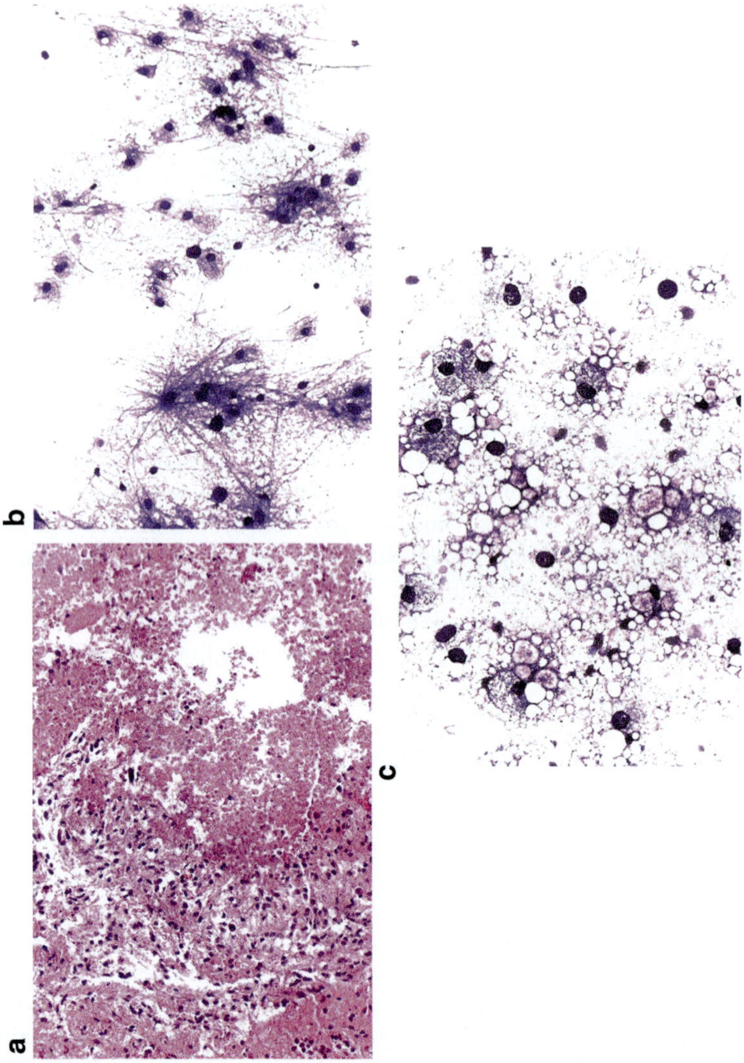

Fig. 20.10 *Evolving infarct.* (**a**) Histology. The admixture of reactive astrocytes and the cellularity of the process particularly in the edge of an organized infarct may result in a misdiagnosis of glioma (H&E stain). Smears consist of lipid-laden macrophages and some stellate reactive astrocytes (**b**), in a granular-vacuolated background with lipid droplets (**c**). Unlike active demyelinating lesions, infarcts usually lack lymphocytes (**b, c**; Romanowsky)

Toxoplasmosis

Up to the explosive spread of AIDS in the 1980s, cerebral toxoplasmosis used to be a rare process affecting newborns or related to immunosuppression. Since then, its incidence has increased to the point of becoming a common disease and the leading cause of space-occupying intracranial lesions in HIV-1-seropositive individuals (before the introduction of HAART therapy, almost half of seropositive patients developed the disease). The causative agent is the intracellular protozoan *Toxoplasma gondii*, which is present in cats, the definitive host. Humans are the intermediate host and become infected by ingesting oocyst-contaminated soil and water, undercooked red meats containing encysted organisms, or congenitally. The trophozoites are released in the human intestine and are carried within macrophages in the circulation in the form of tachyzoites (fast multiplying forms) to other organs (i.e., brain) where they subsequently develop into tissue cysts bradyzoites (slow multiplying forms) that remain for long periods of time. Reactivation of dormant infection associated with immunosuppression evokes symptomatic and progressive neurologic disease. Cerebral toxoplasmosis commonly presents as solitary or multifocal necrotic abscesses in any part of the brain. This consists of a central mass of necrotic cellular debris surrounded by edematous and inflamed brain tissue, typically exhibiting conspicuous vascular abnormalities (i.e., thrombosis and fibrinoid necrosis). It differs from bacterial abscesses because it lacks the normal sea of polys and is more coagulative than liquefactive; it is within the perimeter zone that *Toxoplasma* are most numerous, with the necrotic core often being devoid of identifiable organisms (Fig. 20.11a). The intraoperative diagnosis is based on the identification of specific – free and/or encysted – organisms in a nonspecific necrotic-inflammatory background, which usually includes lymphocytes, macrophages, some polys, and granular necrotic debris. The organisms are best seen in Romanowsky-stained preparations: *cysts* are thin-walled, bag-like structures filled with numerous bradyzoites (Fig. 20.11b), whereas *tachyzoites* may be recognized in the form of small aggregates, even though it is easy to confuse them with cellular debris. The organisms measure 4–8 mμ by 2–4 mμ and exhibit a crescentic "banana-shaped" profile – the Greek *toxon* means bow or arc – with eccentrically placed hyperchromatic nuclei (Fig. 20.11c). Encysted forms have less obvious crescent shape, and the organisms appear blunted or even round and may be confused with chromosomes of a granular mitosis. Differentiation is simple, because chromosomes, in contrast to bradyzoites, usually remain confined to the center of the cell and do not reach the external cell border. In spite of this, the intraoperative diagnosis of toxoplasmosis is often challenging and, although the dirty necrosis and mixed inflammation suggest *Toxoplasma* encephalitis, the parasites are easily overlooked (pattern can be reported as "chronic active encephalitis"). In such cases, deferred immunohistochemistry is mandatory in confirm (or exclude) toxoplasmosis.

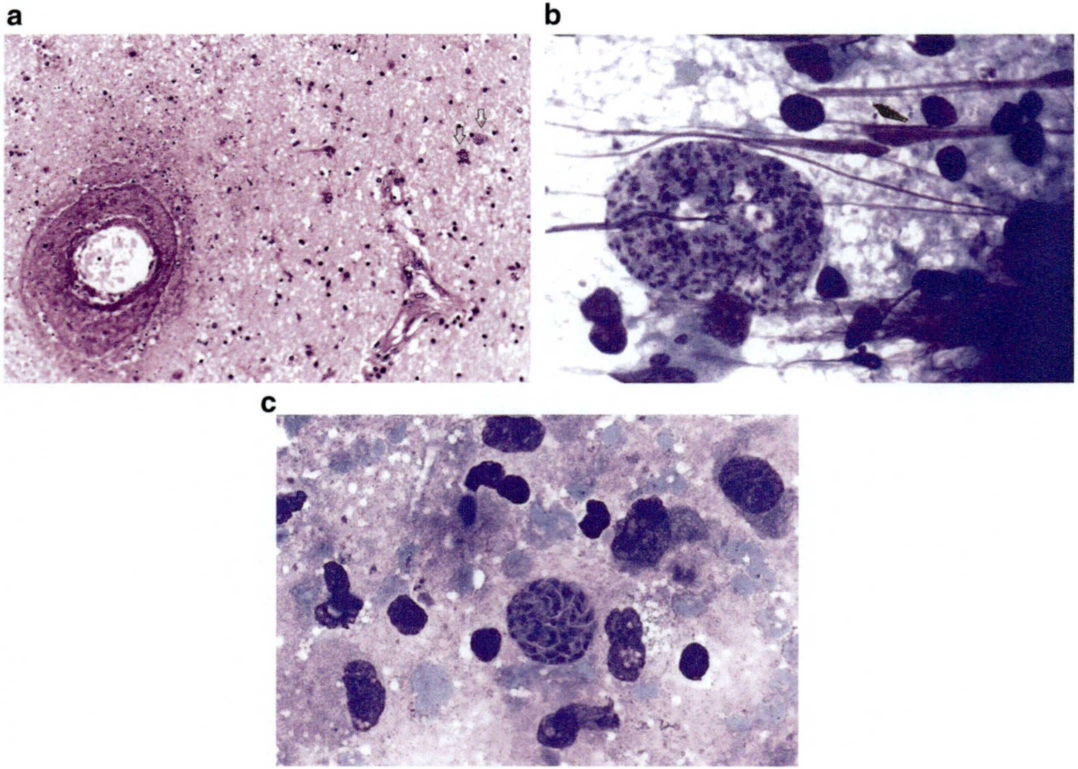

Fig. 20.11 *Toxoplasmosis.* (**a**) Histology. Typical toxoplasma abscess with a necrotic center and distinctive vascular fibrinoid necrosis. Note two bradyzoite-filled cysts (*arrows*) at the edge of the lesion. Diagnostic cytologic preparations consist of granular debris with a polymorphous inflammatory infiltrate, in which bradyzoites filled cysts (**b**) and tachyzoites with a crescentric profile (**c**) can be identified (**b, c**; Smears, Romanowsky)

Progressive Multifocal Leukoencephalopathy

Described by Aström et al. (1958) as a neurologic complication in patients with chronic lymphocytic leukemia and Hodgkin's disease, progressive multifocal leukoencephalopathy (PML) used to be a rare disease until the expansion of the AIDS pandemic. However, in HIV-seropositive patients, the incidence is high (about 5%) and may be the presenting manifestation of the disease. PML can also occur in patients treated with the monoclonal antibodies natalizumab, efalizumab, and rituximab. This is an opportunistic infectious demyelination caused by the ubiquitous *JC polyomavirus* (named JC after 1971 virus isolation from autopsied brain of patient John Cunningham), with only exceptional cases linked to the related *SV-40.* Although JC virus infects most of us at sometimes during our life – approximately 80% of the adult population is seropositive – it produces disease only in the significantly immunocompromised host. Once the dormant JC virus is reactivated, it gains access to the central nervous system, where it lytically infects oligodendroglial cells and non-lytically infects astrocytes, determining the progressive development of a myriad of small foci of demyelinization with infiltration by lipid-laden macrophages and atypical astrocytic hyperplasia (Fig. 20.12a). The spotty nature of the process leads to a multiplicity of symptoms such as focal neurologic deficits, speech or visual deficits, cognitive abnormalities, and signs of cerebellar and brainstem dysfunction. The imaging findings are quite characteristic: T_2-hyperintense, nonenhancing white-matter foci, most commonly in the cerebral hemispheres – with a predilection for the parietal-occipital regions – cerebellar peduncles, and corpus callosum (Fig. 20.12b). In such circumstances, PCR amplification of JC virus DNA sequences from CSF is the diagnostic method of choice (newer ultrasensitive techniques for CSF PCR have demonstrated greater than 95% sensitivity). However, in equivocal cases – PCR testing is not 100% sensitive – stereotactic brain biopsy provides a definitive diagnosis. Intraoperative smears show an appearance quite similar to that observed in TLDLs – lipid-laden macrophages and reactive astrocytes – but with two highly significant differences: the presence of inclusion-bearing oligodendrocytes and of greatly enlarged astrocytes with bizarre nuclear abnormalities (Fig. 20.13a). Productive infection of oligodendrocytes results in progressive enlargement of their nuclei with dissolution of their compacted chromatin and its replacement by homogeneous, dense, amphophilic material (Fig. 20.13b). On their part, infected astrocytes develop a neoplastic morphology including unusually large and hyperchromatic nuclei (Fig. 20.13c). Unlike most other viral infections,

a b

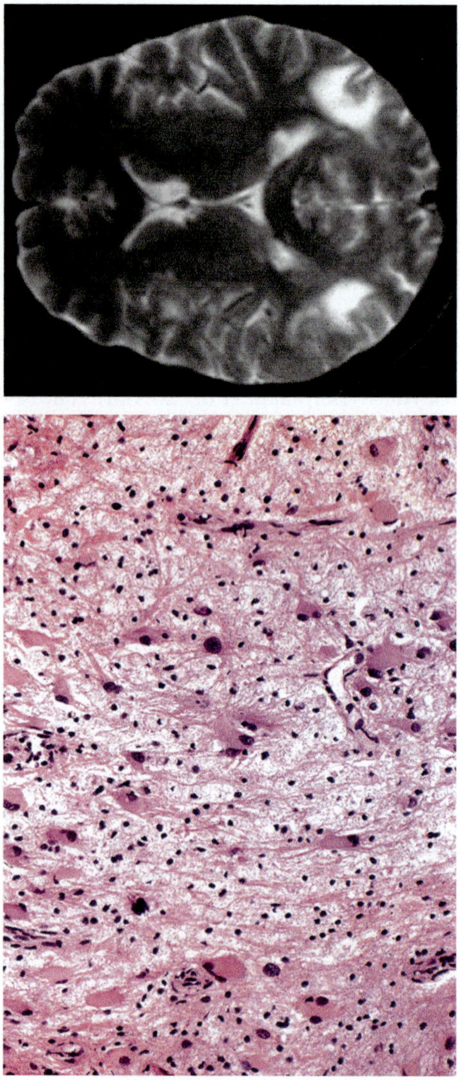

Fig. 20.12 *Progressive multifocal leukoencephalopathy (PML).* (**a**) The tissue pattern of PML is one of active demyelination. The marked astrocytic atypia can lead to a mistaken diagnosis of a high-grade astrocytoma unless the accompanying macrophages and viral inclusions are recognized. (**b**) This axial MRI shows T2-hyperintense, bilateral parieto-occipital lesions in an AIDS patient with PML

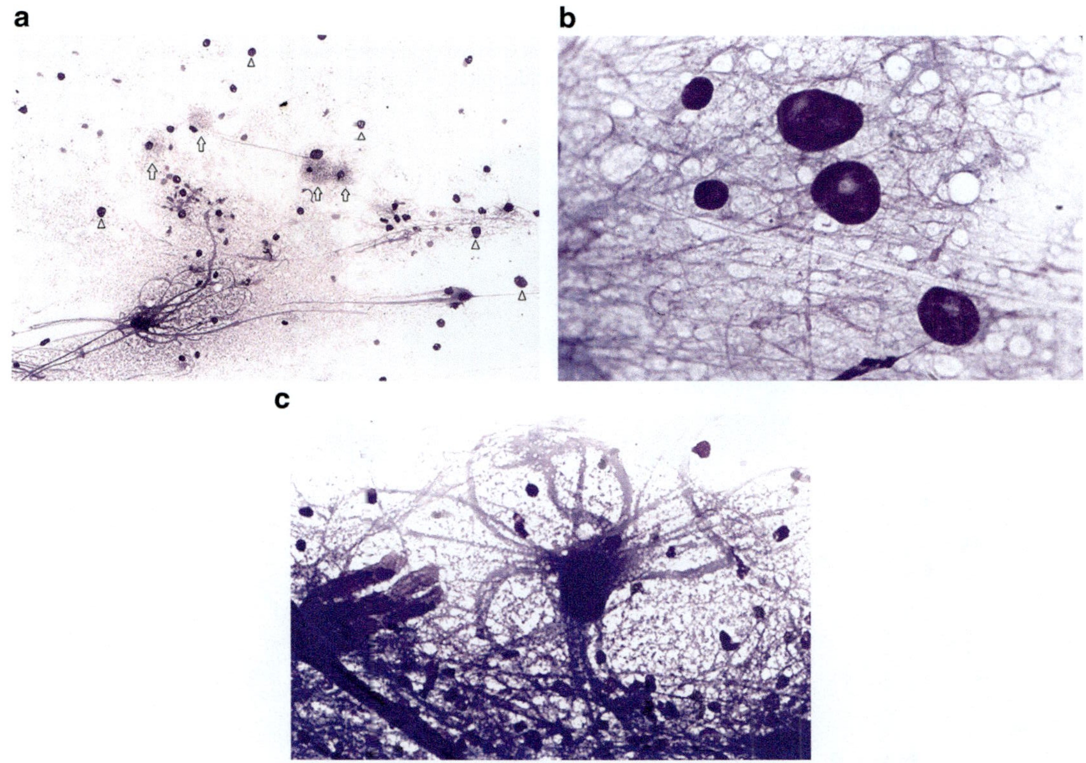

Fig. 20.13 *Progressive multifocal leukoencephalopathy, cytologic features.* (**a**) This preparation shows lipid-laden macrophages (*arrows*), large infected oligodendrocytes (*arrowheads*), and atypical reactive astrocytes. (**b**) Infected oligodendrocytes exhibit partial chromatin dissolution and replacement by homogeneous "ground glass" material. Compare the nuclear size of infected cells with that of normal-appearing oligodendrocytes. Also note a granular-vacuolated background of disintegrated neuropil. (**c**) Impressive enlargement and grotesque cytologic alterations may result from infection of astrocytes by the JC virus (**a–c**; Smears, Romanowsky)

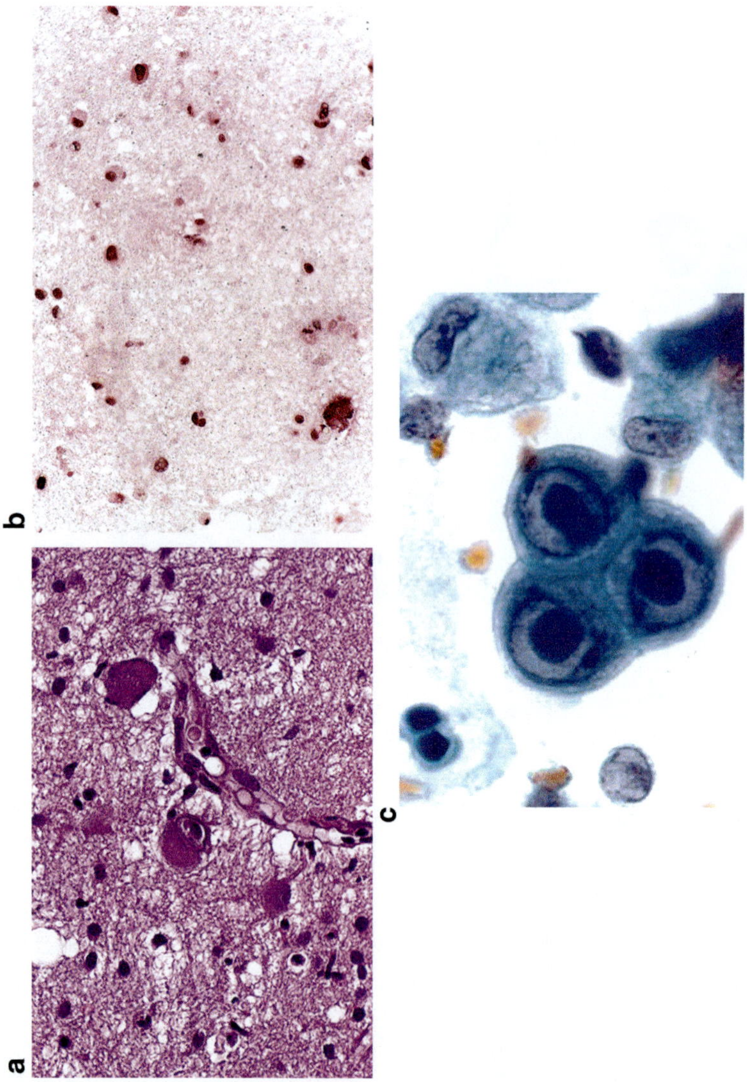

Fig. 20.14 *Cytomegalovirus (CMV) encephalitis*. (**a**) This tissue section displays enlarged infected astrocytes, with one of them exhibiting a distinctive "owl's eye" nucleus. (**b**) Immunostain for viral antigen showing many positive cells not seen with conventional stains. (**c**) The viral cytopathic effect is similar to CMV infection of other body sites. Note a group of three infected cells with distinct intranuclear inclusions and peripheral halos (Smear, Papanicolaou)

lymphocytes and lymphocytic cuffs are typically uncommon or absent. However, as treatment for AIDS reconstitutes the damaged immune system, the appearance of PML will evolve to show more lymphocytes and fewer diagnostic, infected cells – a change referred to as the immune reconstitution inflammatory syndrome (IRIS). Principal *differential diagnostic considerations* include noninfectious demyelination and glioma (as a result of misinterpretation of enlarged atypical viral nuclei).

Cytomegalovirus Encephalitis

Another opportunistic virus, cytomegalovirus (CMV), may cause chronic and subacute encephalitis of periventricular predominance that are difficult to distinguish, clinically and radiologically, from the pictures of dementia associated with HIV. CMV nervous system infections can also occur as complications of organ transplantation, especially the bone marrow and hematopoietic stem cell. The diagnosis usually requires PCR amplification of CMV genome from CSF, but in equivocal cases, stereotactic brain biopsy should be considered. The morphological diagnosis is based on the identification of the cytopathic changes that are characteristic of the virus: the cells, of large size, display a voluminous nuclear basophilic inclusion surrounded by a clear halo due to margination of host chromatin ("owl's eye" nucleus); at the same time, less well-defined small intracytoplasmic inclusions may be seen. This cytopathic action is ubiquitous and may involve the whole range of brain tissue cells: neurons, astrocytes, oligodendrocytes, ependymal cells, endothelial cells, and even macrophages. The identification of infected cells is made easier by specific immunostaining, revealing positive immunoreactivity even in cells in which the viral cytopathic effect is not fully developed (Fig. 20.14a–c).

Suggested Reading

Agnihotri SP, Singhal T, Stern BJ, Cho TA. Neurosarcoidosis. Semin Neurol. 2014;34:386–94.

Aström KE, Mancall EL, Richardson EP Jr. Progressive multifocal leuko-encephalopathy; a hitherto unrecognized complication of chronic lymphatic leukaemia and Hodgkin's disease. Brain. 1958;81:93–111.

Berger JR, Khalili K. The pathogenesis of progressive multifocal leukoencephalopathy. Discov Med. 2011;12:495–503.

Cação G, Branco A, Meireles M, Alves JE, et al. Neurosarcoidosis according to Zajicek and scolding criteria: 15 probable and definite cases, their treatment and outcomes. J Neurol Sci. 2017;779:84–8.

Chun CH, Johnston JP, Hofstetter M, Raff MJ. Brain abscess: a study of 45 consecutive cases. Medicine. 1986;65:415–31.

Elmore SA, Jones JL, Conrad PA, Patton S, Lindsay DS, Dubey JP. Toxoplasma gondii: epidemiology, feline clinical aspects, and prevention. Trends Parasitol. 2010;26:190–6.

Feiden W, Bise K, Steude U, Pfister HW, Möller AA. The stereotactic biopsy diagnosis of focal intracerebral lesions in AIDS patients. Acta Neurol Scand. 1993;87:228–33.

Fink MC, Penalva de Oliveira AC, Milagres FA, Vidal JE, et al. JC virus DNA in cerebrospinal fluid samples from Brazilian AIDS patients with focal brain lesions without mass effect. J Infect. 2006;52:30–6.

Hsu CC, Tokarz R, Briese T, Tsai HC, Quan PL, Lipkin WI. Use of staged molecular analysis to determine causes of unexplained central nervous system infections. Emerg Infect Dis. 2013;19:1470–7.

Jansen M, Corcoran D, Bermingham N, Keohane C. The role of biopsy in the diagnosis of infections of the central nervous system. Ir Med J. 2010;103:6–8.

Kepes JJ. Large focal tumor-like demyelinating lesions of the brain: intermediate entity between multiple sclerosis and acute disseminated encephalomyelitis? A study of 31 patients. Ann Neurol. 1993;33:18–27.

Kleinschmidt-DeMasters BK, Miravalle A, Schowinsky J, Corboy J, Vollmer T. Update on PML and PML-IRIS occurring in multiple sclerosis patients treated with natalizumab. J Neuropathol Exp Neurol. 2012;71:604–17.

Landry ML, Eid T, Bannykh S, Major E. False negative PCR despite high levels of JC virus DNA in spinal fluid: implications for diagnostic testing. J Clin Virol. 2008;43:247–9.

Levy RM, Russell E, Yungbluth M, Hidvegi DF, Brody BA, Dal Canto MC. The efficacy of image-guided stereotactic brain biopsy in neurologically symptomatic acquired immunodeficiency syndrome patients. Neurosurgery. 1992;30:186–90.

Louis DN, Frosch MP, Mena H, Rushing EI, Judkins AR. Non-neoplastic diseases of the central nervous system. AFIP atlas of nontumor pathology. First series. Washington DC: ARP press; 2009.

Mathisen GE, Johnson JP. Brain abscess. Clin Infec Dis. 1997;25:763–81.

Menkü A, Kurtsoy A, Tucer B, Yildiz O, Akdemir H. *Nocardia* brain abscess mimicking brain tumor in immunocompetent patients: report of two cases and review of the literature. Acta Neurochir. 2004;146:411–4.

Menon S, Bharadwaj R, Chowdhary AS, Kaundinya DV, Palande DA. Tuberculous brain abscesses: case series and review of literature. J Neurosci Rural Pract. 2011;2:153–7.

Meyding-Lamadé U, Strank C. Herpesvirus infections of the central nervous system in immunocompromised patients. Ther Adv Neurol Disord. 2012;5:279–96.

Miralles P, Berenguer J, Lacruz CR, Cosín J, et al. Inflammatory reactions in progressive multifocal leukoencephalopathy after highly active antiretroviral therapy. AIDS. 2001;15:1900–2.

Moazzam AA, Rajagopal SM, Sedghizadeh PP, Zada G, Habibian M. Intracranial bacterial infections of oral origin. J Clin Neurosci. 2015;22:800–6.

Morrison A, Gyure KA, Stone J, Wong K, McEvoy P, Koeller K, Mena H. Mycobacterial spindle cell pseudotumor of the brain: a case report and review of the literature. Am J Surg Pathol. 1999;23:1294–9.

Pawate S, Moses H, Sriram S. Presentations and outcomes of neurosarcoidosis: a study of 54 cases. QJM. 2009;102:449–60.

Peterson K, Rosenblum MK, Powers JM, Alvord E, Walker RW, Posner JB. Effect of brain irradiation on demyelinating lesions. Neurology. 1993;43:2015–2.

Plesec TP, Prayson RA. Frozen section discrepancy in the evaluation of nonneoplastic central nervous system samples. Ann Diagn Pathol. 2009;13:359–66.

Raisanen J, Goodman HS, Ghougassian DF, Harper CG. Role of cytology in the intraoperative diagnosis of central demyelinating disease. Acta Cytol. 1998;42:907–12.

Silver SA, Arthur RR, Erozan YS, Sherman ME, McArthur JC, Uematsu S. Diagnosis of progressive multifocal leukoencephalopathy by stereotactic brain biopsy utilizing immunohistochemistry and the polymerase chain reaction. Acta Cytol. 1995;39:35–44.

Strigle SM, Rarick MU, Cosgrove MM, Martin SE. A review of the fine-needle aspiration cytology findings in human immunodeficiency virus infection. Diagn Cytopathol. 1992;8:41–52.

Suri V, Kakkar A, Sharma MC, Padma MV, Garg A, Sarkar C. Primary angiitis of the central nervous system: a study of histopathological patterns and review of the literature. Folia Neuropathol. 2014;52:187–96.

Swinburne NC, Bansal AG, Aggarwal A, Doshi AH. Neuroimaging in central nervous system infections. Curr Neurol Neurosci Rep. 2017;17:49.

Thomas G, Murphy S, Staunton H, O'Neill S, Farrell MA, Brett FM. Pathogen-free granulomatous diseases of the central nervous system. Hum Pathol. 1998;29:110–5.

Withley RJ. Viral encephalitis. New Engl J Med. 1990;323:242–50.

Wu M, Huang F, Jiang X, Fan Z, et al. Herpesvirus-associated central nervous system diseases after allogeneic hematopoietic stem cell transplantation. PLoS One. 2013;8:e77805.

Yu GH, Hidvegi DF, Cajulis RS, Brody BA, Levy RM. Cytomorphology of progressive multifocal leukoencephalopathy (PML): review of sixteen cases occurring in HIV-positive patients. Diagn Cytopathol. 1996;14:4–9.

Zagzag D, Miller DC, Kleinman GM, Abati A, Donnenfeld H, Budzilovich GN. Demyelinating disease versus tumor in surgical neuropathology: clues to a correct pathological diagnosis. Am J Surg Pathol. 1993;17:537–45.

Part IV
Regions

Chapter 21
Pineal Region

The pineal region is comprised by the pineal gland, posterior third ventricle, tela choroidea, and velum interpositum. The regional approach to processes of the pineal area is justified by common symptomatology and the peculiar anatomic relationships in the region of the pineal gland – at the base of the brain – that usually preclude open surgery. Pineal region-related tumors comprise from 0.5% to 1% of all brain tumors in adults and from 5% to 10% of brain tumors in children. Despite its low frequency, these neoplasms often pose a diagnostic dilemma due to the wide diversity of pathologic types. The majority of pineal region neoplasms belong to the germ cell group, mainly *germinoma* (over a half of pineal tumors) and *teratoma*, followed by *pineal parenchymal tumors* and tumors arising from the adjacent anatomical structures, including *glial tumors* originating from the tectum (tectal plate gliomas) and *meningiomas* originating from the falcotentorial junction. *Papillary tumor of the pineal region* is a rare neuroepithelial tumor that occurs exclusively in this specific localization. *Metastases* to the pineal gland are very rare and most often result from lung and breast carcinomas. Other tumor types that may occasionally occur in this region are *atypical teratoid/rhabdoid tumor*, *pineal anlage tumor*, *rhabdomyosarcoma*, *embryonal tumor with abundant neuropil and true rosettes*, *rosette-forming glioneuronal tumor*, and *craniopharyngioma*. Also *pineal cysts* and other nonneoplastic lesions should be included in this group of "tumors" of the pineal region, because they may be confused with neoplasms (Table 21.1).

Of all of these processes, roughly 25% may be subjected to primary surgery, being benign, well-demarcated, and radioresistant; for the remaining 75%, a conservative approach is preferable, because they are malignant and chemo−/radiosensitive. Therefore, distinguishing the histologic types of these various lesions remains a main goal for the improvement of treatment planning. As the morbidity and mortality rates for open surgical procedures of pineal region are as high as 50%, the intraoperative consultation of pineal region lesions is often made using very small stereotactic or neuroendoscopic biopsy specimens. Under these circumstances, cytological preparations can be of distinct diagnostic utility.

C. R. Lacruz et al., *Central Nervous System Intraoperative Cytopathology*, Essentials in Cytopathology 13, https://doi.org/10.1007/978-3-319-98491-9_21

Table 21.1 Lesions in the pineal region

Expected	Uncommon	Rare
Germinoma	PTPR	Metastases
Teratoma	NGGCTs	Pineal anlage tumor
PPTs	Choroid plexus tumors	Rhabdomyosarcoma
Gliomas	AT/RT	ETANTR
Meningioma	Arachnoid cyst	RGNT
Pineal cyst	Vascular malformations	Craniopharyngioma

PPTs pineal parenchymal tumors, *PTPR* papillary tumor of the pineal region, *NGGCTs* nongerminomatous germ cell tumors (yolk sac tumor, embryonal carcinoma, choriocarcinoma, mixed germ cell tumors), *AT/RT* atypical teratoid/rhabdoid tumor, *ETANTR* embryonal tumor with abundant neuropil and true rosettes, *RGNT* rosette-forming glioneuronal tumor

Pineocytoma

Pineocytoma is a slowly growing neoplasm composed of well-differentiated pineocytes with a generally favorable prognosis (WHO grade I tumor). It accounts for about 20% of PPTs and most commonly affects adults, with a mean patient age at diagnosis of 43 years.

Pineocytoma usually remains localized in the pineal region and grows compressing neighboring structures giving rise to the symptomatology characteristic of tumors in this region: increased intracranial pressure, diplopia, and hypothalamus-based dysfunction. In neuroimaging, pineocytoma appears as a well-demarcated mass centered in the pineal gland that displaces the normal pineal calcifications peripherally and generally shows a strong homogeneous contrast enhancement.

Macroscopically, it is a circumscribed lesion with a grayish-tan, homogeneous or granular cut surface. Degenerative changes (calcification and cyst formation) can be present, but necrosis is absent.

Microscopically, pineocytoma is a moderately cellular neoplasm composed of uniform, mature-appearing pineocytes. It grows in sheets or ill-defined lobules and often features nucleus-free spaces filled with a network of fine neuritic processes (pineocytomatous rosettes). Characteristically, such rosettes are larger and more irregular than neuroblastic rosettes and are frequently found in confluent arrangements (Fig. 21.1). Ganglion cell differentiation and prominent nuclear – prognostically insignificant – pleomorphism may occasionally be encountered. Pineocytoma strongly expresses neuronal markers (i.e., synaptophysin, neurofilament protein), both within rosettes and individual cell cystoplasm.

Gross total resection is the most appropriate treatment and should be attempted whenever possible. The 1- and 5-year progression-free survival rates for patients that underwent resection are 97% and 90%, respectively. Radiotherapy administration to subtotally resected tumor is not associated with either increased tumor control or survival.

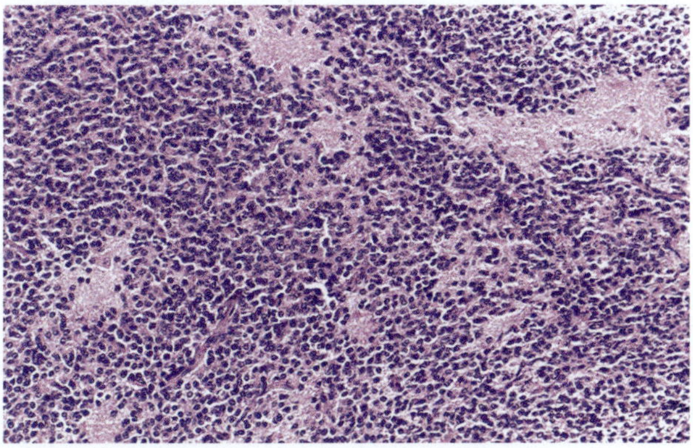

Fig. 21.1 *Pineocytoma.* Typical histology featuring a sheet of small tumor cells with large, irregular pineocytomatous rosettes. Unlike ependymoma, the pineocytomatous rosettes lack central vessels

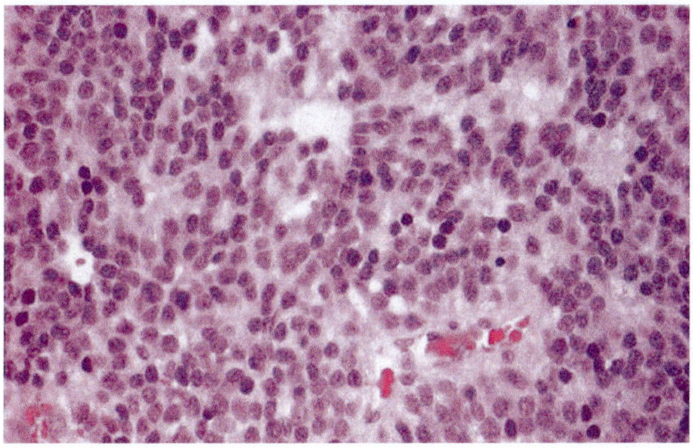

Fig. 21.2 *Pineal parenchymal tumor of intermediate differentiation.* Characteristic histologic features include sheet-like architecture and hypercellularity, but nuclei are relatively uniform with slight anisokaryosis and denser chromatin. Note small pseudorosettes, but larger pseudorosettes, as seen in pineocytomas, are not observed

The current WHO grading system recognizes a *PPT of intermediate differentiation (PPTID)* that may correspond to grade II or III. PPTID represents a tumor that is transitional between pineocytoma and pineoblastoma, featuring moderate to high cellularity and increased mitotic activity but mild to moderate nuclear atypia (Fig. 21.2).

- Grade II criteria: lessthan6 mitoses/10 HPF; positive immunoreactivity for neurofilament protein
- Grade III criteria: ≥6 mitoses/10HPF or lessthan6 mitoses but absence of immunoreactivity for neurofilament protein

The potential for local infiltration and CSF dissemination is significant, making these tumors more aggressive than pineocytoma. PPTIDs account for approximately 45% of all PPTs and may occur at any age (mean patient's age: 41 years).

Cytologic Features

Pineocytoma displays a discohesive pattern of uniform cells with round nuclei, stippled chromatin, and inconspicuous nucleoli. The cytoplasm is sparse with occasional delicate processes, which have a tendency to group together forming ill-defined, fibrillary nucleus-free areas (pineocytomatous rosettes). Occasionally, nuclear pleomorphism and gangliogliomatous differentiation may be present; but necrosis, mitosis, and apoptotic bodies are absent (Fig. 21.3a, b).

PPTID cases usually show higher cellularity and greater nuclear atypia than does pineocytoma. Small rosettes may also be present (Fig. 21.4a, b).

Differential Diagnosis Considerations

Given its location and the good degree of cellular differentiation, the main differential diagnosis of pineocytoma is native pineal parenchyma. Increased cellularity and pineocytomatous rosettes are the hallmark of the neoplastic nature of the process. Pathologists should also be aware not to mistake pineocytoma with large ganglion cells with germinoma or pineocytoma with nuclear pleomorphism with anaplastic astrocytoma (Table 21.2).

Pineoblastoma

Pineoblastoma is a poorly differentiated embryonal neoplasm arising in the pineal gland and represents the most primitive and malignant of the pineal parenchymal tumors (WHO grade IV). It accounts for approximately 35% of all PPTs and typically occur in the childhood and adolescence (mean patient age: 18 years), but they may occur at any age, and no gender preference is apparent. Pineoblastoma has been found in patients with hereditary bilateral retinoblastomas, an association known as "trilateral retinoblastoma," in the setting of *RB1* (retinoblastoma 1 gene) mutation. Recently, a subset of pineoblastomas has been noted with mutations of the *DICER1* gene, including germline examples.

The clinical presentation is similar to that of other pineal-region tumors but with a markedly rapid and aggressive progression (the interval between initial symptoms and surgery may be lessthan1 month). Neuroimaging shows a large and relatively poorly demarcated solid mass with heterogeneous contrast enhancement (Fig. 21.5a). Because of common CSF spread before surgery, including spinal cord seeding, the initial staging should include MRI of the spine and examination of the CSF.

Macroscopically, these are soft and friable masses with common infiltration of surrounding structures. Necrosis and hemorrhagic foci are frequent.

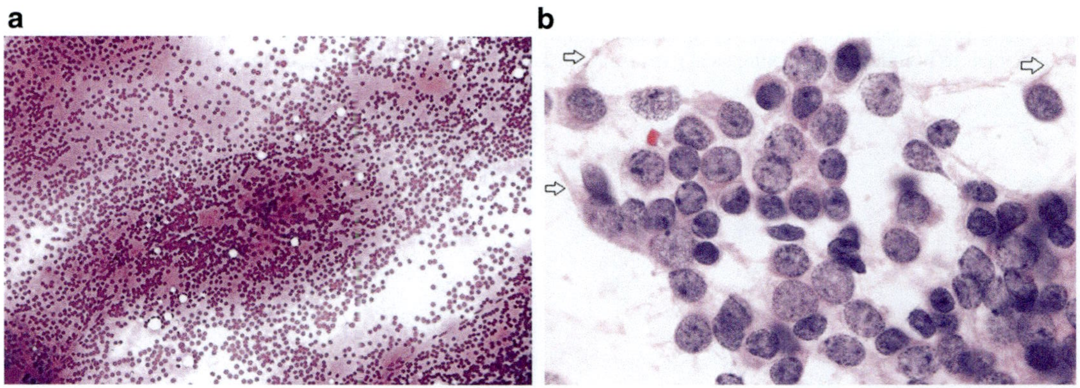

Fig. 21.3 *Pineocytoma, cytologic features*. (**a**) Discohesive pattern of uniform, round cells intermixed with irregular pineocytomatous rosettes. Characteristically, the nuclei surrounding rosettes are not regimented (Smear, Romanowsky). (**b**) Uniform tumor cells resembling pinealocytes. Note the ill-defined, cytoplasmic processes (*arrows*) and "salt-and-pepper" chromatin (Smear, H&E)

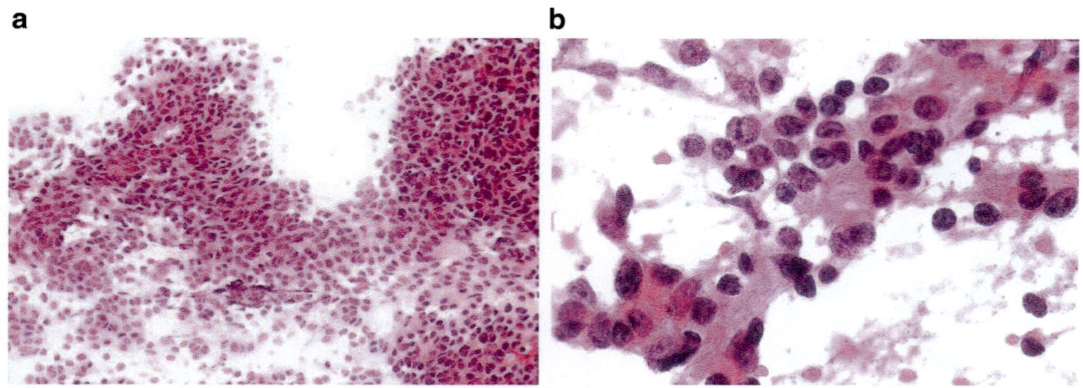

Fig. 21.4 *Pineal parenchymal tumor of intermediate differentiation, cytologic features*. (**a**) These tumors are composed of cells that are cytologically less anaplastic than those of pineoblastoma but more closely disposed than those of pineocytoma. (**b**) The tumor cells have nuclear features intermediate between pineoblastoma and pineocytoma (**a, b**; Smears, H&E)

Table 21.2 Characteristics of pineocytoma

Cytologic features
Well spread smear with a discohesive cell pattern
Uniform, round cells with stippled chromatin
Delicate cytoplasmic processes
Ill-defined rosettes
Differential diagnosis and pitfalls
Native pineal gland
Pineocytoma with ganglion cell differentiation versus germinoma
Pineocytoma with nuclear pleomorphism versus anaplastic astrocytoma

Microscopically, pineoblastoma is a densely packed, primitive-looking, small-cell neoplasm resembling other CNS embryonal tumors, mainly medulloblastoma. Homer-Wright and Flexner-Wintersteiner rosettes may occasionally be found (Fig. 21.5b). In pineoblastomas, immunolabeling of neuronal markers is variable. *Pineal anlage tumor* is often considered a peculiar variant of pineoblastoma, characterized by a combination of neuroectodermal (pineoblastoma-like) and heterologous ectomesenchymal (melanocytic, cartilaginous, and rhabdomyoblastic) components.

Despite multimodal therapy, the prognosis is poor with rapid recurrence and cerebrospinal dissemination. Currently, the median postsurgical survival time is about 4 years.

Cytologic Features

The smear pattern of pineoblastoma is similar to that of CNS embryonal tumors (mainly medulloblastoma), including highly cellular preparations with discohesive sheets of small, primitive-looking cells. Nuclear molding, mitotic figures, and frequent apoptotic bodies are common findings. Just as in medulloblastoma, the degree of atypia and anaplasia is variable from tumor to tumor, but nuclear polymorphism is usually prominent with round to variable angulated or indented nuclei. A thin rim of cytoplasm with monopolar processes is occasionally visible in some cells. Homer-Wright or Flexner-Wintersteiner rosettes may also be observed (Fig. 21.6a–c).

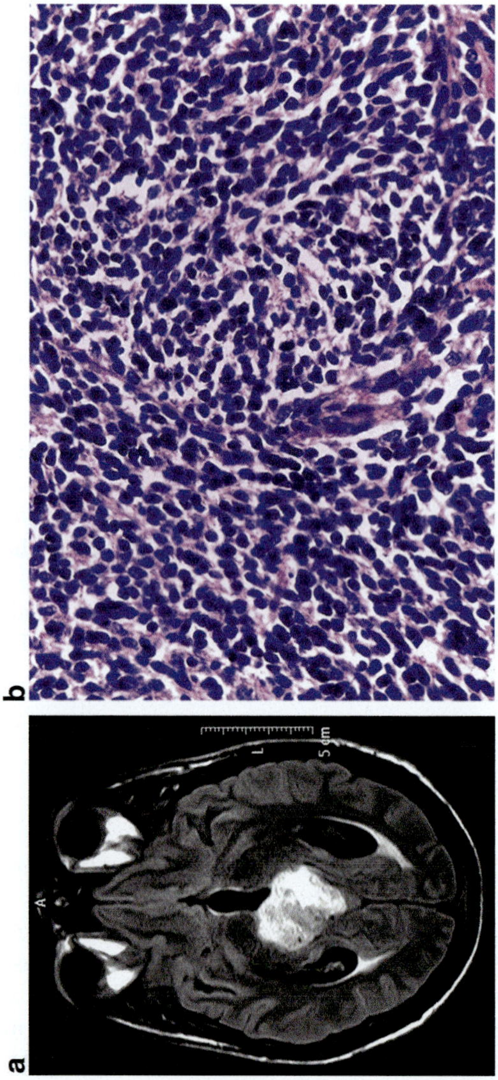

Fig. 21.5 *Pineoblastoma.* (**a**) An axial T1-weighted image with gadolinium reveals a large, enhancing mass in the pineal region affecting adjacent structures. (**b**) Marked proliferation of undifferentiated neoplastic cells with high nuclear-to-cytoplasmic ratios are characteristic histologic features

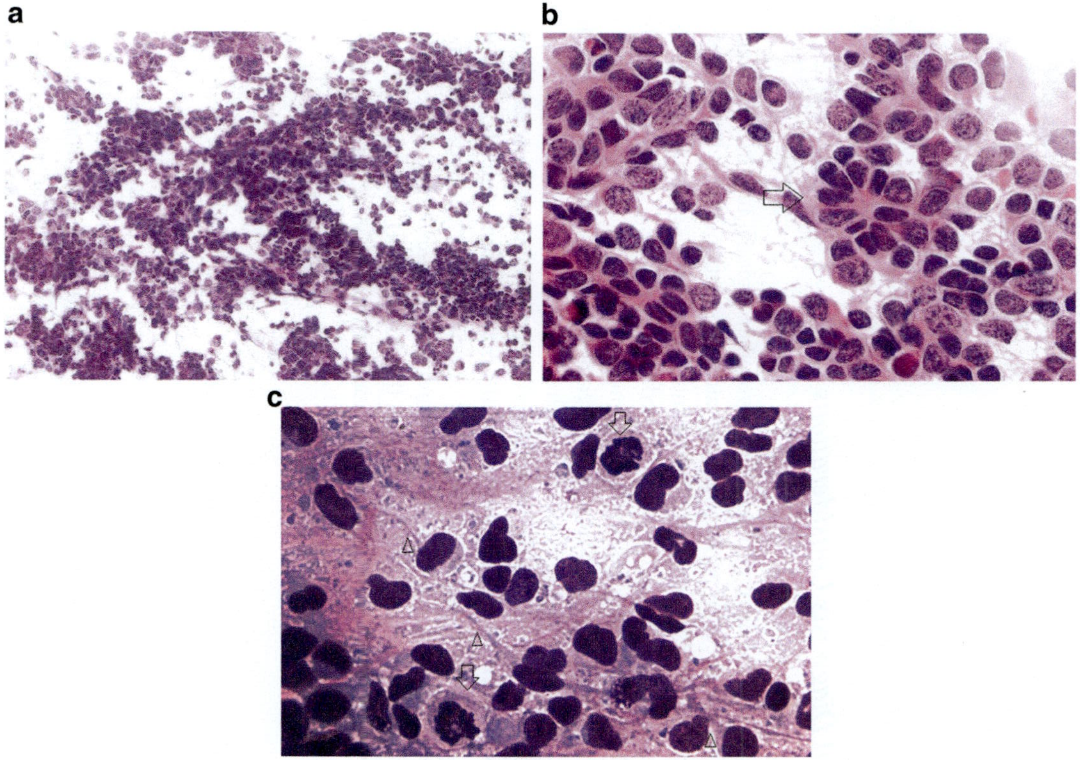

Fig. 21.6 *Pineoblastoma, cytologic features.* (**a**) Highly cellular preparation displaying loosely cohesive sheets and isolated small, undifferentiated cells (Smear, H&E). (**b**) A discohesive pattern of small, hyperchromatic cells shows nuclear molding and angulations that are characteristic of malignancy. Note the presence of a Flexner-Wintersteiner rosette (*arrow*) as a reminder of the photoreceptor origin of the pineal gland (Smear, H&E). (**c**) Higher magnification showing nuclear polymorphism and frequent mitotic figures (*arrows*). Note monopolar cytoplasmic processes (*arrowheads*) in some tumor cells (Smear, Romanowsky)

Table 21.3 Characteristics of pineoblastoma

Cytologic features
Highly cellular smears
Small, hyperchromatic cells
Nuclear moldings and angulations
Homer-Wright and Flexner-Wintersteiner rosettes
Differential diagnosis and pitfalls
Germinoma
Pineal parenchymal tumor of intermediate differentiation
Atypical teratoid/rhabdoid tumor

Differential Diagnosis Considerations

Pineoblastoma must be differentiated from two other regional tumors: germinoma and PPTID. With respect to germinoma, we already mentioned that this diagnosis may be problematic in frozen sections, but not in smears – germinoma shows a characteristic dual cell population and a striped "tigroid" background. On the other hand, PPTID shows neither the highly malignant nor the primitive appearance of pineoblastoma, but due to the fact that stereotactic- or neuroendoscopic-guided biopsies are small and may be associated with sampling problems, the differentiation between both tumors should be rendered in permanent sections of a larger sample. AT/RT – occasionally encountered in the pineal region – must be also taken into account, and in cases with predominance of small-cell (primitive) component, an intraoperative accurate diagnosis may be unreliable (suggest report these cases as "high-grade, malignant small-cell tumor"). In this respect, INI1 nuclear expression is retained in pineoblastoma enabling distinction from AT/RT in permanent sections (Table 21.3).

Papillary Tumor of the Pineal Region

Papillary tumor of the pineal region (PTPR) is a rare neuroepithelial tumor that occurs exclusively in the pineal region, mainly in young adults (mean age: 35 years), with a guarded prognosis. As its name implies, PTPR does not arise from the pineal gland itself, being the cell of origin thought to be specialized ependymocytes of the subcommissural organ. Symptoms are nonspecific and include headache and other signs related to increased intracranial pressure due to obstructive hydrocephalus; local recurrence and/or CSF dissemination is frequent. In neuroimaging, PTPRs appear as well-circumscribed, relatively large (2–4 cm diameter), pineal region enhancing masses with an occasional cystic element; the tumors may demonstrate intrinsic T1 hyperintensity. Microscopic evaluation often demonstrates a papillary tumor with evidence of epithelial and ependymal differentiation, including true rosettes and tubes, thought regions of solid growth are frequently apparent. Focal expression of pancytokeratins and more diffuse immunopositivity for cytokeratin 18 are useful markers, since they are not expressed in PPTs. The most consistent genetic finding in PTPRs is the whole loss of a copy of chromosome 10 (present in almost all cases); loss of chromosome 10, thus one allele of *PTEN*, may be in concert with deletion or mutation of the other allele of *PTEN*, causing an activation of the PI3K/AKT/mTOR signaling pathway that increases proliferation and cell growth. Gross total excision is the treatment of choice, with complementary radiation commonly employed.

Cytologic Features and Differential Diagnosis

PTPRs typically have a much more epithelioid appearance than PPTs. Smears are hypercellular displaying papillary tissue fragments and single cells, with papillary arrangements often exhibiting an inner vascular core. Tumor cells have plump oval or infolded nuclei and stippled chromatin. Smooth cell borders lend a distinctive epithelial quality, but some processes that are shorter and thicker than those of ependymoma may also be seen. The background looks clear or granular-vacuolated, but no fibrillary (Fig. 21.7a–c).

With a so well-defined epithelioid and papillary morphology, the main *differential diagnoses* arise with choroid plexus tumors and metastatic papillary carcinoma – considering possibility of PTPR if the patient is a young adult with a mass located in the posterior commissure or pineal region, particularly if a pre-contrast T1 hyperintensity is noticed.

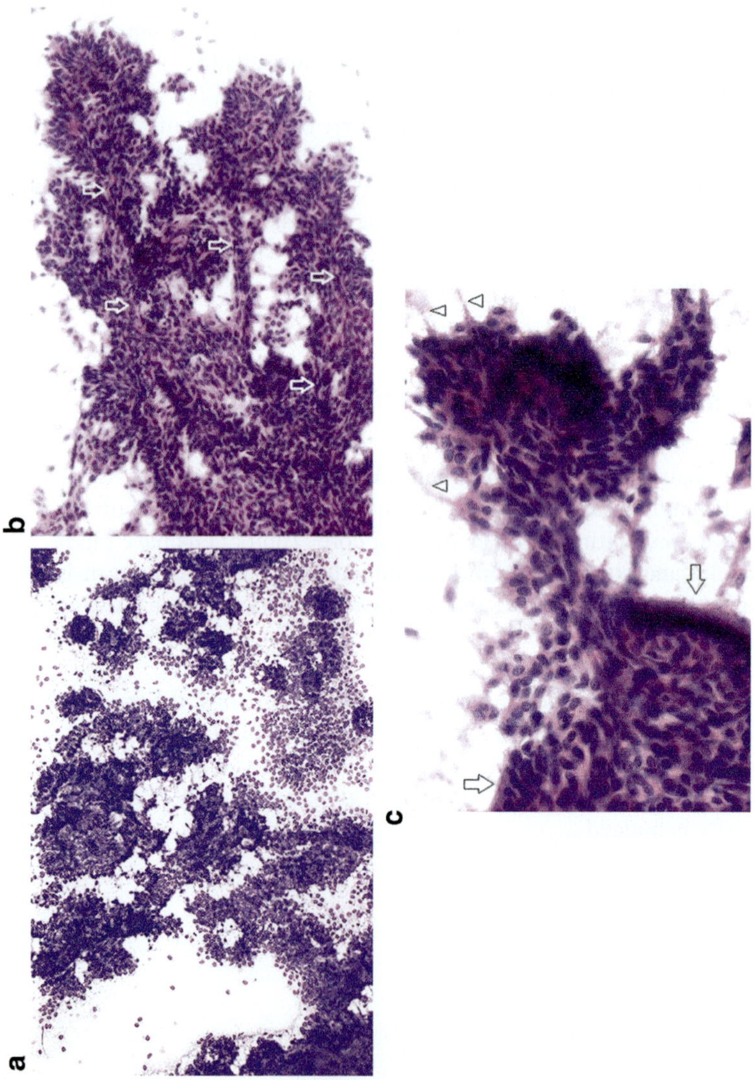

Fig. 21.7 *Papillary tumor of the pineal region (PTPR), cytologic features*. (**a**) When evaluating preparations of a pineal tumor in an adult, the presence of papillary structures and numerous single cells should raise the possibility of PTPR (Smear, Romanowsky). (**b**) Orientation to a vessel (*arrows*) creates a cytological equivalent to the histological perivascular formations. Note that the background is clear, not fibrillary. (**c**) The cytoplasmic appearance is variable, with smooth-epithelial (*arrows*) or frayed-glial (*arrowheads*) cell boundaries (**b, c**; Smears, H&E)

Suggested Reading

Chang AH, Fuller GN, Debnam JM, Karis JP, et al. MR imaging of papillary tumor of the pineal region. Am J Neurodiol. 2008;29:187–9.
Clark AJ, Ivan ME, Sughrue ME, Yang I, et al. Tumor control after surgery and radiotherapy for pineocytoma. J Neurosurg. 2010;113:319–24.
De Kock L, Sabbaghian N, Druker H, Weber E, et al. Germ-line and somatic *DICER1* mutations in pineoblastoma. Acta Neuropathol. 2014;128:583–95.
Fauchon F, Jouvet A, Paquis P, Saint-Pierre G, et al. Parenchymal pineal tumors: a clinicopathological study of 76 cases. Int J Radiat Oncol Biol Phys. 2000;46:959–68.
Fèvre-Montange M, Szathmari A, Champier J, Mokhtari K, et al. Pineocytoma and pineal parenchymal tumors of intermediate differentiation presenting cytologic pleomorphism: a multicenter study. Brain Pathol. 2008;18:354–9.
Goschzik T, Gessi M, Denkhaus D, Pietsch T. *PTEN* mutations and activation of the PI3K/Akt/mTOR signaling pathway in papillary tumors of the pineal region. J Neuropathol Exp Neurol. 2014;73:747–51.
Heim S, Sill M, Jones DT, Vasiljevic A, et al. Papillary tumor of the pineal region: a distinct molecular entity. Brain Pathol. 2016;26:199–205.
Jiménez-Heffernan JA, Bárcena C, Gordillo C, Cañizal JM. Cytologic features of papillary tumor of the pineal region: a case report showing tigroid background. Diagn Cytopathol. 2016;44:1098–101.
Jouvet A, Fauchon F, Liberski P, Saint-Pierre G, et al. Papillary tumor of the pineal region. Am J Surg Pathol. 2003;27:505–12.
Kreth FW, Schätz CR, Pagenstecher A, Faist M, Volk B, Ostertag CB. Stereotactic management of lesions of the pineal region. Neurosurgery. 1996;39:280–91.
Kumar P, Tatke M, Sharma A, Singh D. Histological analysis of lesions of the pineal region: a retrospective study of 12 years. Pathol Res Pract. 2006;202:85–92.
Lau SK, Cykowski MD, Desai S, Cao Y, Fuller GN, Bruner J, Okazaki I. Primary rhabdomyosarcoma of the pineal gland. Am J Clin Pathol. 2015;143:728–33.
Maiti TK, Arimappamagan A, Mahadevan A, Yasha TC, Pandey P, Santosh V. Rare pathologies in the posterior third ventricular region in children: case series and review. Pediatr Neurosurg. 2015;50:42–7.
Mena H, Armonda RA, Ribas JL, Ondra SL, Rushing EJ. Nonneoplastic pineal cysts: a clinicopathologic study of twenty-one cases. Ann Diagn Pathol. 1997;1:11–8.
Murali R, Scheithauer BW, Chaseling RW, Owler BK, Ng T. Papillary tumour of the pineal region: cytological features and implications for intraoperative diagnosis. Pathology. 2010;42:474–9.
Parwani AV, Baisden BL, Erozan YS, Burger PC, Ali SZ. Pineal gland lesions: a cytopathologic study of 20 specimens. Cancer. 2005;105:80–6.
Raleigh DR, Solomon DA, Lloyd SA, Lazar A, et al. Histopathologic review of pineal parenchymal tumors identifies novel morphologic subtypes and prognostic factors for outcome. Neuro-Oncology. 2017;19:78–88.
Regis J, Bouillot P, Rouby-Volot F, Figarella-Branger D, Dufour H, Peragut JC. Pineal region tumors and the role of stereotactic biopsy: review of the mortality, morbility, and diagnostic rates in 370 cases. Neurosurgery. 1996;39:907–12.
Shimada K, Nakamura M, Kuga Y, Taomoto K, Ohnishi H, Konishi N. Cytologic feature by squash preparation of pineal parenchyma tumor of intermediate differentiation. Diagn Cytopathol. 2008;36:749–53.
Varikatt W, Dexter M, Mahajan H, Murali R, Ng T. Usefulness of smears in intra-operative diagnosis of newly described entities of CNS. Neuropathology. 2009;29:641–8.

Chapter 22
Sellar Region

In spite of its reduced dimensions, the sellar region is a complex crossroad where a diversity of skeletal, meningeal, vascular, endocrine, and cerebral structures converges. This is why this region can host such a numerous and heterogeneous group of neoplastic and nonneoplastic processes (Table 22.1). Many of these lesions, while infrequent, may clinically and radiologically mimic pituitary adenomas, and so we must take them into account in order to avoid mistakes during intraoperative consultation. Common indications for intraoperative assessment to diagnose lesions of the sellar region include the following: (1) ensure appropriate tissue allocation and processing for accurate diagnosis, (2) confirm the presence of pituitary adenoma, (3) distinguish pituitary adenoma from other regional lesions, and (4) identify an unexpected lesion. Due to the peculiar location of the pituitary gland, just above the sphenoid sinus, a transnasal surgical approach is the rout by which biopsy or excision of most pituitary lesions is performed. Because the specimens obtained for this technique are slippery tiny fragments, cytologic preparations play a crucial role on pituitary intraoperative assessment.

Pituitary Adenoma

Pituitary adenoma is derived from adenohypophyseal cells and represents the third most common tumor in the CNS (10–20% of all primary intracranial tumors in most neurosurgery practices). These are much more frequent in adults than in children, with a peak incidence between 30 and 50 years, and approximately twice more common in females than in males. The vast majority of cases are sporadic, whereas familial adenomas account for 5% or less of all adenomas. Pituitary adenoma predisposition syndromes include MEN1 (gene *MEN1*, results in all pituitary tumor types), Carney complex (gene *PPKR1A*, associated with GH- or PRL-secreting adenomas), MEN4 (gene *CDKN1B*, too few patients described to be certain of

C. R. Lacruz et al., *Central Nervous System Intraoperative Cytopathology*,
Essentials in Cytopathology 13, https://doi.org/10.1007/978-3-319-98491-9_22

Table 22.1 Lesions in the pituitary gland and sellar region

Neoplastic	Nonneoplastic
Pituitary adenoma	Pituitary apoplexy
Craniopharyngioma	Rathke cleft cyst
Pituicytoma	Epidermoid cyst
Granular cell tumor	Dermoid cyst
Spindle cell oncocytoma	Pituitary abscess
Pituitary blastoma	Lymphocytic hypophysitis
Chiasmatic astrocytoma	Granulomatous hypophysitis
Meningioma	Sellar xanthogranuloma
Germinoma	Hypothalamic hamartoma
Chordoma	Sarcoidosis
Hematolymphoid tumors	Inflammatory pseudotumor
Paraganglioma	Aneurysms
Metastases	Cavernous angioma
Atypical teratoid/rhabdoid tumor[a]	Mucocele

[a]in adult females

adenoma type), and familial isolated pituitary adenomas (gene *AIP*, all pituitary tumor types).

In about 70% of cases, there is evidence of a characteristic hypersecretory syndrome, with Cushing's disease (corticotrophic adenomas), acromegaly/gigantism (growth hormone cell adenomas), and galactorrhea/amenorrhea (prolactin cell adenomas) being the most frequents. The remaining third of cases are endocrinologically silent, but some patients may have symptoms of gradual hypopituitarism with a significant impact on quality of life. If a tumor reaches a sufficiently large size to expand beyond the limits of the sella turcica, it may cause symptoms related to local mass effect, usually visual disturbances and hypothalamus-based dysfunction. Due to pituitary stalk compression, there is often a mild elevation in serum prolactin concentration (usually less than 200 ng/ml) known as "stalk effect." Spontaneous hemorrhagic infarction of pituitary adenoma – *pituitary apoplexy* – often leads to surgical emergency. Following gadolinium administration, the normal gland shows increased contrast uptake that delineates it from the adenoma that shows less and delayed contrast enhancement. On plain skull radiographs, some cases show ballooning and erosion of the bony fossa.

Macroscopically, pituitary adenomas are discrete, soft, tan-red masses. The size is very variable, from a few millimeters (microadenomas lessthan10 mm) to several centimeters (macroadenomas greaterthan10 mm). Microadenomas are intrasellar, whereas macroadenomas may balloon the sella and extend upward to the suprasellar region filling the chiasmatic cistern and even the third ventricle, laterally to the cavernous sinus or the temporal lobes, and downward to the paranasal sinuses. This extrasellar extension occurs in about 15% of cases. Cystic change is not rare, particularly in macroadenomas, which is why cystic pituitary adenoma and craniopharyngioma are the most common sellar/suprasellar cystic lesions.

Microscopic features are variable from tumor to tumor, both in cellular appearance and pattern of growth. This is characterized by the disruption of the nesting pattern of normal anterior pituitary, due to the proliferation of fairly monomorphic cells forming sheets, follicles, trabeculae, or papillae. Tumor cells show typical features of a neuroendocrine neoplasm with round nuclei, delicate chromatin, and inconspicuous nucleoli. Occasional bi−/multinucleation and nuclear pleomorphism may occur without correlation with aggressiveness of the tumor (Fig. 22.1a, b). The cytoplasm may be acidophilic, basophilic, or chromophobic, but classification of pituitary adenomas based on tinctorial characteristics of tumor cells is no longer used. The current most widely accepted classification is based primarily on clinical evidence of hormone hypersecretion and immunostaining profile, with selective ultrastructural analyses. About 25% of adenomas will be nonsecretory (null cell adenomas including oncocytomas), whereas a small percentage of adenomas will secrete more than one hormone (plurihormonal adenomas). Pathologists should too beware that dopamine agonists therapy for PRL-secreting adenomas (i.e., bromocriptine, Parlodel) induce tumoral fibrosis and cellular shrinkage (cells may resemble lymphocytes or small-cell carcinoma-like), which could lead to an erroneous intraoperative diagnosis. Locally infiltrating tumors invading dural sinuses, the sellar floor bone, and/or the sellar diaphragm are designated as *invasive adenomas*. The new 2017 WHO classification system acknowledges that parameters in addition to invasiveness may be of prognostic significance in pituitary adenomas, including MIB1 labeling indices, tumor size, and clinical presentation, as well as IHC, but the term *atypical adenoma* is no longer used. On the other hand, the term *pituitary carcinoma* (an exceedingly rare disorder) is defined as a pituitary neoplasm, usually hormone secreting (prolactin secreting and corticotropin secreting more common), which has undergone craniospinal dissemination or systemic metastases. Carcinomas usually evolve from invasive aggressive adenomas over several years than presenting de novo as previously undiagnosed metastasizing tumors.

All adenomas are immunoreactive for synaptophysin (even when they are clinically nonfunctional null cell adenomas) and cytokeratins 8/18 (i.e., CAM 5.2) but are negative or exhibit only rare cytokeratin 7-positive cells. On the other hand, the use of a full immunohistochemical panel of pituitary antibodies for hormones (PRL, GH, FSH, LH, TSH, ACTH) and transcription factors (SF-1, Pit-1) has made electron microscopy infrequently necessary for classification.

Most pituitary tumors are relatively benign, but incompletely resected adenomas tend to recur locally (macroadenomas and invasive adenomas are more likely to recur). The rare cases of pituitary carcinoma have a poor prognosis despite multimodal therapy (temozolomide therapy may be efficacious).

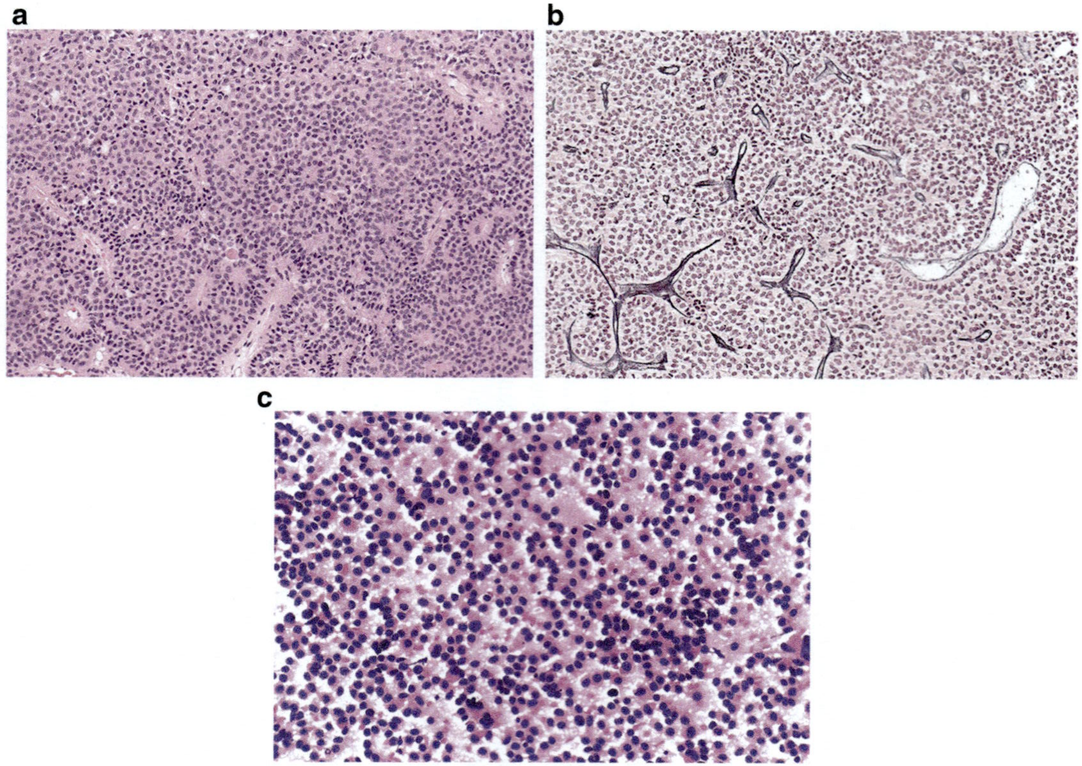

Fig. 22.1 *Pituitary adenoma*. (**a**) Histology. Many pituitary adenomas are composed of sheets of cells interrupted only by a delicate fibrovascular network. Tumor cells have rounded nuclei and indistinct cytoplasmic borders. Also note perivascular pseudorosettes. (**b**) In contrast to the acinar pattern in normal pituitary gland, reticulin fibers are almost entirely lost except around vessels. (**c**) Myriad of monomorphous cells with round nuclei is the characteristic feature of pituitary adenoma in cytologic preparations. Cytoplasmic contents from ruptured cells make up most of the background (Smear, H&E)

Cytologic Features

Due to scant reticulin most *pituitary adenomas* have soft texture and smear easily displaying an astonishing cellular abundance at low power. The most frequent presentation is a thin film of small-to-medium-sized cells that are evenly distributed without molding against each other (Fig. 22.1c). Follicles, small clusters, short chains, and papillary structures may also be present, which represent the cytological counterparts of histologic patterns (follicular, solid, trabecular, and papillary). Nuclei are uniformly round with stippled chromatin and small "peppery" nucleoli that lend a distinctive endocrine quality. The cytoplasm is fragile, with the result that many bare nuclei are seen in a granular background due to spilled cytoplasmic contents. When preserved, the cytoplasm looks well-defined with an oval or round morphology without processes. This feature, together with the frequent nuclear eccentric position, creates a plasmacytoid cellular morphology of great diagnostic usefulness. Cytoplasmic staining properties range from clear to pale to densely granulated, depending of the type and functional state of the tumor (Fig. 22.2a–c). Nuclear pleomorphism is uncommon and without connotations of malignant behavior but may be particularly conspicuous in some cases, especially in Crooke's cell adenoma (aggressive variant of ACTH cell adenoma) and sparsely granulated GH adenoma. Rarely, smears may show an additional ganglion cell population (*mixed pituitary adenoma-gangliocytoma*). Following *tumor apoplexy* (hemorrhage and tumor infarction) the smears may show only tumor cell necrosis, bloody background, and neutrophilic infiltrate.

Pituitary carcinoma can show distinct nuclear atypia and mitotic activity (Fig. 22.3), but also cases with "bland-appearing" cytomorphology may have an aggressive behavior.

Differential Diagnosis Considerations

The major differential diagnostic consideration of intrasellar adenomas is normal pituitary gland tissue, but tumors with large suprasellar extension may be mistaken for oligodendroglioma, ependymoma, germinoma, craniopharyngioma, meningioma, or lymphoma. In skull base-invasive cases, chordoma should also be taken into account. Normal pituitary tissue is substantially more difficult to smear in comparison to soft adenomas, and smears are less cellular featuring small clusters of different cell types. Preparations from oligodendroglioma exhibit round cells with scant and wispy cytoplasm and no epithelial features. Smears from ependymomas have a fibrillary background and perivascular pseudorosettes. Germinomas are recognized by a dual cell population in a striped "tigroid" background. Craniopharyngiomas are characterized by flattened epithelial cells sheets, nodules of "wet keratin," and a granular cystic content with cholesterol crystals. Smears from meningiomas show syncytial-like cell clusters and whorls. Malignant lymphomas are characterized by

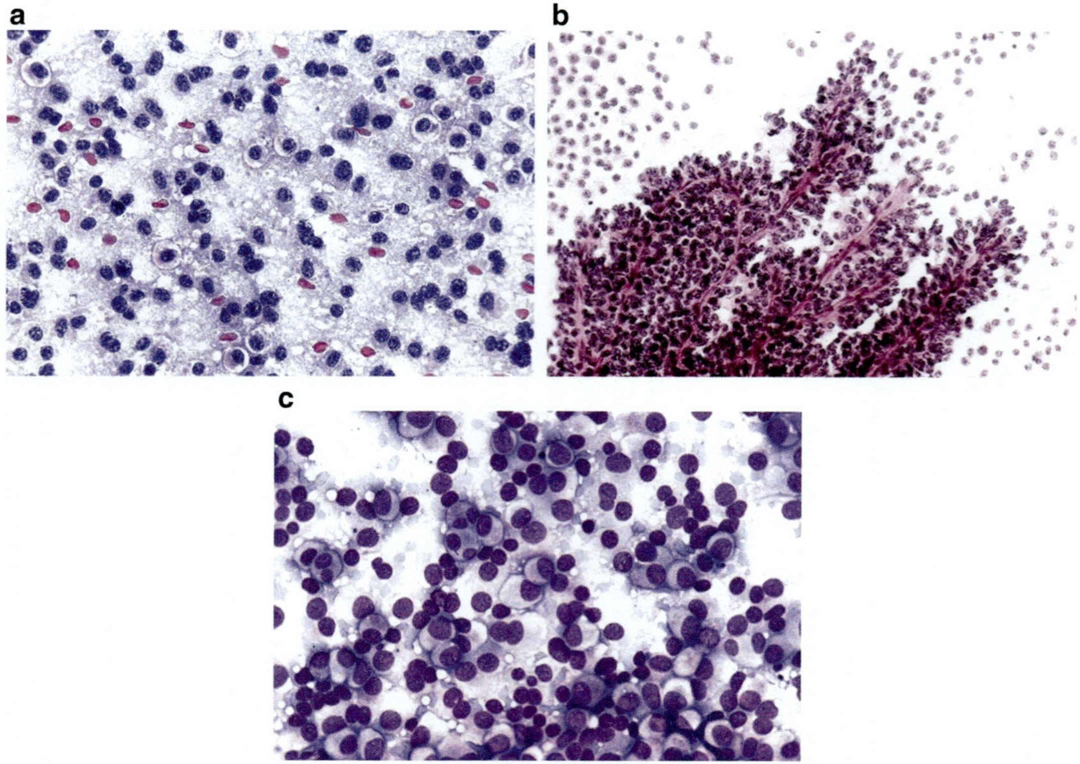

Fig. 22.2 *Pituitary adenoma*. (**a**) Discohesive pattern of small cells and numerous bare nuclei. Note characteristic speckled chromatin and small nucleoli (Smear, Papanicolaou). (**b**) Vascular-core papillary structures with tumor cell aggregations are a frequent finding in gonadotrophic adenomas (Smear, H&E). (**c**) In this preparation many cells exhibit plasmacytoid features with oval cytoplasm and eccentric nuclei (Smear, Romanowsky)

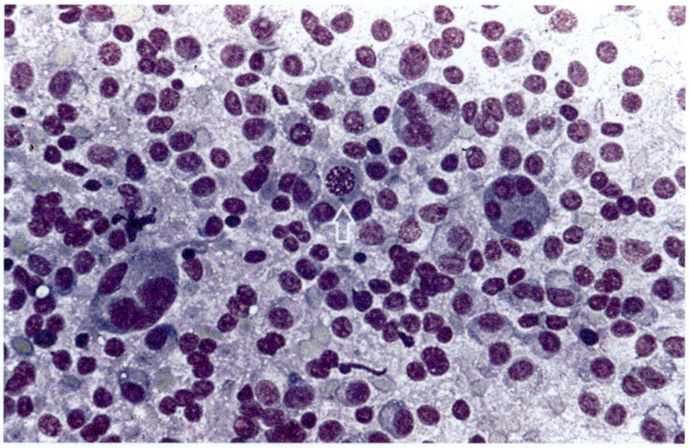

Fig. 22.3 *Pituitary carcinoma*. This pituitary tumor displays conspicuous pleomorphism, including multinucleated cells and mitotic figures (*arrow*). The patient had wide tumor spread through CSF, but an undoubted diagnosis of malignancy can't be done neither by cytology nor histology (Smear, Romanowsky)

Table 22.2 Characteristics of pituitary adenoma

Cytologic features
Highly cellular smears
Discohesive monolayer pattern
Round nuclei with stippled chromatin
Plasmacytoid cell appearance
Granular background with many bare nuclei
Beware of sparse cellularity following
Bromocriptine therapy
Tumor apoplexy
Differential diagnosis and pitfalls
Normal pituitary tissue
Oligodendroglioma
Ependymoma
Germinoma
Craniopharyngioma
Meningioma
Lymphoma
Metastatic carcinoma
Chordoma

nuclear anaplasia and lymphoglandular bodies without cell clusters. Chordomas include a dense myxoid matrix, and their cellular features are quite different from those of pituitary adenoma. Likewise, pituitary involvement by metastatic carcinoma is not rare, and some neoplasms like neuroendocrine carcinoma (stippled chromatin) may cause confusion requiring careful clinical correlation (Table 22.2).

Craniopharyngioma

Craniopharyngioma is a benign, but locally invasive, epithelial neoplasm that arises from the pituitary stalk or gland and develops in the sellar and suprasellar region. It accounts for between 2% and 5% of all primary intracranial neoplasms, but in children it constitutes 10% of brain tumors. The most common location is the suprasellar cistern with frequent extension to neighboring structures, including the optic pathway and the pituitary; some cases (mainly the papillary variant) are also found in the third ventricle. Sphenoid sinus, cerebellopontine angle, and pineal region are rare primary sites. Craniopharyngioma has a bimodal distribution with peaks occurring during childhood (5–15 years) and latter in adulthood (45–60 years); the papillary variant occurs almost exclusively in adults. No gender preference is apparent.

Clinical features include raised intracranial pressure, endocrine deficiencies, diabetes insipidus, visual deficits, and psychological abnormalities. In neuroimaging, they appear as complex and partially enhancing tumors intermixed with non-enhancing cysts. Unlike cerebral spinal fluid, these cholesterol-laden cysts will be T1-bright. Calcification is a frequent finding, especially in long-standing lesions.

Grossly, these tumors are lobulated, solid masses with a variable cystic component and frequently calcified. Cysts are filled with a turbid, dark, viscous fluid resembling motor oil. Papillary craniopharyngiomas are well-circumscribed, solid masses most often present in the third ventricle and, unlike the adamantinomatous type, when cystic the fluid content is clear.

Histologically, most tumors are *adamantinomatous or pediatric type*, featuring solid epithelial nests with peripheral palisading alternating with cystic areas. Nodules of "wet keratin" composed of squamoid nests containing ghost-like cells and associated dystrophic calcification are frequent (Fig. 22.4a). Xanthogranulomatous inflammation with cholesterol clefts and foreign body-type giant cell reaction is more common in recurrent lesions. When craniopharyngiomas impinge upon brain tissue, they evoke an intense gliotic reaction with prominent Rosenthal fibers (piloid gliosis), not infrequently coupled with fibrosis. Adamantinomatous craniopharyngioma shows *CTNNB1* mutations and aberrant IHC nuclear expression of β-catenin. The *papillary variant or adult type* (about 10% of cases) is composed by monomorphic masses of well-differentiated, pseudopapillary squamous epithelium (without surface keratinization) resembling oropharyngeal mucosa. Goblet cells and individual keratinization can be present, but palisades, "wet keratin" collections, and calcification are absent (Fig. 22.4b). This variant shows *BRAF* V600E mutations in 85–95% of cases, which can be detected by BRAF VE1 immunoreactivity.

The prognosis for patients with craniopharyngioma is favorable – both adamantinomatous and papillary types correspond to WHO grade I, but recurrence takes place in more than 20% of cases. The most significant factors associated with recurrence are tumor size and incomplete excision (more than 5 cm and/or subtotal resection carrying a worse prognosis). Papillary craniopharyngioma may response to targeted therapies (vemurafenib) due to *BRAF* V600E mutation.

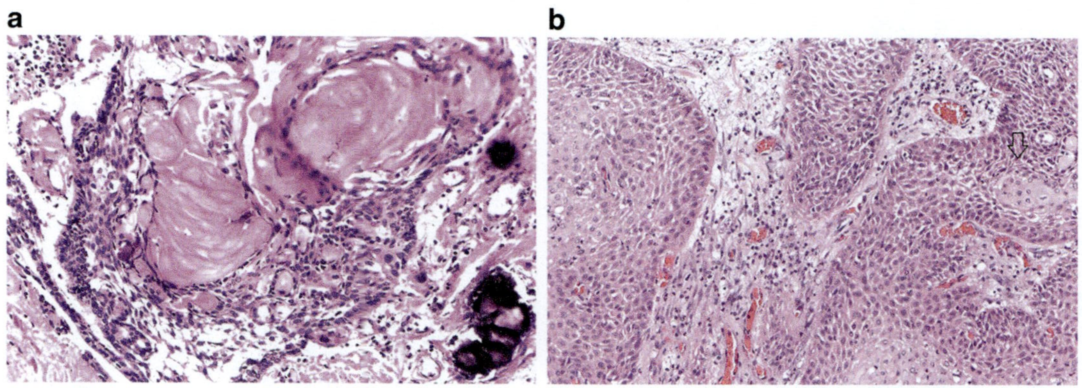

Fig. 22.4 *Craniopharyngioma, histology*. (**a**) *Adamantinomatous type*. A complex epithelium ranges from compact with peripheral palisading to loose knit (stellate reticulum). Also note the presence of "wet" keratin nodules and focal calcification. (**b**) *Papillary type*. This variant consists of sheets of well-differentiated squamous epithelium associated with fibrous stroma. Epithelial whorls (*arrow*) are not uncommon in papillary craniopharyngiomas, but unlike the adamantinomatous type, it is devoid of keratin, ghost cells, or calcification

Cytologic Features

Although *adamantinomatous craniopharyngioma* is not easy to smear, preparations generally reveal cohesive sheets of flattened epithelial cells, either polygonal or basaloid, and nodules of keratinized cells with ghost nuclei ("wet keratin") which are sufficient for diagnosis (Fig. 22.5a). The presence of cholesterol crystals (leached from degenerated cell membranes) admixed with keratinous debris and macrophages from the cystic fluid provides additional support for the diagnosis. Cholesterol crystals dissolve in alcohol and must be looked for in air-dried Romanowsky-stained preparations or in unfixed wet smears under polarized light; they appear as crystalline, polygonal notched plates (Fig. 22.5b, c). Clusters of parakeratotic cells, calcification, multinucleated giant cells, and reactive "piloid" gliosis may also be present. Smears from *papillary craniopharyngioma* show cohesive sheets of squamous epithelial cells. Goblet cells and individual cell keratinization may occasionally be found, but unlike adamantinomatous craniopharyngioma nodules of "wet keratin," calcification and cholesterol crystals are absent (Fig. 22.6). However, differentiating these two tumors in an intraoperative smear is challenging and generally unnecessary.

Differential Diagnosis Considerations

A fluid cyst alone with macrophages, cholesterol crystals, and keratinous debris is compatible with a craniopharyngioma, but it is not diagnostic and may be seen in other cystic sellar and suprasellar lesions, such as epidermoid/dermoid cysts, mature cystic teratoma, or Rathke cleft cyst with xanthogranulomatous degeneration. Additional cytology preparations or biopsy specimens must include the adamantinomatous zones to be diagnostic. On the other hand, the ragged interface with the adjacent brain is usually typified by florid reactive gliosis simulating a low-grade astrocytoma. Awareness of this potential pitfall, along with the presence of small clumps of epithelial cells or nodules of "wet keratin" between the gliotic tissue fragments, will prevent a misdiagnosis (Fig. 22.7a). In some craniopharyngiomas, degenerative atypia with hyperchromatic parakeratotic cells and even keratin "pearls" may occur, making their distinction from metastatic squamous carcinoma difficult on pure morphologic grounds (Fig. 22.7b). Once again, this does not constitute a problem with a careful clinical correlation. Table 22.3 summarizes the characteristic of craniopharyngioma.

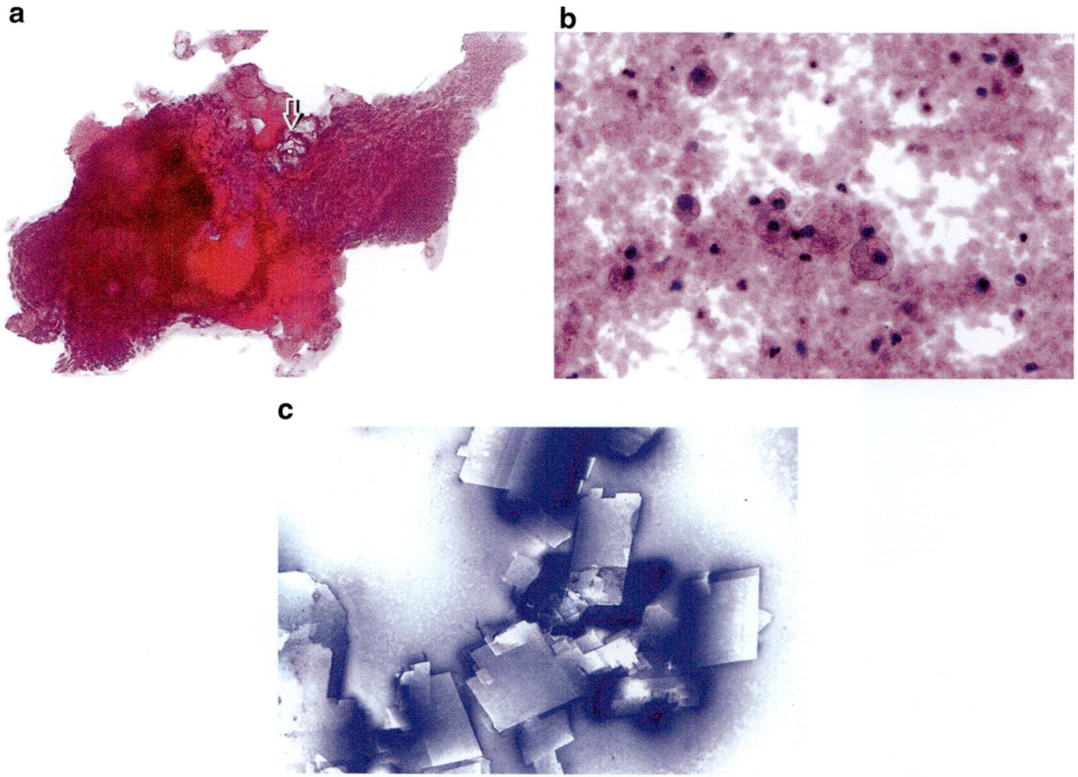

Fig. 22.5 *Adamantinomatous craniopharyngioma, cytologic features*. (**a**) This large, cohesive epithelial cell sheet has intermixed nodules of "wet" keratin and jagged edges. Calcium (*arrow*) is usually deposited on keratin nodules (Smear, H&E). (**b**) Granular debris and foamy macrophages from the cystic fluid content (Smear, H&E). (**c**) Cholesterol crystals in air-dried preparations appear as negative three-dimensional images (Smear, Romanowsky)

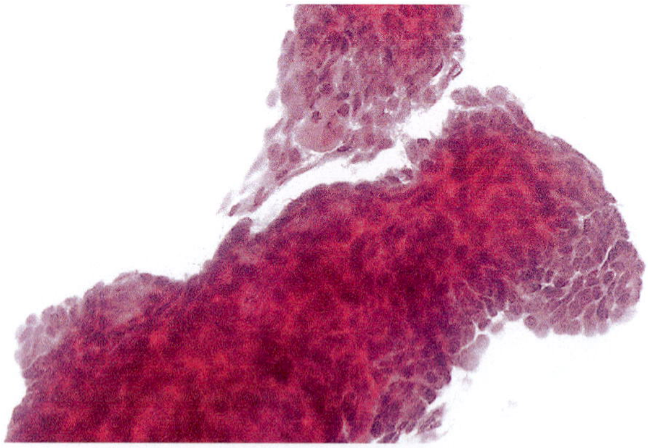

Fig. 22.6 *Papillary craniopharyngioma, cytologic features.* This preparation reveals papillary sheets of benign squamous epithelium with a caracteristic "paving stone" appearance, but neither the basaloid epithelium nor the wet keratin nodules of the adamantinomatous type are present (Smear, H&E)

Other Lesions of the Sellar Region

We have already seen that the sellar region may host many masses, of a very different nature, other than pituitary adenoma and craniopharyngioma (Table 22.1).

Neoplastic Lesions

The neurohypophysis can spawn pituicytoma, spindle cell oncocytoma, and granular cell tumor. These three rare WHO grade I neoplasms are now recognized to be derivatives of normal pituicytes expressing positive nuclear TTF-1 immunoexpression like the normal posterior gland. To refine the classification of these lesions, the terminologies "oncocytic pituicytoma" and "granular cell pituicytoma" have been proposed.

Pituicytoma is a spindle cell tumor composed of plump cells arranged in fascicles. Smears show plump spindle cells with elongated nuclei and moderate cytoplasm with distinct cytoplasmic borders. It can be misinterpreted as meningioma but lacks whorls, nuclear pseudoinclusions, and calcifications.

Spindle cell oncocytoma is essentially a pituicytoma with epithelioid cells and oncocytic features due to mitochondrial accumulation.

Granular cell tumor of the sellar region has an identical morphology to granular cell tumor elsewhere in the body. However, as we have already mentioned, it is thought to arise from TTF-1 expressing pituicytes rather than Schwann cells. Smears are characterized by loose clusters of swollen, histiocytic-like cells with granular – lysosomal-rich – cytoplasm and small eccentric nuclei with inconspicuous nucleoli. This monomorphic, bland nature of granular cell tumor may cause considerable confusion with pituitary adenomas in frozen sections, but not in smears (Fig. 22.8).

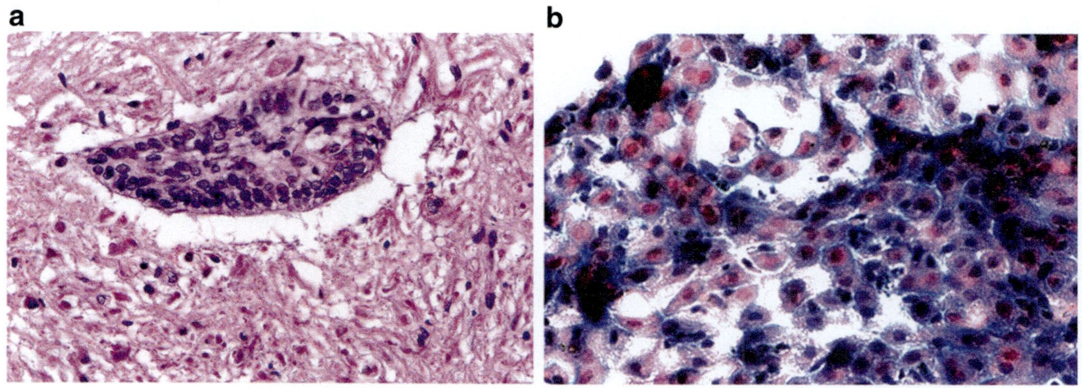

Fig. 22.7 *Craniopharyngioma, pitfalls*. (**a**) Craniopharyngiomas are locally invasive evoking a vigorous reactive gliosis with Rosenthal fiber formation that may be misinterpreted as pilocytic astrocytoma. (**b**) Parakeratotic cells with eosinophilic cytoplasm and hyperchromatic nuclei mimicking epidermoid carcinoma (Smear, Papanicolaou)

Table 22.3 Characteristics of craniopharyngioma

Cytologic features	
	Sheets of polygonal and/or basaloid epithelial cells
	Nodules of "wet keratin"
	Calcifications
	Fluid cystic content:
	Macrophages, cholesterol crystals, keratinous debris
	Piloid gliosis
	Papillary type
	Sheets of monomorphic squamous cells
	Goblet cells (occasional)
	Individual keratinization (occasional)
Differential diagnosis and pitfalls	
	Epidermoid/dermoid cysts
	Mature teratoma
	Rathke cleft cyst
	Metastatic squamous carcinoma
	Pilocytic astrocytoma

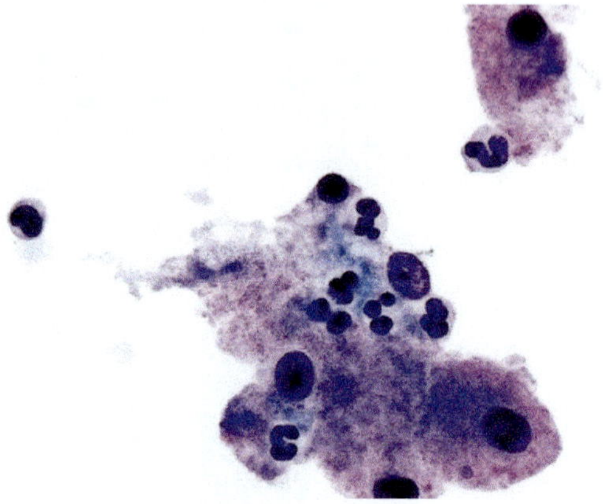

Fig. 22.8 *Granular cell tumor*. Cluster of plump cells with round nuclei and abundant granular cytoplasm due to lysosomal accumulation. Compare the cell size with that of admixed neutrophils (Smear, Papanicolaou)

Pituitary blastoma is a neonatal pituitary tumor exhibiting differentiation to Rathke epithelium and adenohypophysial – folliculostellate and secretory – cell types, and should be differentiated from pituitary adenoma and immature teratomas.

Other CNS tumors, particularly *meningiomas* and *germinoma*, may arise in the sellar region, but smears from these lesions are quite different from those of pituitary adenoma or craniopharyngioma.

The pituitary gland, via hematogenous spread or – more frequently – by direct sellar extension, may be a site of *metastasis* in the context of advanced systemic cancer, with breast, lung, prostate, and gastrointestinal tract as the most frequent primary sites. In smear preparations, the presence of cellular anaplasia and cohesive cell groups – typical of metastatic carcinoma – are useful differential features, but clinical workup is essential.

Adult women may develop *atypical teratoid/rhabdoid tumors* in the sellar region. Thus, this characteristic childhood neoplasm should be included in the differential diagnosis of regional masses in adult females.

Lastly, since occasional intrasellar examples have been described in the literature, it is also necessary to consider *paraganglioma* in the differential diagnosis of sellar region masses.

Nonneoplastic Lesions

Epithelial remnants of pituitary development can produce *Rathke cleft cyst.* This lesion may cause, as we have already mentioned, considerable confusion with craniopharyngioma when the primitive columnar lining epithelium is destroyed or substituted by metaplastic squamous epithelium.

Xanthogranuloma of the sellar region is considered to be a reactive lesion, most often to remnants of Rathke cleft cyst, and can also be mistaken for craniopharyngioma. It is composed of cholesterol clefts, xanthomatous macrophages, multinucleated giant cells, chronic inflammation, necrotic debris, and hemosiderin deposits, but adamantinomatous epithelium is absent.

Hypothalamic hamartomas (HHs) are rare developmental malformative masses, which arise from the hypothalamus and tuber cinereum. They are typically composed of nodules or sheets of small, well-differentiated neurons embedded within a glial matrix. The main differential diagnosis is ganglioglioma, but HHs are composed of a cytologically normal neuronal population, which differs from the large dysplastic ganglion cells of ganglioglioma (Fig. 22.9).

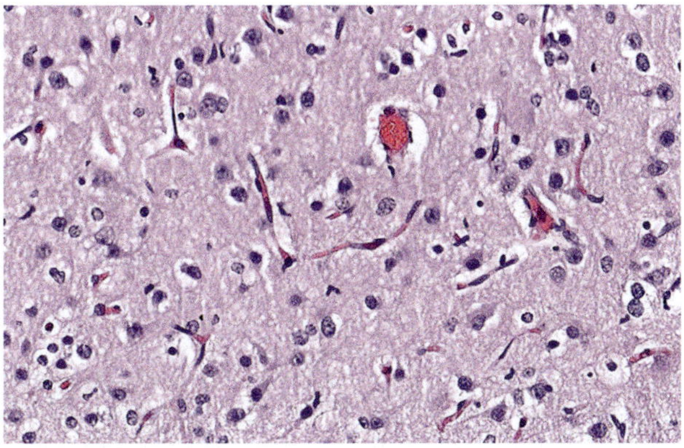

Fig. 22.9 *Hypothalamic hamartoma.* In contrast with ganglion cell tumors, this lesion is composed of cytologically normal small to midsize neurons embedded within a glial matrix. Note a plexus of slim capillaries (resection specimen from a 1-year-old boy suffering gelastic seizures)

Hypophysitis is an inflammatory infiltrate of the pituitary gland but is not a single disorder and may be either primary or secondary (i.e., sarcoidosis, Sjögren syndrome, Wegener granulomatosis). Primary hypophysitis was originally thought to affect almost exclusively women during pregnancy or early postpartum period, but more recent studies show less association with pregnancy and indicate that males and females are nearly equally affected. Primary hypophysitis is most commonly divided into lymphocytic, granulomatous, and xanthomatous types. The chronic inflammatory infiltrate of lymphocytic hypophysitis should be differentiated from infiltrations by malignant lymphoma (cytologic preparations can help distinguish among both processes).

Inflammatory pseudotumor or plasma cell granuloma can involve the sella turcica and parasellar tissues mimicking a neoplastic process. This lesion is composed of a mixed inflammatory infiltrate (lymphoid aggregates, plasma cells, and macrophages), often containing fibrosis and granulation tissue. The mature plasmacytic infiltrate of this lesion must not be mistaken for atypical plasma cells of plasmacytoma/myeloma.

Sphenoid sinus mucoceles are epithelium-lined cystic masses that usually are filled with a thick mucoid material. Extension beyond the confines of the sinus into the orbit may produce exophthalmos, whereas more centrally directed lesions may compress cranial nerves and pituitary gland itself. Therefore, these types of mucoceles should be included in the differential diagnosis of regional cystic masses.

Suggested Reading

Aylwin SJ, Bodi I, Beaney R. Pronounced response of papillary craniopharyngioma to treatment with vemurafenib, a BRAF inhibitor. Pituitary. 2016;19:544–6.

Boari N, Losa M, Mortini P, Snider S, Terreni MR, Giovanelli M. Intrasellar paraganglioma: a case report and review of the literature. Acta Neurochir. 2006;148:1311–4.

Brastianos PK, Taylor-Weiner A, Manley PE, Jones RT, et al. Exome sequencing identifies BRAF mutations in papillary craniopharyngiomas. Nat Genet. 2014;46:161–5.

Brat DJ, Scheithauer BW, Staugaitis SM, Holtzman RN, Morgello S, Burger PC. Pituicytoma: a distinctive low-grade glioma of the neurohypophysis. Am J Surg Pathol. 2000;24:362–8.

Buslei R, Nolde M, Hofmann B, Meissner S, et al. Common mutations of beta-catenin in adamantinomatous craniopharyngiomas but not in other tumours originating from the sellar region. Acta Neuropathol. 2005;109:589–97.

Ceyhan K, Yagmurlu B, Dogan BE, Erdogan N, Bulut S, Erekul S. Cytopathologic features of pituitary carcinoma with cervical vertebral bone metastasis: a case report. Acta Cytol. 2006;50:225–30.

Chen KT. Crush cytology of pituicytoma. Diagn Cytopathol. 2005;33:255–7.

Cohen-Gadol AA, Pichelmann MA, Link MJ, Scheithauer BW, et al. Granular cell tumor of the sellar and suprasellar region: clinicopathologic study of 11 cases and literature review. Mayo Clin Proc. 2003;78:567–75.

Coons SW, Rekate HL, Prenger EC, Wang N, et al. The histopathology of hypothalamic hamartomas: study of 57 cases. J Neuropathol Exp Neurol. 2007;66:131–41.

Daneshbod Y, Monabati A, Kumar PV, Taghipoor M, Bedayat GR. Intraoperative cytologic crush preparation findings in craniopharyngioma. A study of 12 cases. Acta Cytol. 2005;49:7–10.

Devi S, Ganger A, Sharma S, Saxena R. Sphenoid mucocele with unusual panhypopituitarism. BMJ Case Rep. 2016;2016:pii: bcr2015214218. https://doi.org/10.1136/bcr-2015-214218.

Gomez-Hernandez K, Ezzat S, Asa SL, Mete Ö. Clinical implications of accurate subtyping of pituitary adenomas: perspectives from the treating physician. Turk Patoloji Derg. 2015;31(Suppl 1):4–17.

Hagel C, Buslei R, Buchfelder M, Fahlbusch R, et al. Immunoprofiling of glial tumours of the neurohypophysis suggests a common pituicytic origin of neoplastic cells. Pituitary. 2017;20:211–7.

Hansen I, Petrossians P, Thiry A, Flandroy P, et al. Extensive inflammatory pseudotumor of the pituitary. J Clin Endocrinol Metab. 2001;86:4603–10.

He W, Chen F, Dalm B, Kirby PA, Greenlee JD. Metastatic involvement of the pituitary gland: a systematic review with pooled individual patient data analysis. Pituitary. 2015;18:159–68.

Heaney AP. Pituitary carcinoma: difficult diagnosis and treatment. J Clin Endocrinol Metab. 2011;96:3649–60.

Hölsken A, Sill M, Merkle J, Schweizer L, et al. Adamantinomatous and papillary craniopharyngiomas are characterized by distinct epigenomic as well as mutational and transcriptomic profiles. Acta Neuropathol Commun. 2016;4:20.

Inagawa H, Ishizawa K, Mitsuhashi T, et al. Giant invasive pituitary adenoma extending into the sphenoid sinus and nasopharynx. Report of a case with intraoperative cytologic diagnosis. Acta Cytol. 2005;49:452–6.

Kim JS, Lee YS, Jung MJ, Hong YK. The predictive value of pathologic features in pituitary adenoma and correlation with pituitary adenoma recurrence. J Pathol Transl Med. 2016;50:419–25.

Kleinschmidt-DeMasters BK, Lopes MB. Update on hypophysitis and TTF-1 expressing sellar region masses. Brain Pathol. 2013;23:495–514.

Kleinschmidt-DeMasters BK, Lopes MB, Prayson RA. An algorithmic approach to sellar region masses. Arch Pathol Lab Med. 2015;139:356–72.

Kontogeorgos G, Bassiouka I, Giannou P, Vamvassakis E, Rologis D, Orphanidis G. Diagnosis of pituitary adenomas on touch preparations assisted by immunocytochemistry. Acta Cytol. 1995;39:141–52.

Kontogeorgos G, Mourouti G, Kyrodimou E, Liapi-Avgeri G, Parasi E. Ganglion cell containing pituitary adenomas: signs of neuronal differentiation in adenoma cells. Acta Neuropathol. 2006;112:21–8.

Lee TJ, Li SP, Fu CH, Huang CC, et al. Extensive paranasal sinus mucoceles: a 15-year review of 82 cases. Am J Otolaryngol Head Neck Med Surg. 2009;30:234–8.

Liu JK, Patel J, Eloy JA. The role of temozolomide in the treatment of aggressive pituitary tumors. J Clin Neurosci. 2015;22:923–9.

Madhavan M, George J, Jafri JA, Idris Z. Intraventricular squamous papillary craniopharyngioma. Report of a case with intraoperative imprint cytology. Acta Cytol. 2005;49:431–4.

McDonald WC, Banerji N, McDonald KN, Ho B, Macias V, Kajdacsy-Balla A. Steroidogenic factor 1, Pit-1, and adrenocorticotropic hormone: a rational starting place for the immunohistochemical characterization of pituitary adenoma. Arch Pathol Lab Med. 2017;141:104–12.

Mete O, Lopes MB, Asa SL. Spindle cell oncocytomas and granular cell tumors of the pituitary are variants of pituicytoma. Am J Surg Pathol. 2013;37:1694–9.

Murakami K, Muraishi K, Ikeda H, Yoshimoto T. Plasma cell granuloma of the pituitary gland. Surg Neurol. 2001;56:247–51.

Ng H-K. Smears in the diagnosis of pituitary adenomas. Acta Cytol. 1998;42:614–8.

Nguyen G-K, Johnson ES, Mielke BW. Comparative cytomorphology of pituitary adenomas and oligodendrogliomas in intraoperative crush preparations. Acta Cytol. 1992;36:661–7.

Parwani AV, Taylor DC, Burger PC, Erozan YS, Olivi A, Ali SZ. Keratinized squamous cells in fine needle aspiration of the brain. Cytopathologic correlates and differential diagnosis. Acta Cytol. 2003;47:325–31.

Paulus W, Honegger J, Keyvani K, Fahlbusch R. Xanthogranuloma of the sellar region: a clinicopathological entity different from adamantinomatous craniopharyngioma. Acta Neuropathol. 1999;97:377–82.

Pegolo G, Buckwalter JG, Weiss MH, Hinton DR. Pituitary adenomas. Correlation of the cytologic appearance with biologic behavior. Acta Cytol. 1995;39:887–92.

Pernicone PJ, Scheithauer BW, Sebo TJ, Kovacs KT, et al. Pituitary carcinoma: a clinicopathologic study of 15 cases. Cancer. 1997;79:804–12.

Piccirilli M, Maiola V, Salvati M, D'Elia A, et al. Granular cell tumor of the neurohypophysis: a single-institution experience. Tumori. 2014;100:160e–4e.

Policarpio-Nicolas ML, Le BH, Mandell JW, Lopes MB. Granular cell tumor of the neurohypophysis: report of a case with intraoperative cytologic diagnosis. Diagn Cytopathol. 2008;36:58–63.

Roque A, Odia Y. BRAF-V600E mutant papillary craniopharyngioma dramatically responds to combination BRAF and MEK inhibitors. CNS Oncol. 2017;6:95–9.

Salame K, Ouaknine GE, Yossipov J, Rochkind S. Paraganglioma of the pituitary fossa: diagnosis and management. J Neuro-Oncol. 2001;54:49–52.

Sav A, Rotondo F, Syro LV, Di Ieva A, Cusimano MD, Kovacs K. Invasive, atypical and aggressive pituitary adenomas and carcinomas. Endocrinol Metab Clin N Am. 2015;44:99–104.

Scheithauer BW, Horvath E, Abel TW, Robital Y, et al. Pituitary blastoma: a unique embryonal tumor. Pituitary. 2012;15:365–73.

Schneiderhan TM, Beseoglu K, Bergmann M, Neubauer U, et al. Sellar atypical teratoid/rhabdoid tumours in adults. Neuropathol Appl Neurobiol. 2001;37:326–9.

Sekine S, Shibata T, Kokubu A, et al. Craniopharyngiomas of adamantinomatous type harbor beta-catenin gene mutations. Am J Pathol. 2002;161:1997–2001.

Sibal L, Ball SG, Connolly V, James RA, et al. Pituitary apoplexy: a review of clinical presentation, management and outcome in 45 cases. Pituitary. 2004;7:157–63.ç.

Simms NM, Brown WE, French LA. Mucocele of the sphenoid sinus presenting as an intrasellar mass. Case report. J Neurosug. 1970;32:708–10.

Smith AR, Elsheikh TM, Silverman JF. Intraoperative cytologic diagnosis of suprasellar and sellar cystic lesions. Diagn Cytopathol. 1999;20:137–47.

Sy J, Ang LC. Cytomorphologic spectrum of mixed pituitary adenoma-gangliocytomas. A report of two cases. Acta Cytol. 2010;54:981–4.

Tena-Suck M, Salinas-Lara C, Vega-Orozco R, Rembao-Bojorquez D, Gelista N. Crush intraoperatory analysis in craniopharyngioma. Diagn Cytopathol. 2012;40:865–70.

Wang H, Liang J, Yong WH, Sullivan P. Metastatic pituitary carcinoma to cervical lymph node: diagnosis by fine needle aspiration and review of the literature. Acta Cytol. 2017;61:242–6.

Zada G, Lin N, Ojerholm E, Ramkissoon S, Laws ER. Craniopharyngioma and other cystic epithelial lesions of the sellar region: a review of clinical, imaging, and histopathological relationships. Neurosurg Focus. 2010;28:E4.

Chapter 23
Spine and Epidural Space

Neurologic function becomes extremely vulnerable as it funnels through the slender spinal cord. Thus, neoplastic and nonneoplastic processes of the spine and epidural space often give rise to severe backache, radiculopathy, sensorimotor disturbances, loss of sphincter control, and even paraplegia. This clinical scenario, which may appear suddenly, requires an accurate diagnosis that will make proper patient management possible. Depending on the severity of the symptomatology, the diagnostic approach may be a percutaneous image-guided needle biopsy or an intraoperative consultation in the course of a decompressive laminectomy. In both diagnostic procedures, cytologic studies are especially valuable, both for the initial differentiation between neoplastic and nonneoplastic processes and for identifying the neoplasms most frequently found in this region (Table 23.1).

Neoplastic Lesions

Spinal cord compression from epidural metastases is the most common neurological complication of cancer after brain metastases, being the nature of the primary tumor and the degree of the neurological deficit the most important factors affecting survival. The most common tumors associated with epidural spinal cord compression are lung and breast cancers, followed by lymphoma, myeloma, and prostate cancer. Other tumors that must be also taken into consideration are chordoma (selective location in the axial skeleton) and neurofibroma (frequent location in the paraspinal space). Cytologic preparations can help distinguish among all of these neoplasias.

C. R. Lacruz et al., *Central Nervous System Intraoperative Cytopathology*,
Essentials in Cytopathology 13, https://doi.org/10.1007/978-3-319-98491-9_23

Table 23.1 Mass lesions in the spine and epidural space

Neoplastic	Nonneoplastic
Metastatic carcinoma	Prolapsed disc
Lymphoma	Epidural abscess
Myeloma	Tuberculosis (Pott's disease)
Chordoma	Other infectious spondilodiscitis
Other bone tumors	Facet joint synovial cyst
Neurofibroma	Postoperative scar
Lipoma	Vascular malformations
Hemangioma	Extramedullary hematopoiesis

Metastatic Carcinoma

Metastatic bone disease is not uncommon in the spine and sacrum, being the spine the third most common site for cancer cells to metastasize, following the lung and the liver. Penetration into the epidural space is a frequent complication, with neoplastic cells commonly entering the spinal canal via the bony foramina traversed by vertebral veins. In the chapter on metastatic tumors, we saw how lung, breast, and prostate carcinomas are the ones that most frequently involve the spinal epidural space, followed by neoplasms arising in the digestive tract (i.e., colon) and kidney. From the clinical point of view, they may behave as an extension of an already diagnosed tumor or else be the first expression of a hidden tumor – when bone metastasis is the first manifestation of a malignant tumor, the spine is involved in about 80% of cases. The latter scenario, which represents a greater diagnostic challenge, is especially frequent in renal, pulmonary, and prostatic carcinomas. In such cases, percutaneous image-guided biopsy is useful to establish a definitive diagnosis. The characteristic cytologic picture of metastatic carcinoma, cohesive clumps of atypical cells with epithelial features (Fig. 23.1a), allows a clear differentiation from the other neoplasms most frequently found in this region (lymphoma and plasma cell tumors).

Lymphoma

Epidural lymphomas comprise 9% of all spinal epidural tumors, with an epidural location for lymphoma observed in 0.1–6.5% of all lymphomas. The most common region of involvement is the thoracic spine, followed by the lumbar and cervical spine. Any form of Hodgkin or non-Hodgkin lymphoma may be encountered, although most tumors are B-cell lymphomas of intermediate and high grade. Distinction between subtypes is not necessary intraoperatively, but it is indeed necessary to differentiate high-grade lymphomas from metastatic carcinoma and low-grade lymphomas from nonneoplastic inflammatory processes. Differentiating *high-grade lymphomas* from metastatic carcinoma, as we have already seen, is not

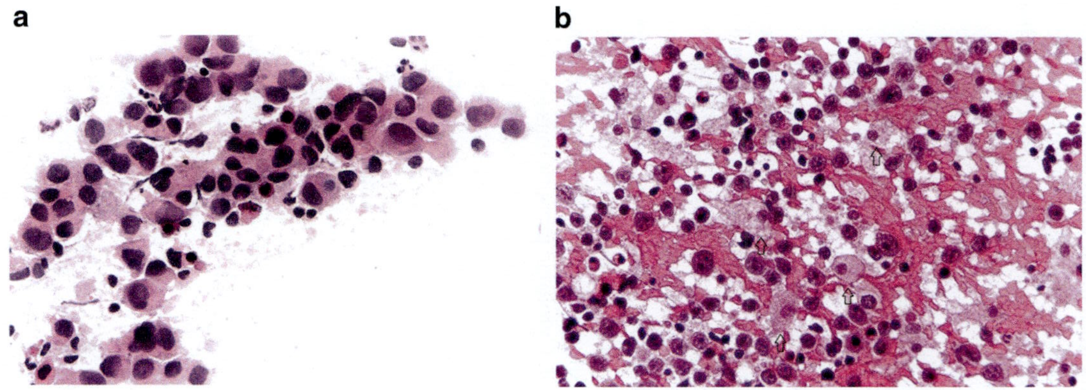

Fig. 23.1 *Metastatic carcinoma* versus *lymphoma, CT-guided needle aspiration biopsy.* (**a**) Metastasis from a lung primary showing characteristic cohesive clumps of cells and epithelial features. (**b**) This preparation from a diffuse large B-cell lymphoma displays a single cell pattern of atypical lymphoid cells. Note macrophages (*arrows*) and numerous apoptotic bodies (**a**, **b**; Smears, H&E)

difficult (Fig. 23.1b). Appropriate handling of some difficult cases, i.e., small-cell lung carcinoma in adults and "small round blue cell tumors" – neuroblastoma, Ewing sarcoma, and rhabdomyosarcoma – in children, can be made by deferring the specific diagnosis to the performance of ancillary techniques in permanent sections. On the other hand, distinguishing a *low-grade lymphoma* from a chronic inflammatory lesion may be particularly difficult. It is necessary to examine the sample carefully in order to find the characteristic polymorphism and cellular variety of the inflammatory lesions. However, we may have to resort to testing the monoclonality of the process in order to have a conclusive diagnosis.

Myeloma

Myeloma is the most common primary tumor of the spine, representing 20% of neoplasms in this location. Pain of an increasing nature is the most common complaint, and it is often centered in the lumbar or thoracic spinal regions. Also neurologic symptoms, usually from disease of spinal cord or nerve roots secondary to pathologic fracture or epidural extraosseous extension of the neoplastic tissue, are frequently observed. Radiologically, they most often present as ill-defined lytic lesions that can be either multiple (*myeloma*) or solitary (*plasmacytoma*). Due to cortical bone destruction, plasma cell neoplasms are often amenable to needle aspiration, and the cell yield is rich. Cytologic preparations show variable differentiation from all most normal-appearing plasma cells to highly pleomorphic (bi- or multinucleated) cells. Occasionally, cells with plasmablastic morphology (immunoblast-like cells with prominent central nucleoli) may be seen (Fig. 23.2a, b).

Chordoma

Although considered not to possess significant metastatic potential, chordomas are locally aggressive, leading to neurologic compromise and lytic destruction of bone. About two-third of cases occur along the spinal cord, with the sacrum being the most common location. Sacral and non-sacral spinal tumors often present with back pain, pathologic fractures, and motor or sensory losses in lower extremities, and scans show heterogeneous bulky masses that destroy bone. Neuroimaging-guided FNA is the preferred method for establishing the preoperative morphologic diagnosis of chordoma (due to cortical bone destruction, chordomas are often easy to needle aspiration). Aspirates are cellular, with groups and single cells in a rich myxoid matrix. The diagnostic cell is the *physaliphorous* one (from Greek *physalis*, meaning *bubble*): these cells rarely mold and have different shapes with well-defined cytoplasmic boundaries. The cytoplasm is occupied by a single or multiple vacuoles giving it a bubbly appearance. Nuclei are round and uniform with small to inconspicuous nucleoli (Fig. 23.3a, b).

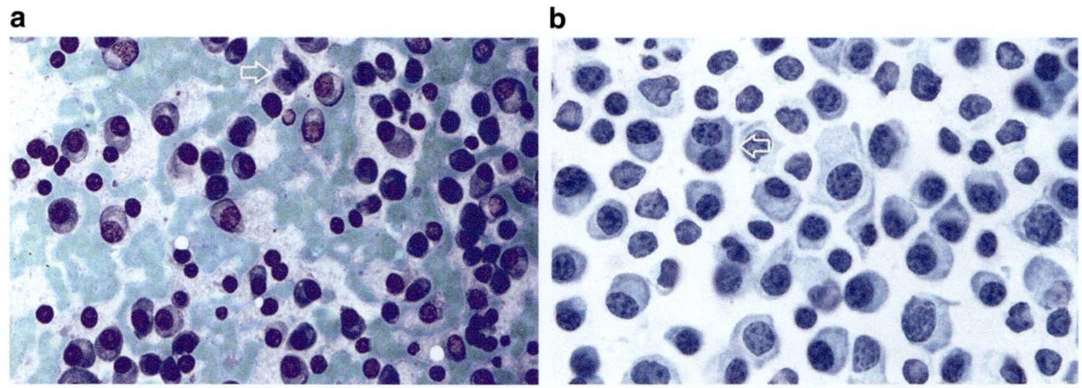

Fig. 23.2 *Myeloma, CT-guided needle aspiration biopsy.* (**a**) Smear preparation displaying dispersed slightly atypical, neoplastic plasma cells with occasional mitotic figures (*arrow*; Romanowsky). (**b**) ThinPrep preparation showing atypical plasma cells including binucleation (*arrow*; Papanicolaou)

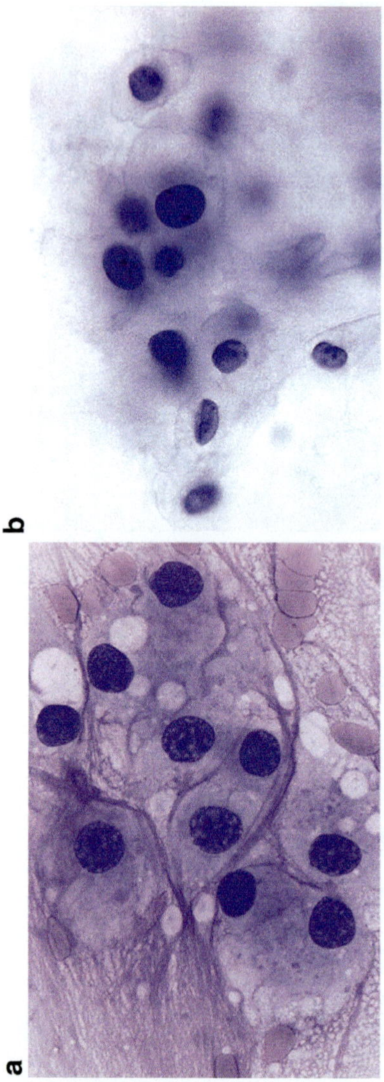

Fig. 23.3 *Chordoma, CT-guided needle aspiration biopsy.* (**a**) Typical "physaliphorous" cells featuring bubbly cytoplasm and round nuclei in a metachromatic myxoid matrix (Smear, Romanowsky). (**b**) This stain enhances nuclear features, but the myxoid background and bubbly cytoplasm are not clearly seen (Smear, Papanicolaou)

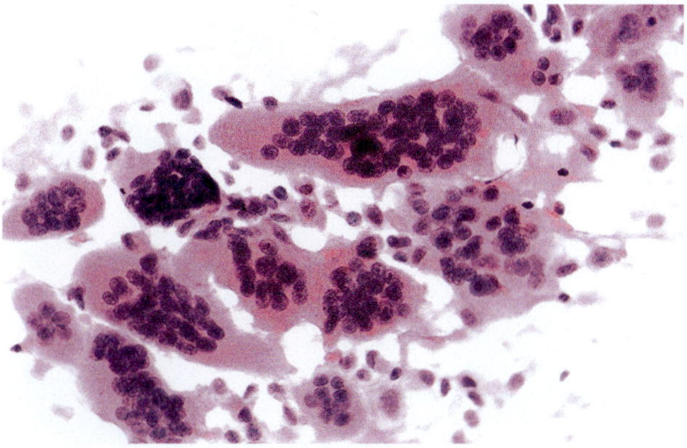

Fig. 23.4 *Giant cell tumor of the bone, intraoperative smear*. A 42-year-old woman suffered sudden paraplegia, and a destructive lesion of thoracic vertebra T9 with vertebral collapse was seen on scans. This H&E stained, intraoperative smear – performed in the course of emergency decompressive laminectomy – shows numerous osteoclast-like giant cells and round-to-ovoid single cells; both cell types share nuclear features and are characteristic of this tumor

Other Regional Tumors

The *giant cell tumor of the bone* can involve the spine with a particular predilection for the vertebral bodies. It can cause severe spinal cord compression due to extension into the spinal canal or due to pathologic fracture and subsequent vertebral collapse. In such circumstances the mainstay of therapy is surgery (decompressive laminectomy), in the course of which an intraoperative assessment can be solicited (Fig. 23.4).

Neurofibroma and *lipoma* (covered in previous chapters) should also be taken into account, as they may involve the epidural space and cause spinal cord compression.

The *vertebral hemangioma* (VH) is an aggregate of thin-walled blood vessels with qualities more hamartomatous than neoplastic. Most often these vascular lesions are incidental radiographic findings (a lucency defect with vertical septations) and do not cause neurological symptoms. However, VH may rarely present with a rapid onset of myelopathic symptoms. Therefore, this lesion should also be included in the differential diagnosis of regional processes that can produce spinal cord compression.

Nonneoplastic Lesions

Prolapsed disc, epidural abscess, and tuberculosis are the most common regional nonneoplastic lesions; but other infectious spondilodiscitis (i.e., brucellosis) and extramedullary hematopoiesis may also be considered. Cytologic preparations can help distinguish among all of them.

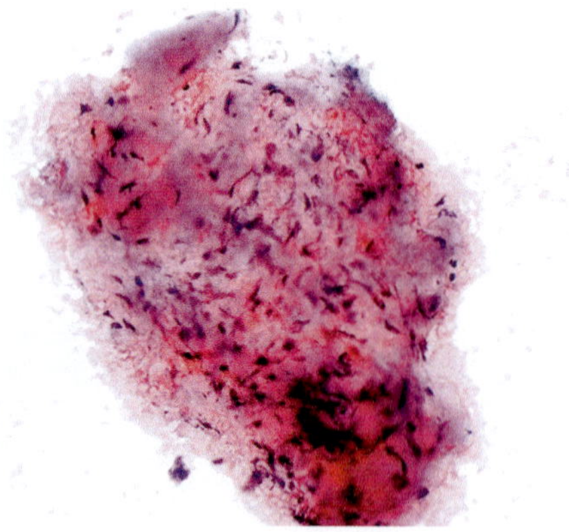

Fig. 23.5 *Herniated disc, CT-guided needle aspiration biopsy.* This preparation shows a small fragment of the herniated disc with characteristic myxoid degeneration of fibrocartilage (Smear, Papanicolaou)

Prolapsed Disc

One of the most frequent causes of spinal cord compression is the herniation of the nucleus pulposus of an intervertebral disc into the epidural space. Lumbar lesions far exceed those at other levels, followed by the cervical and lastly the thoracic spine. In certain clinical situations, this process may require differential diagnosis with vertebral tumors, in which case the performance of a CT-guided needle aspiration biopsy is indicated. The specimen smears poorly, but characteristic small fragments of degenerating fibrocartilage from the herniated disc may usually be recognized. The background is clean, and no other cellular components either inflammatory or neoplastic can be seen (Fig. 23.5).

Epidural Abscess

Spinal epidural abscesses (SEA) are more common than their intracranial counterparts, and their incidence has increased in the past decade. They are a potentially life-threatening condition that can cause paralysis by the accumulation of purulent material in the epidural space. Approximately one-third of spinal epidural abscesses arise without any apparent cause. The remainder are secondary localizations of contiguous (vertebral osteomyelitis, disc infection, decubitus ulcers) or distant infectious foci, or else they are related to invasive regional procedures, including spinal surgery, lumbar puncture, and epidural catheterization. Intravenous drug abuse, alcoholism, and diabetes mellitus are also significant risk factors. Once SEA is suspected radiographically, direct sampling of the infected fluid or tissue via image-guided needle biopsy should be performed to help confirm the diagnosis and direct antimicrobial therapy. Anterior tethering of the dura to adjacent vertebral bodies presumably accounts for the fact that most epidural abscesses are posteriorly or

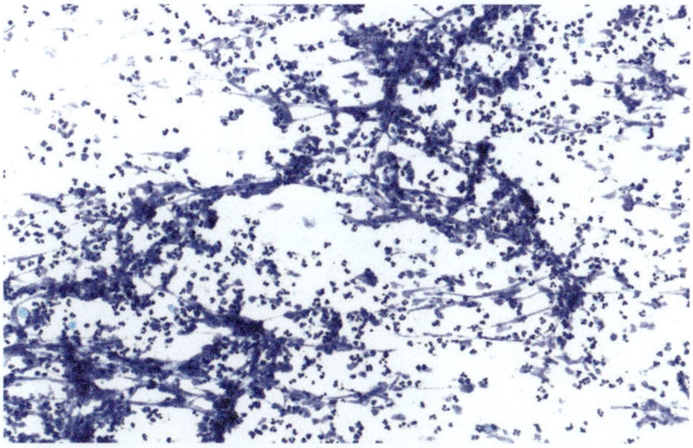

Fig. 23.6 *Epidural abscess, CT-guided needle aspiration biopsy***.** Preparation from the purulent content displaying hypersegmented neutrophils and fibrin strands (Smear, Papanicolaou)

posterolaterally positioned, facilitating the performance of an imaging-guided needle biopsy. Smears show a dirty background with sheets of neutrophils and associated granular debris (this pattern can be reported as "abscess contents, favor bacterial") (Fig. 23.6). Triaging tissue to document organisms is essential, and just as in intracranial locations, bacteria are responsible for the majority of SEA. *Staphylococcus aureus* accounts for the majority of cases (60–90%) – with methicillin-resistant *S. aureus* accounting for an increasing number – distantly trailed by gram-negative aerobes such as *E. coli* and *Pseudomonas aeruginosa*, streptococci, and various anaerobes.

Tuberculosis

The vertebral column is the most common site of osseous involvement by disseminated tuberculosis, which usually involves the thoracic segment and has its highest incidence in the first three decades of life. Although *Mycobacterium tuberculosis* is among the more common agents of spinal epidural abscess, especially among intravenous drug abusers, the lesion it produces is typically granulomatous and caseating rather than suppurative ("cold abscess"). This usually arises by extension from contiguous foci of tuberculous vertebral osteomyelitis and disc infection, giving rise to complex lesions with involvement of the vertebral column and the epidural space (Pott's disease). Common clinical manifestations include constitutional symptoms, back pain, and spinal tenderness. Without adequate treatment, subsequent vertebral collapse, spinal deformities (marked angular kyphosis), paraplegia, and tuberculous meningitis are serious complications. Neuroimaging-guided needle biopsy from the affected site is the gold standard technique for early histopathological diagnosis. Smears show the same features (necrotic or granulomatous) described previously in the intracranial tuberculomas (Figs. 23.7a, b).

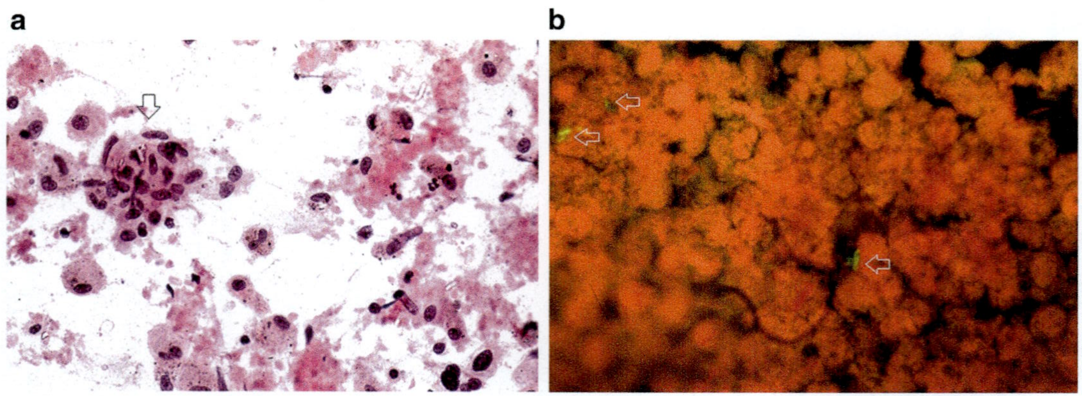

Fig. 23.7 *Vertebral tuberculosis, CT-guided needle aspiration biopsy*. (**a**) This preparation displays a clump of epithelioid cells (*arrow*), macrophages, chronic inflammatory infiltrate, and necrotic granular debris (Smear, H&E). (**b**) Fluorescence microscopy with fluorochrome dyes is more sensitive and specific than acid-fast stains. Mycobacteria fluoresce green-yellow (*arrows*) in a reddish background under ultraviolet light (Smear, auramine-rhodamine stain)

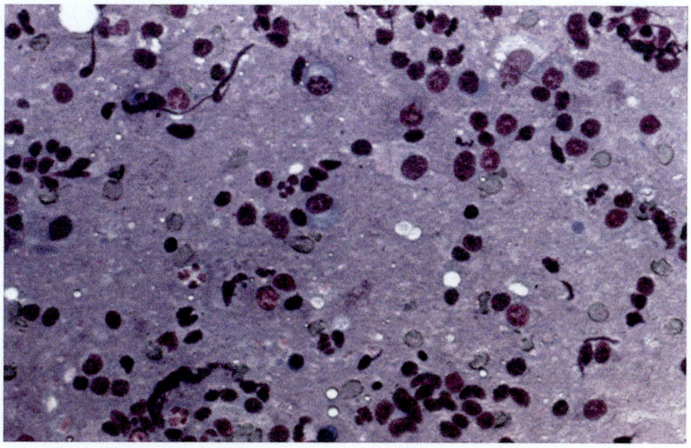

Fig. 23.8 *Vertebral brucellosis, CT-guided needle aspiration biopsy.* This preparation shows a mixed inflammatory infiltrate with mature lymphocytes, plasma cells, some neutrophils, and histiocytes. These features confirm the nonneoplastic, inflammatory nature of the process (Smear, Romanowsky)

Other Regional Nonneoplastic Processes

Brucellosis (*Malta's fever*) is a systemic disease and may affect many organ systems with frequent musculoskeletal focal complications. Involvement of the spine is one of the most common localized forms of human brucellosis, especially spondylodiscitis of the lumbar vertebrae with sacroiliitis, although no part of the spine is spared. Spinal brucellosis is a destructive disease that requires a correct and early diagnosis and immediate treatment. In certain clinical situations, this process may require differential diagnosis with other inflammatory processes or vertebral tumors, in which case the performance of a neuroimaging-guided needle biopsy is indicated. Smears show a characteristic mixed inflammatory component (mature lymphocytes, well-defined plasma cells, polymorphonuclear cells, and histiocytes) ruling out the possibility of neoplasia (Fig. 23.8). Likewise, triaging tissue to document organisms is essential; a diagnosis of brucellosis is definitive when *Brucella* organisms are recovered from blood, bone marrow, or other tissue.

Extramedullary hematopoiesis (EMH) is a rare noncancerous proliferation of hematopoietic tissue outside the bone marrow that may occur in response to chronic severe anemia, most often secondary to hematologic diseases like thalassemia or myelofibrosis. The most frequent sites of EMH are the liver, spleen, and lymph nodes but may be found in unusual sites, which include the spinal epidural space. This unexpected location may lead to mistakes in the interpretation of a neuroimaging-guided needle biopsy or during an intraoperative consultation, by confusing extramedullary hematopoietic tissue with more expected regional lesions, like malignant lymphoid processes or metastatic cancer. However, the cytologic diagnosis is very simple: we have to consider only this possibility and pay attention to the presence of elements from the three hematopoietic lineages – erythroid, myeloid, and megakaryocytic (Fig. 23.9).

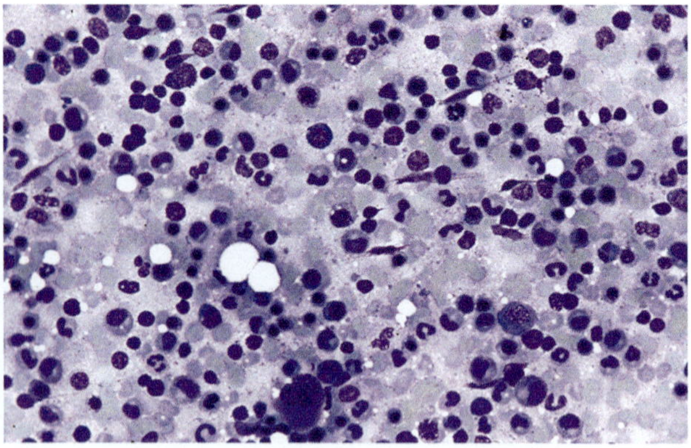

Fig. 23.9 *Extramedullary hematopoiesis, intraoperative smear.* This preparation, from a mass occupying the spinal epidural space, displays a cellular single cell pattern with myeloid, erythroid, and megakaryocytic features (Smear, Romanowsky)

Suggested Reading

Aithala JP. Role of percutaneous image guided biopsy in spinal lesions: adequacy and correlation with MRI findings. J Clin Diagn Res. 2016;10:RC11–5.

Akhtar I, Flowers R, Siddiqi A, Heard K, Baliga M. Fine needle aspiration biopsy of vertebral and paravertebral lesions: retrospective study of 124 cases. Acta Cytol. 2006;50:364–71.

Alp E, Doganay M. Current therapeutic strategy in spinal brucellosis. Int J Infect Dis. 2008;12:573–7.

Bilsky MH, Lis E, Raizer J, Lee H, Boland P. The diagnosis and treatment of metastatic spinal tumor. Oncologist. 1999;4:459–69.

Bond A, Manian FA. Spinal epidural abscess: a review with special emphasis on earlier diagnosis. Biomed Res Int. 2016;2016:1614328.

Chakraborti C, Miller KL. Multiple myeloma presenting as spinal cord compression: a case report. J Med Case Rep. 2010;4:251.

Cristallini EG, Ascani S, Paganelli C, Peciarolo A, Bolis GB. Role of fine-needle aspiration biopsy in the assessment of sacrococcygeal masses. Diagn Cytopathol. 1991;7:618–21.

Cugati G, Singh M, Pande A, Ramamurthi R, et al. Primary spinal epidural lymphomas. J Craniovertebr Junction Spine. 2011;2:3–11.

Darouiche RO. Spinal epidural abscess. N Engl J Med. 2006;355:2012–20.

Ezenekwe AM, Collins BT, Ponder TB. Fine needle aspiration biopsy of precursor B-cell lymphoblastic lymphoma presenting as a sacral mass. A case report. Acta Cytol. 2004;48:239–42.

Garg RK, Somvanshi DS. Spinal tuberculosis: a review. J Spinal Cord Med. 2011;34:440–54.

Ghelman B, Lospinuso MF, Levine DB, O'Leary PF, Burke SW. Percutaneous computed-tomography-guided biopsy of the thoracic and lumbar spine. Spine. 1991;16:736–9.

Gupta S, Takhtani D, Gulati M, Khandelwal N, et al. Sonographically guided fine needle aspiration biopsy of lytic lesions of the spine: technique and indications. J Clin Ultrasound. 1999;27:123–9.

Kay PA, Nascimento AG, Unni KK, Salomão DR. Chordoma. Cytomorphologic findings in 14 cases diagnosed by fine needle aspiration. Acta Cytol. 2003;47:202–8.

Kelley SP, Ashford RU, Rao AS, Dickson RA. Primary bone tumors of the spine: a 42-year survey from the Leeds Regional Bone Tumor Registry. Eur Spine J. 2007;16:405–9.

Monti L, Romano DG, Gozzetti A, Di Pietro G, Miracco C, Cerase A. Myelodysplasia presenting as a thoracic spinal epidural extramedullary hematopoiesis: a rare treatable cause of spinal cord myelopathy. Skelet Radiol. 2012;41:611–4.

Ozerdemoglu RA, Transfeldt EE, Thompson RC. Lumbosacral chordoma: prognostic factors and treatment. Spine. 1999;24:1639–45.

Perrin RG, Laxton AW. Metastatic spine disease: epidemiology, pathophysiology, and evaluation of patients. Neurosurg Clin N Am. 2004;15:365–73.

Phadke DM, Lucas DR, Madan S. Fine-needle aspiration biopsy of vertebral and intervertebral disc lesions: specimen adequacy, diagnostic utility, and pitfalls. Arch Pathol Lab Med. 2001;125:1463–8.

Saad RS, Clary KM, Liu Y, Silverman JF, Raab SS. Fine needle aspiration biopsy of vertebral lesions. Acta Cytol. 2004;48:39–46.

Saenz-Santamaria J, Catalina-Fernandez I. Fine needle aspiration diagnosis of extramedullary hematopoiesis resembling mediastinal and paravesical tumors. Acta Cytol. 2004;48:95–8.

Salehi SA, Koski T, Ondra SL. Spinal cord compression in beta-thalassemia: case report and review of the literature. Spinal Cord. 2004;42:117–23.

Sanjay BK, Sim FH, Unni KK, McLeod RA, Klassen RA. Giant cell tumors of the spine. J Bone Joint Surg Br. 1993;75:148–54.

Spinazzé S, Caraceni A, Schrijvers D. Epidural spinal cord compression. Crit Rev Oncol Hematol. 2005;56:397–406.

Stoker DJ, Kissin CM. Percutaneous vertebral biopsy: a review of 135 cases. Clin Radiol. 1985;36:569–77.

Syed R, Bishop JA, Ali SZ. Sacral and presacral lesions: cytopathologic analysis and clinical correlates. Diagn Cytopathol. 2012;40:7–13.

Tehranzadeh J, Tao C, Browning CA. Percutaneous needle biopsy of the spine. Acta Radiol. 2007;48(8):860–8.

Tekkök IH, Berker M, Ozcan OE, Ozgen T, Akalin E. Brucellosis of the spine. Neurosurgery. 1993;33:838–44.

Templin CR, Stambough JB, Stambough JL. Acute spinal cord compression caused by vertebral hemangioma. Spine J. 2004;4:595–600.

Wang A, Carberry N, Solli E, Gillick J, Islam H, Hillard V. Spinal cord compression secondary to extramedullary hematopoiesis: case report and review of the literature. Case Rep Oncol. 2016;9:290–7.

Appendix A: Diagnoses that May Change the Surgical Approach

It is well known that during neurosurgical intraoperative consultation, the main role of the pathologist is to confirm that a diagnostic tissue sample has been obtained, but in the course of a craniotomy or laminectomy, there are occasions when the diagnosis does impact on the surgical approach. Therefore, in such scenario, attempt to respond the following questions also are necessary:

- Is the disease process a neoplasm of a type that is amenable to a total resection?
- Or, by the contrary, further resection could actually be potentially detrimental for the patient?

The following list summarizes the role of the surgery in various CNS tumors:

1. *Tumors for which surgical resection is the treatment of choice*

   Well-demarcated gliomas

   - Pilocytic astrocytoma
   - Ependymoma (any grade)
   - Myxopapillary ependymoma
   - Subependymoma
   - Pleomorphic xanthoastrocytoma
   - Subependymal giant cell astrocytoma
   - Focal and dorsally exophytic brainstem gliomas
   - Chordoid glioma

   Meningioma
   Nerve sheath tumors
   Pituitary adenoma
   Craniopharyngioma

C. R. Lacruz et al., *Central Nervous System Intraoperative Cytopathology*,
Essentials in Cytopathology 13, https://doi.org/10.1007/978-3-319-98491-9

Neuronal and mixed neuronal-glial tumors
Hemangioblastoma
Teratoma
Choroid plexus papilloma
Paraganglioma of the filum terminale
Pineocytoma
Angiocentric glioma

2. *Malignant tumors with improved prognosis after total resection/debulking*

Medulloblastoma
Atypical teratoid/rhabdoid tumor
Choroid plexus carcinoma
Solitary metastasis

3. *Representative tumors treated with radiation therapy or chemotherapy rather than aggressive surgical resection*

Diffuse gliomas
Lymphoma (primary or metastatic)
Germinoma
Metastatic small-cell lung carcinoma

All of the group 1 neoplasms are usually associated with a favorable or improved prognosis post resection; thus, surgery should be pursued to avoid harmful adjuvant therapies. On the contrary, a radical surgical approach may be more harmful than beneficial in the case of group 3 processes.

Appendix B: Troubleshooting with CNS Intraoperative Consultation

During intraoperative consultation special care should be taken to avoid the following pitfalls:

- Failure to consider that the biopsy may not be representative of the lesion (evaluation of the microscopic findings in the clinico-radiologic setting is critical to avoid this)
- Failure to consider nonneoplastic processes
- Overgrading of neoplastic lesions

The following list summarizes the most characteristics intraoperative diagnostic dilemmas/pitfalls with reference to the page/s in the text where they are discussed.

Troubleshooting with CNS intraoperative consultation

Diagnostic dilemma/pitfall	Page/s
Low-grade astrocytoma vs reactive gliosis	68–74
Pilocytic astrocytoma vs diffuse astrocytoma (any grade)	106
Pilocytic astrocytoma vs pilocytic gliosis	71–74, 110
Glioblastoma vs metastatic carcinoma vs lymphoma	95, 276, 305
PXA vs high-grade diffuse astrocytoma	115
SEGA vs high-grade diffuse astrocytoma	111
Oligodendroglioma vs diffuse astrocytoma vs oligoastrocytoma	125
Ependymoma vs diffuse astrocytoma	134
Anaplastic ependymoma vs embryonal tumors	134–138, 197
Choroid plexus papilloma vs papillary ependymoma	160
Choroid plexus carcinoma vs metastatic adenocarcinoma vs AT/RT	160–163
Embryonal tumors vs lymphoma vs metastatic small-cell carcinoma	197–199, 276
Meningioma vs metastatic carcinoma	228–230

(continued)

C. R. Lacruz et al., *Central Nervous System Intraoperative Cytopathology*, Essentials in Cytopathology 13, https://doi.org/10.1007/978-3-319-98491-9

(continued)

Diagnostic dilemma/pitfall	Page/s
Hemangioblastoma vs metastatic renal cell carcinoma	234–236
Schwannoma vs fibrous meningioma vs SFT	239, 286
Craniopharyngioma (surrounding gliosis) vs pilocytic astrocytoma	382
Germinoma vs pineoblastoma vs lymphoma	258
Ganglioglioma vs glioma infiltrating gray matter	179–182
Cerebral abscess vs glioblastoma	332–334
Tumefactive demyelination vs glioma	341–345
Cerebral infarction vs glioma	345
Normal cerebellar cortex vs medulloblastoma	65, 197–199
Normal white mater vs low-grade glioma	61–62
Normal gray matter vs glioneural mixed tumors	62–64
Normal choroid plexus vs choroid plexus papilloma	65, 160
Normal leptomeninges vs meningioma	68
Normal pineal gland vs pineocytoma	68, 362
Normal pituitary gland vs pituitary adenoma	377

PXA pleomorphic xanthoastrocytoma, *SEGA* subependymal giant cell astrocytoma, *AT/RT* atypical teratoid/rhabdoid tumor, *SFT* solitary fibrous tumor

Index

A
Abt-Letterer-Siwe disease, 277
Accuracy
    absolute precision, 7
    CNS intraoperative cytopathology, 5, 6
    stereotactic biopsy, 6
Acute bacterial infection, 332
Acute inflammatory-cell-rich lesions
    brain abscesses, 332, 334
    epidural abscess, 334
    polymorphonuclear leukocytes, 332
    subdural empyema, 334
Acute tissue destruction, 332
Adamantinomatous/pediatric type, 380–383
Adenohypophyseal cells, 373
Adult pineal gland, 68
Aicardi syndrome, 155, 324
Algorithmic approach
    background and related processes, 44, 46
    blood vessels, 46
    cell types, 48, 52
    general-category interpretation
        abnormal, 57
        glial *vs.* non-glial, 59
        low- *vs.* high-grade, 59
        neoplastic, 57
        non-neoplastic, 59
    intraoperative diagnosis, 59
    neurosurgeon's primary interest, 59
    sample triage, 41–42
    smear evaluation, 42, 43
    smearing, type of, 44
    specific cell groups and tumors types, 48, 51
    specific cellular elements, 48, 51, 57
Anaplastic astrocytoma, 3, 8, 89
    characteristics, 89, 91
    cytologic features, 89, 90
    differential diagnosis, 89, 91
    histology, 80, 82
    IDH1/2 genes, 80, 82
Anaplastic ependymoma, 129, 132, 134, 137, 138
Anaplastic hemangiopericytoma, 237
Anaplastic medulloblastoma, 186, 192
Anaplastic meningiomas, 208, 222
Anaplastic oligodendroglioma, 120, 122
    cytologic features, 125, 126
    differential diagnosis, 125, 127
    IDH gene family mutation, 120
Anaplastic pilocytic astrocytoma, 105
Anaplastic PXA, 113
Ancient neurofibroma, 286, 288, 293
Angiocentric glioma
    characteristics, 150
    cytologic features, 148, 150
    descriptions, 147
    differential diagnosis, 148, 150
    histology, 149
    MRI, 147
Angiomatous meningioma, 218
Antoni B component, 284
Arachnoid cyst, 325, 326
Astroblastoma
    characteristics, 148
    cytologic features, 147, 148
    description, 145
    differential diagnosis, 147, 148
    histologic groups, 145
    histologic pattern, 145

C. R. Lacruz et al., *Central Nervous System Intraoperative Cytopathology*,
Essentials in Cytopathology 13, https://doi.org/10.1007/978-3-319-98491-9

Astroblastoma (*cont.*)
histology, 146
MRI, 145
prognosis, 145
Astrocytes, 343
Astrocytic tumors
diffuse, 79
astrocytoma (*see* Diffuse astrocytoma)
midline glioma, 100
nondiffuse, 79
Astrocytoma
anaplastic, 80, 82
diagnostics, 82, 84
diffuse (*see* Diffuse astrocytoma)
gliomatosis, 100, 102–104
PA (*see* Pilocytic astrocytoma (PA))
PMA, 105
protoplasmic, 84
PXA (*see* Pleomorphic xanthoastrocytoma (PXA))
SEGAs (*see* Subependymal giant cell astrocytomas (SEGAs))
Atypical adenoma, 375
Atypical choroid plexus papilloma, 160
Atypical meningioma, 215, 223
Atypical mycobacteria infection, 337, 342
Atypical papilloma, 156
Atypical teratoid/rhabdoid tumor (AT/RT), 160, 163, 197, 387
cytologic features, 204, 205
differential diagnosis, 203, 205
histology, 202
malignant polyphenotypic neoplasm, 199
symptoms, 199
tumors, 199

B

Benign cystic lesions
classification, 319
columnar to cuboidal epithelium-lined cysts, 322–325
differential diagnosis, 319
epithelial-lining cysts, 319
neuraxis, 319, 320
neuroaxis, 320
non-epithelial-lining cysts, 319, 325–327
squamous epithelium-lined cysts, 319–322
Blood vessels, 43, 46, 47
Bone pathology, 17
BRAF V600E mutations, 380
Brain abscesses, 331–334
Brain biopsies, 42
Brain lesions
genetic disorders and CNS tumors, 18
neuroimaging evaluation (*see* Neuroimaging evaluation)
topography and symptoms and signs, 16–17
Brain neoplasm
genetic disorders and CNS tumors, 17–18
history of, 16
"M-rule", differential diagnosis, 25
Brain tumors
classification, 8
cytologic method, 5
initial study, 4
smear diagnosis, brain biopsies, 5
Breast carcinoma, 305, 310
Brucellosis (Malta's fever), 401
Butterfly lesions, 80

C

Carcinoma, 156
Carney complex, 290
Cellular schwannoma, 284, 286, 288
Central Brain Tumor Registry of the United States (CBTRUS), 233
Central nervous system (CNS)
acute inflammatory cell-rich lesions, 332–334
brain lesions, 331
clinico-radiologic correlation, 15
cytologic method, 331
epithelioid-cell-rich lesions (*see* Epithelioid-cell-rich lesions)
frozen sections, 1, 2
infectious-inflammatory lesions in AIDS (*see* Infectious-inflammatory lesions in AIDS)
intraoperative consultation, 407
macrophage-rich lesions (*see* Macrophage-rich lesions)
neoplasia, types of, 7
non-neoplastic disorders, 331
perivascular chronic inflammatory cell-rich lesions, 334–336
role of surgery, 405, 406
smear technique (*see* Smear technique)
troubleshooting, 407, 408
tumors, WHO classification, 7–9
vasculitis, 331, 335, 336
Central neurocytoma
cerebellar liponeurocytoma, 172
cytologic features, 175

extraventricular location, 172
neuroimaging, 172
Cerebellar cortex, 65, 66
Cerebellar liponeurocytoma, 172
Cerebral ganglioneuroblastoma, 194, 195, 197, 199, 201
Cerebral infarction, 345, 346
Cerebral neuroblastoma, 194, 195, 197, 198, 201
Cerebritis, 332
Chordoid glioma
characteristic, 152
cytologic features, 150, 152
description, 150
differential diagnosis, 152
histology, 151
optimal treatment, 150
symptoms, 150
tumor cells, 150
Chordoid meningioma, 222, 224
Chordoma, 248–250, 391, 394, 396
Choriocarcinoma, 263, 266, 267
Choroid plexus, 65, 67
Choroid plexus carcinomas (CPCs), 156, 160, 163
Choroid plexus cyst, 324
Choroid plexus papillomas (CPPs), 156, 160
Choroid plexus tumors (CPTs)
Aicardi syndrome, 155
characteristics, 163
choroid plexus neoplasms, 155
CPPs (*see* Choroid plexus papillomas (CPPs))
cytologic features, 163
differential diagnosis, 163
Li-Fraumeni syndrome, 155
in neuroimaging, 155
prevalence, 155
supratentorial cases, 155
surgical resection, 156
types, 156
Chronic active encephalitis, 347
Circumscribed astrocytomas, 103
Clear cell ependymoma, 132, 133, 136
Clear cell meningioma, 207, 225
Clinical approach
age and location, 16
family history, 17–18
focal clinical signs, 16
lesional topography and symptoms/signs, 17
medical history, 16
CNS ganglioneuroblastoma, 39
CNS lymphoma, 34
CNS metastasis
characteristics, 315
in children, 301
craniospinal bone, 302
cytology, 304, 305
diagnosis, 304
meningeal, 302
parenchymal, 302
Coagulative necrosis, 100
Colloid cyst, third ventricle, 322–324
Colonic carcinoma, 305
Columnar to cuboidal epithelium-lined cysts
choroid plexus cyst, 324
colloid cyst, 322–324
cytologic features, 324, 325
differential diagnosis, 324, 325
endodermal (enterogenous) cyst, 323
ependymal cyst, 323–324
Rathke cleft cyst, 322, 323, 325
Computed tomography (CT)
calcification and hemorrhage, 19
emergency CT scans, 19
interpretation/terminology, 19
intravenous iodinated contrast, 20
as screening tool, 19
Contaminants, 74, 75
Conventional schwannoma, 284
Craniopharyngioma, 377, 380, 382, 383
adamantinomatous/pediatric type, 380, 381
bimodal distribution, 380
characteristics, 382, 385, 386
clinical features, 380
cytologic features, 382–384
differential diagnosis, 382, 385, 386
papillary variant/adult type, 380, 381
sellar and suprasellar region, 380
solid masses, 380
sphenoid sinus, 380
xanthogranulomatous, 380
Cytokeratins 8/18, 375
Cytologic method, 4, 5
Cytology
angiocentric glioma, 148, 150
astroblastoma, 147, 148
AT/RT, 203, 205
brain biopsies, 5, 42
central neurocytomas, 175
chordoid glioma, 150, 152
chordoma, 248
CNS metastasis, 305
CNS PNETs, 194, 201
CPTs, 156, 160, 163
cytologic method, 4
cytological preparations, 32

Cytology (*cont.*)
DIA/DIG, 172
DNTs, 166
ependymomas, 132, 134, 138
EWS, 245
fibrosarcomas, 248
ganglion cell tumors, 169
general-category interpretation, 57
germinomas, 258, 259
hemangioblastoma, 236
LCH, 278
lipoma, 241
medulloblastoma, 189
meningiomas
common meningioma variants, 211
extracranial meningiomas, 228
grade II meningiomas, 215, 222
grade III meningiomas, 222
uncommon meningioma variants, 211, 215
myxopapillary ependymoma, 141, 143
osteosarcoma, 250
paraganglioma, 179
preparation, 3
RGNTs, 175
rhabdomyosarcoma, 243
schwannomas, 284
SFT, 237, 239
stains, 5
subependymomas, 139, 141
Cytomegalovirus (CMV) encephalitis, 345, 352, 353

D

Demyelinating disorders, 331, 332
Dermoid cysts, 320, 321
Desmoplastic infantile astrocytoma and ganglioglioma (DIA/DIG)
cytologic features, 172
description, 169
manifestations, 169
molecular profile, 172
Desmoplastic medulloblastoma, 186, 191, 201
DICER1 gene, 362
Diffuse astrocytoma
butterfly lesions, 80
characteristics, 88
cytologic features, 84
dedifferentiation/malignancy, 80
diagnostics, 82, 84
differential diagnosis, 88
fibrillary/gemistocytic features, 80
fibrillary variant, 84, 85
gemistocytic variant, 84, 86
glioblastoma, 79, 80, 83
histology, 80, 81
IDH1/2 genes, 80, 82
ill-delimited neoplasms, 80
MGMT, 82
MRI, 80
protoplasmic variant, 84, 87
symptoms, 80
Diffuse gliomas, 119, 120, 125, 127
Diffuse large B-cell type (DLBCL), 270
histology, 270
lymphoma, 272
prominent nucleoli, 273
stereotactic biopsy, 274
Diffuse midline glioma, 100
Diffusion-weighted imaging (DWI), 21
Dopamine agonists therapy, 375
Dysembryoplastic neuroepithelial tumors (DNTs)
cytologic features, 166
multinodular neoplasms, 165
neuroimaging, 165
specific glioneural element, 165
temporal lobe, 165

E

Embryonal carcinoma, 256, 258, 263, 266, 267
Embryonal rhabdomyosarcoma, 244
Embryonal tumor with abundant neuropil and true rosettes (ETANTR), 189, 193
Embryonal tumor with multilayered rosettes (ETMR), 189, 193, 194, 197
Encephalitis, 331, 334–336, 345, 347, 352, 353
Endocrinologically silent, 374
Endodermal (enterogenous) cyst, 323
Eosinophilic granuloma of bone, 277
Ependymal cyst, 323, 324
Ependymal tumors
ependymoma, 129, 130 (*see also* Ependymoma)
histologic types, 129
myxopapillary ependymoma (*see* Myxopapillary ependymoma)
subependymoma (*see* Subependymoma)
Ependymoblastoma, 194, 197
Ependymoma
anaplastic, 132
characteristics, 129, 130, 138
classic, 130
clear cell, 132
cytologic features, 132, 134
differential diagnosis, 134

of fourth ventricle, 130
histologic features, 130
immunohistochemical staining pattern, 132
molecular groups, 129
neuroimaging, 130
papillary, 132
"placenta-like" borders, 130
supratentorial, 130
tanycytic, 132
and variants, 129
Epidermoid cyst, 319–321
Epidural abscess, 397–399
Epidural lymphomas, 392
Epithelioid-cell-rich lesions, *see* Granulomatous inflammation
Epithelioid glioblastoma, 95, 99
Erdheim-Chester disease, 276, 278
Ewing sarcoma (EWS), 243, 245, 246
Extracranial meningioma, 228
Extramedullary hematopoiesis (EMH), 397, 401, 402

F
Familial tumor syndromes, 17–18
Fast staining methods
hematoxylin and eosin method, 35–37
modified fast Romanowsky stain, 37–38
Papanicolaou method, 37
toluidine blue method, 38–39
Felt-like neuropil, 71
Fibrillary variant, 84, 85
Fibrosarcomas, 245, 247, 248
Fibrous meningioma, 208, 209, 211, 214
Fluid-attenuated inversion recovery (FLAIR), 21

G
Gangliocytic paraganglioma, 179
Gangliocytoma
dysmorphic ganglion cells, 169
and ganglioglioma, 169
histology, 168
with minimal glial component, 166
Ganglioglioma
brainstem, 169
cytologic features, 171
desmoplastic infantile, 173
DIA/DIG, 169
dysmorphic ganglion cells, 169
imaging features, 181
vs. infiltrating glioma, 182
malignant transformation, 169
neuroimaging, 166
neuronal component, 166
Ganglion cell tumors
cytologic features, 169
description, 166
gangliogliomas, 169
neuroimaging, 166
Ganglioneuromas, 297, 298
Gemistocytic variant, 84, 86
General-category interpretation, 58
abnormal, 57
glial *vs.* non-glial, 59
low- *vs.* high-grade, 59
nonneoplastic, 59
and smear evaluation, 41
Germ cell group, 359
Germinomas, 255, 359, 362, 368, 377
characteristics, 261
cytology, 258, 259
differential diagnosis, 258
histology, 257
iGCTs, 256
immature teratoma, 260
inflammatory reaction, 260
prognosis, 256
Giant cell glioblastoma, 95, 97, 111, 113
Giant cell tumor of bone, 397
Glial cyst, 326
Glial neoplasms, 145, 147
Glioblastoma, 47, 48, 79, 80
cell types, 95, 96
characteristics, 102
cytology, 89, 92
differential diagnosis, 95, 100–102
epithelioid, 95, 99
fibrillary, 91
giant cell, 95, 97
gliosarcoma, 95, 98
histology, 80, 83
morphologic variants, 95
necrosis, 91, 93
necrotic-fibrillary, 91
vascular changes, 91, 94
Gliomatosis
clinicoradiologic pattern, 100
cytologic features, 103, 104
differential diagnosis, 103
histologic pattern, 102
symptoms, 102
Gliosarcoma, 95, 98, 115
Gliosis
astrocytoma, 68
contaminants, 74, 75
diagnosis, 71

Gliosis (*cont.*)
felt-like neuropil, 71
vs. low-grade astrocytoma, 68, 71, 74
piloid, 71, 74
reactive, 71–73
stereotypic tissue, 68
Goblet cells, 380
Granular cell pituicytoma, 384
Granular cell tumor, 384, 386
Granulomatous inflammation
classification, 336
CNS, 336
mycobacterial infections, 337, 339–341
neurosarcoidosis, 337, 338
Gray matter, 62, 64
Growing teratoma syndrome, 266
Gyriform calcification, 119

H
Hand-Schüller-Christian disease, 277
Hemangioblastoma, 233–235, 237
Hemangiopericytoma (HPC), 238
cytologic features, 239
differential diagnosis, 239, 241
12q13 locus, 237
Herniated disc, 398
High-grade lymphomas, 392
Highly active antiretroviral therapy (HAART), 269
Histiocytic sarcoma, 276, 278, 280
Histogenesis, 145
Historical background, 4–5
Hodgkin/non-Hodgkin lymphoma, 392
Homer-Wright/Flexner-Wintersteiner rosettes, 365, 367
Hyperchromatism, 113
Hypersecretory syndrome, 374
Hypophysitis, 388
Hypothalamic hamartomas (HHs), 374, 387

I
Immune reconstitution inflammatory syndrome (IRIS), 336, 353
Infant pineal gland, 68
Infectious encephalitis, 335
Infectious-inflammatory lesions in AIDS
CMV encephalitis, 352, 353
lymphoma, 345
PML, 349–351, 353
toxoplasmosis, 345, 347, 348
Infiltrating astrocytoma, 80
Inflammatory pseudotumor/plasma cell granuloma, 388
Intracranial germ cell tumors (iGCTs), 255, 256, 258, 261
Intracranial histiocytic tumors, 277
Intraoperative assessment, 397
Intraoperative brain assessment, 248, 258, 266, 271, 295, 301, 373
algorithmic approach (*see* Algorithmic approach)
CPTs (*see* Choroid plexus tumors (CPTs))
embryonal tumor (*see* Embryonal tumor)
ependymal tumors (*see* Ependymal tumors)
meningiomas, 207
Intraoperative consultation, 1, 7
Intraparenchymal metastases, 302, 303
Invasive adenomas, 375
Isocitrate dehydrogenase-1 or -2 (*IDH1/2*) genes, 80, 82

J
JC polyomavirus, 349
Juvenile xanthogranuloma, 278

K
Keratin, 48, 54, 57

L
Langerhans cell histiocytosis (LCH), 276, 278
Large-cell/anaplastic medulloblastoma, 186, 192
Leptomeninges, 65, 68, 69
Leptomyelolipomas, 241
Li-Fraumeni syndrome, 155
Lipoma, 239, 241, 242, 397
Lipomeningocele, 239
Low-grade lymphoma, 394
Lymphocytic hypophysitis, 388
Lymphoma, 301, 345, 392–394
Lymphoplasmacyte-rich meningioma, 219

M
Macrophage-rich lesions
authentic rarities, 341
definitive diagnosis, 341, 343
nonneoplastic disorder, 341
TLDLs, 341, 343–345
Magnetic resonance imaging (MRI)
CNS lymphoma, 23

ependymoma, 20
glioblastoma, WHO grade IV, 22
interpretation/terminology, 20
metastasis, 21, 24
multiplanar capability, 21
sequences, 21
T1-weighted, 21
T2-weighted, 21
Magnetic resonance spectroscopy (MRS), 22, 23, 25
Malignant peripheral nerve sheath tumors (MPNSTs), 288, 295–297
MALT-lymphoma, dura, 276
Medulloblastoma, 365
characteristics, 188
cytologic features, 189
diagnostic approach, 189
etiology, 186
macroscopically, 186
microscopically, 186
symptoms, 186
Medulloepithelioma, 189, 193, 194
Melanin, 43, 48, 51, 55, 57
Melanotic schwannoma (MS), 284, 289–292
Meningeal carcinomatosis, 301
Meningioma
characteristics, 230
cytologic features (*see* Cytology)
differential diagnosis, 228, 229
"en plaque" meningioma, 208
immunomarkers, 210
mutations, 207
neuroaxis, 207
in neuroimaging, 207
prevalence, 207
symptoms, 207
tumor cells, 208
WHO 2016 classification scheme, 208
WHO 2016 grading criteria, 210
Meningothelial meningioma, 208, 209
Metastasis
adenocarcinoma, 307
breast carcinoma, 310
carcinoma, 306
CNS (*see* CNS metastasis)
colonic adenocarcinoma, 313
melanoma, 314
renal cell carcinoma, 311
small-cell carcinoma, 309
squamous carcinoma, 308
urothelial cell carcinoma, 312
Metastatic brain tumors
clinical symptoms, 301
cytology, 305
diagnosis, 304
differential diagnosis, 305, 315
histology, 304
imaging features, 303
intraparenchymal metastases, 303
Metastatic carcinoma vs. lymphoma, 393
Metastatic tumors, 392, 393
Microadenomas, 374, 375
Microbiopsy, 32
Microcalcifications, 120
Microcystic meningioma, 215, 217
Microvascular proliferation (MVP), 46
Minimally invasive neurosurgical techniques, 5
Mixed germ cell tumor, 258, 261
Mixed glioneural tumors, 165
Morris method, 5
Mucin, 48, 56, 57
Mucosa-associated lymphoid tissue (MALT), 270
Multiple sclerosis (MS), 341
Mycobacterial infections, 337, 339–341
Mycobacterial pseudotumor, 337
Mycobacterium tuberculosis, 399
Myeloma, 391, 394, 395
Myxopapillary ependymoma, 36
characteristics, 143
cytologic features, 141, 143
differential diagnosis, 143
histology, 141, 142
in young to middle-age adults, 141

N
Native pineal gland, 68, 70
Necrosis, 304
Neoplastic lesions
sellar region
AT/RT, 387
granular cell tumor, 384, 386
paraganglioma, 387
pituicytoma, 384
pituitary blastoma, 386
spindle cell oncocytoma, 384
spine and epidural space
chordoma, 394, 396
cytologic preparations, 391
giant cell tumor of bone, 397
lymphoma, 392–394
metastatic tumors, 392, 393
myeloma, 394, 395
neurofibroma and lipoma, 397
neurological complication, 391
VH, 397

Neuroaxis, 319, 320
Neurofibroma, 290, 293–295, 397
Neurofibromatosis type 1 (NF-1), 103, 293, 295, 297
Neurofibromatosis type 2 (NF-2), 129, 207, 283, 289
Neuroimaging evaluation
- calcifications and cysts, 25, 28
- contrast enhancement, patterns of, 25–29
- edema, necrosis and bleeding, 25, 28–29
- as gamuts, lesions, 27
- intraparenchymal/intraventricular, 23–25
- multifocality, 25
- neural tissue/brain/cord, 25

Neuroimaging-guided FNA, 394
Neuroimaging modalities, 1
- CT, 19, 20
- MRI, 20, 21
- PET, 23
- principles, 17, 19
- proton MRS, 22, 23, 25
- Thallium-201 SPECT, 23

Neuronal tumors, 165
Neurosarcoidosis, 337, 338
Nodular medulloblastoma, 186, 201
Non-epithelial-lining cysts
- arachnoid cyst, 325, 326
- glial cyst, 326
- pineal cyst, 326, 327

Non-germinomatous germ cell tumors (NGGCTs), 160, 263, 266, 267
Noninfectious perivascular chronic inflammation, 336
Nonkeratinizing squamous metaplasia, 322
Non-Langerhans cell histiocytosis, 277
Non-meningothelial mesenchymal tumors
- benign and malignant, 233, 234
- CNS, 233, 234

Non-neoplastic disorders
- CNS, 331

Non-neoplastic lesions
- sellar region
  - HHs, 387
  - hypophysitis, 388
  - inflammatory pseudotumor/plasma cell granuloma, 388
  - sphenoid sinus mucoceles, 388
  - xanthogranuloma, 387
- spine and epidural space
  - brucellosis (Malta's fever), 401
  - EMH, 401, 402
  - epidural abscess, 398, 399
  - prolapsed disc, 398
  - tuberculosis, 399, 400

Normal brain
- cerebellar cortex, 65, 66
- choroid plexus, 65, 67
- gray matter, 62, 64
- leptomeninges, 65, 68, 69
- and misdiagnosis, 68, 71
- native pineal gland, 68, 70
- pineal pattern, 68, 70
- white matter, 61–63

O

Oligoastrocytoma, 125
Oligodendroglial tumors, *see* Oligodendroglioma
Oligodendroglioma
- anaplastic, 120, 122
- calcification, 119
- category, diffuse gliomas, 119
- characteristics, 127
- cytologic features, 120, 123–125
- diagnosis, 119, 120, 125
- differential diagnosis, 125, 127
- gyriform calcification, 119
- histologic features, 120, 121
- IDH gene family mutation, 120
- macroscopically, 119
- survival times, 120
- symptoms, 119
- white matter, 119

O6-methylguanine-DNA methyltransferase (MGMT), 82
Oncocytic pituicytoma, 384
Osteosarcoma, 250, 251

P

Pancytokeratins, 369
Papillary craniopharyngioma, 380
Papillary ependymoma, 132
- *See also* Myxopapillary ependymoma

Papillary meningioma, 222, 226
Papillary tumor, 359
Papillary tumor of the pineal region (PTPR)
- cytokeratin 18, 369
- cytologic features, 369, 370
- differential diagnosis, 369, 370
- microscopic evaluation, 369
- neuroimaging, 369
- pancytokeratins, 369
- *PTEN*, 369
- symptoms, 368

Papillary variant/adult type, 380, 381

Papilloma, 156
Paraganglioma, 387
Percutaneous image-guided biopsy, 392
Percutaneous image-guided needle biopsy, 391
Perivascular chronic inflammatory cell-rich lesions
  CNS, 334, 335
  infectious encephalitis, 335
  noninfectious, 336
Physaliphorous, 394
Pilocytic astrocytoma (PA)
  anaplastic, 105
  angiocentric arrangement, 106
  biphasic pattern, 105
  bipolar astrocytes, 105
  characteristics, 106–110
  chemotherapy, 105
  in children and young adults, 103
  cytologic features, 106–109
  cytoplasmic processes, 105
  differential diagnosis, 106, 110
  EGBs, 106
  hyalinized and glomeruloid vessels, 106
  intra-/para-tumoral cyst formation, 105
  neuroimaging, 103
  NF-1, 103
  PMA, 105
  prognosis, 105
  RFs, 106
Piloid astroglial tissue, 74
Piloid gliosis, 71, 74
Pilomyxoid astrocytoma (PMA), 105, 147, 148
Pineal cyst, 326, 327, 359
Pineal parenchymal tumors (PPTs), 359–362, 369
Pineal pattern, 68, 70
Pineal region
  brain tumors in adults, 359
  germ cell group, 359
  intraoperative consultation, 359
  metastases, 359
  non-neoplastic lesions, 359, 360
  papillary tumor, 359
  pineoblastoma, 362, 365–368
  pineocytoma (*see* Pineocytoma)
  radioresistant, 359
  regional approach, 359
  treatment planning, 359
Pineoblastoma
  clinical presentation, 362
  cytologic features, 365, 367
  DICER1 gene, 362
  embryonal neoplasm, 362
  macroscopically, 362
  microscopically, 365
  multimodal therapy, 365
  neoplastic cells, 362, 366
  neuroimaging, 362
  PPTs, 362
  RB1 mutation, 362
  trilateral retinoblastoma, 362
Pineocytoma
  characteristics, 360, 362, 365
  cytologic features, 362–364
  differential diagnosis, 362, 365
  macroscopically, 360
  microscopically, 360
  neuroimaging, 360
  neuronal markers, 360
  pineocytomatous rosettes, 360, 361
  PPTID, 361
  radiotherapy, 360
  symptomatology characteristics, 360
  WHO grading system, 361
Pituicytoma, 384
Pituitary adenoma
  adenohypophyseal cells, 373
  atypical adenoma, 375
  characteristics, 379
  classification, 375
  cytokeratins 8/18, 375
  cytologic features, 377–379
  cytoplasm, 375
  differential diagnostics, 377, 379
  endocrinologically silent, 374
  hypersecretory syndrome, 374
  invasive adenomas, 375
  microadenomas, 374, 375
  microscopic features, 375
  pituitary apoplexy, 374
  pituitary carcinoma, 375
  predisposition syndromes, 373
  PRL-secreting adenomas, 375
  sporadic, 373
  stalk effect, 374
  synaptophysin, 375
  tumor cells, 375, 376
  WHO classification system, 375
Pituitary apoplexy, 374
Pituitary blastoma, 386
Pituitary carcinoma, 375, 377, 379
Pituitary neoplasm, 375
Plasmacytoma, 394
Pleomorphic meningioma, 221

Pleomorphic xanthoastrocytoma (PXA)
anaplastic, 113
characteristics, 115
cytologic features, 113, 114
differential diagnosis, 115
EGBs, 113
histology, 113, 114
neuroimaging, 113
temporal lobe, 111
treatment, 113
Polymerase chain reaction assay (PCR), 336
Polymorphonuclear leukocytes, 332
Positron emission tomography (PET), 23
Pott's disease, 399
PPT of intermediate differentiation (PPTID), 361, 362, 364, 368
Primary central nervous system lymphomas (PCNLs)
characteristics, 277
clinical presentation, 270
diagnostic approach, 271
DLBCL, 270
Epstein-Barr virus-related genome, 269
HAART, 269
Primary sarcomas of the brain, 243
Primitive neuroectodermal tumor (PNET)
C19MC-altered, 189, 194
embryonal tumors replacing, 197, 201
ETMR, 189
"other CNS embryonal tumors", 194
PRL-secreting adenomas, 375
Progressive multifocal leukoencephalopathy (PML), 349–351, 353
Prolapsed disc, 397, 398
Protoplasmic astrocytoma, 84
Protoplasmic variant, 84, 87
Psammomatous melanotic schwannoma (PMS), 290
Pyogenic abscess, 332, 333

R

Radiation-induced atypia, 100
Radiation necrosis, 100, 101
Radioresistant, 359
Rathke cleft cyst, 322–325, 382, 387
RB1 (retinoblastoma 1 gene), 362
Reactive astrocytosis, 68
Reactive gliosis, 71–73
Renal cell carcinoma, 305, 311
Rhabdoid meningioma, 222, 227
Rhabdomyosarcoma, 243
Romanowsky-stained preparation, 347
Romanowsky stains, 120
Romanowsky-type stains, 141
Rosai-Dorfman disease, 277–278, 280
Rosenthal fibers (RFs), 71, 74
Rosette-forming glioneural tumors (RGNTs)
BRAF alterations, 175
cytologic features, 175
glial element, 178
microscopically, 175
neurocytic element, 177
in posterior fossa, 175

S

Sacral and non-sacral spinal tumors, 394
Sample triage, 41–42
Sarcoidosis, 337, 338
Schwannomas
cellular, 284, 286
characteristics, 289
conventional, 284
cytology, 284, 288
differential diagnosis, 286, 288
histology, 285
incidence, 283
malignant transformation, 284
MS, 284, 289, 290
NF2, 283
symptoms, 284
Schwannomatosis, 283
Secondary brain tumors, 301, 302
Secretory meningioma, 215, 216
Sellar lesions, 380, 382
Sellar region lesions
craniopharyngioma (*see* Craniopharyngioma)
intraoperative consultation, 373
neoplastic
ATRT/, 387
granular cell pituicytoma, 384
granular cell tumor, 384, 386
meningiomas and germinoma, 386
metastasis, 386
oncocytic pituicytoma, 384
paraganglioma, 387
pituicytoma, 384
pituitary blastoma, 386
spindle cell oncocytoma, 384
non-neoplastic lesions
HHs, 387
hypophysitis, 388
inflammatory pseudotumor/plasma cell granuloma, 388
sphenoid sinus mucoceles, 388
xanthogranuloma, 387

pituitary adenoma (*see* Pituitary adenoma)
and pituitary gland, 373, 374
Sella turcica, 374
Single photon emission computed tomography (SPECT), 23
Skull base-invasive cases, 377
Small-cell carcinoma, 305, 309
Small-cell lung carcinoma, 394
Small round blue cell tumors, 394
Smear evaluation, 42, 43
Smear preparation, 2, 5, 106, 237, 241, 248, 258, 261, 266, 271, 290, 304, 324, 332, 343, 382, 387, 395, 398, 399, 401
angiocentric glioma, 148
astroblastoma, 147
central neurocytomas, 175
chordoid glioma, 150
classic medulloblastoma, 189
CPPs, 156
DIA/DIG, 172
DNTs, 166
ependymoma, 132
ganglion cell tumors, 169
meningioma, 211, 212, 215, 222
paraganglioma, 179
RGNTs, 175
Smear technique, 32, 34
advantages, 2
CNS lesions, 4
disadvantages, 2
and frozen sections, 1
Solitary fibrous tumor (SFT)
cytologic features, 237, 239, 241
differential diagnosis, 239
histology, 238
12q13 locus, 237
Specimens handling and processing
bone curettage, 32
fixation, 34
identification and transportation, 31
macroscopic appearances, 32, 33
normal brain, 32
squash/smear technique, 32, 34
staining methods, 35 (*see also* Fast staining methods)
types of, 32
Sphenoid sinus, 380, 388
Spinal cord compression, 391, 397, 398
Spinal epidural abscesses (SEA), 398, 399
Spinal epidural lipomas, 239, 241
Spinal meningioma, 213
Spinal paraganglioma, 180
clinical symptoms, 179
cytologic features, 179
extra-adrenal paragangliomas, 179
microscopically, 179
radiologically, 179
Spindle cell oncocytoma, 384
Spine and epidural space
mass lesions, 391, 392
neoplastic and non-neoplastic processes, 391
neoplastic lesions (*see* Neoplastic lesions)
nonneoplastic lesions (*see* Non-neoplastic lesions)
Squamous cell carcinoma, 305
Squamous epithelium-lined cysts
cytologic features, 321, 322
dermoid cysts, 320, 321
differential diagnosis, 321, 322
epidermoid cyst, 319–321
Squash preparation, 5, 32, 48, 106, 258, 343
AT/RT, 203
subependymoma, 139
Squash technique, 48
Stalk effect, 374
Staphylococcus aureus, 399
Stereotactic biopsy, 6
Subdural empyema, 334
Subependymal giant cell astrocytomas (SEGAs), 147
characteristics, 111, 113
cytologic features, 111, 112
differential diagnosis, 111, 113
epilepsy, 110
histology, 111, 112
symptoms, 110
TSC, 110, 111
Subependymoma
benign tumors, 139
characteristic histologic features, 140
characteristics, 141
cytologic features, 139, 141
differential diagnosis, 139, 141
microcystic degeneration, 139
and myxopapillary ependymoma, 129
surgical excision, 139
Synaptophysin, 375

T

Teratomas, 258, 261, 263, 265, 359
Tissue sampling, 32
Touch preparation, 32
Toxoplasma gondii, 347
Toxoplasmosis, 345, 347, 348

Transitional meningioma, 49, 209, 210
Trilateral retinoblastoma, 362
Tuberculoma, 337
Tuberculosis, 399, 400
Tuberculous abscesses, 337, 341
Tuberculous mycobacterial infection
  atypical mycobacteria infection, 337, 342
  chronic meningitis, 337
  cytologic features, 337, 340
  histology, 337, 339
  immunosuppression, 337
  tuberculous abscesses, 337, 341
Tuberous sclerosis complex (TSC), 110, 111
Tumefactive demyelination, 345
Tumor-like demyelinating lesions (TLDLs), 341, 343–345
  astrocytes, 343
  cerebral infarction, 345, 346
  characteristics, 343
  cytologic features, 343–345
  cytologic preparations, 343
  histology, 343
  macrophages, 343
  MS, 341
  space-occupying lesions, 341
  subcortical/periventricular white matter, 343
  tumefactive demyelination, 345
Tumors of the pineal region (TPR)
  papillary (*see* Papillary tumor of the pineal region (PTPR))

U
Urothelial cell carcinoma, 305, 312

V
Vascular-core papillary structures, 378
Vertebral brucellosis, 401
Vertebral hemangioma (VH), 397
Vertebral tuberculosis, 399, 400

W
Wet film technique, 5
White matter, 61–63

X
Xanthogranuloma, 387
Xanthogranulomatous, 380

Y
Yolk sac tumor, 258, 263, 266, 267

Printed by Printforce, the Netherlands